Prevention and Treatment of Sarcopenia

Prevention and Treatment of Sarcopenia

Editor

Gianluca Testa

MDPI • Basel • Beijing • Wuhan • Barcelona • Belgrade • Manchester • Tokyo • Cluj • Tianjin

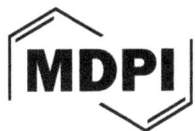

Editor
Gianluca Testa
Dipartimento di Chirurgia
Generale e Specialità
Medico-Chirurgiche
Università degli Studi di Catania
Catania
Italy

Editorial Office
MDPI
St. Alban-Anlage 66
4052 Basel, Switzerland

This is a reprint of articles from the Special Issue published online in the open access journal *Journal of Clinical Medicine* (ISSN 2077-0383) (available at: www.mdpi.com/journal/jcm/special_issues/Prevention_Treatment_Sarcopenia).

For citation purposes, cite each article independently as indicated on the article page online and as indicated below:

LastName, A.A.; LastName, B.B.; LastName, C.C. Article Title. *Journal Name* **Year**, *Volume Number*, Page Range.

ISBN 978-3-0365-1536-6 (Hbk)
ISBN 978-3-0365-1535-9 (PDF)

© 2021 by the authors. Articles in this book are Open Access and distributed under the Creative Commons Attribution (CC BY) license, which allows users to download, copy and build upon published articles, as long as the author and publisher are properly credited, which ensures maximum dissemination and a wider impact of our publications.

The book as a whole is distributed by MDPI under the terms and conditions of the Creative Commons license CC BY-NC-ND.

Contents

About the Editor vii

Preface to "Prevention and Treatment of Sarcopenia" ix

Sophia X. Sui, Kara L. Holloway-Kew, Natalie K. Hyde, Lana J. Williams, Monica C. Tembo, Sarah Leach and Julie A. Pasco
Prevalence of Sarcopenia Employing Population-Specific Cut-Points: Cross-Sectional Data from the Geelong Osteoporosis Study, Australia
Reprinted from: *Journal of Clinical Medicine* 2021, 10, 343, doi:10.3390/jcm10020343 1

Jacobo Á. Rubio-Arias, Raquel Rodríguez-Fernández, Luis Andreu, Luis M. Martínez-Aranda, Alejandro Martínez-Rodriguez and Domingo J. Ramos-Campo
Effect of Sleep Quality on the Prevalence of Sarcopenia in Older Adults: A Systematic Review with Meta-Analysis
Reprinted from: *Journal of Clinical Medicine* 2019, 8, 2156, doi:10.3390/jcm8122156 15

Raquel Fábrega-Cuadros, Agustín Aibar-Almazán, Antonio Martínez-Amat and Fidel Hita-Contreras
Impact of Psychological Distress and Sleep Quality on Balance Confidence, Muscle Strength, and Functional Balance in Community-Dwelling Middle-Aged and Older People
Reprinted from: *Journal of Clinical Medicine* 2020, 9, 3059, doi:10.3390/jcm9093059 29

Julie A. Pasco, Amanda L. Stuart, Sophia X. Sui, Kara L. Holloway-Kew, Natalie K. Hyde, Monica C. Tembo, Pamela Rufus-Membere, Mark A. Kotowicz and Lana J. Williams
Dynapenia and Low Cognition: A Cross-Sectional Association in Postmenopausal Women
Reprinted from: *Journal of Clinical Medicine* 2021, 10, 173, doi:10.3390/jcm10020173 39

Máximo Bernabeu-Wittel, Raquel Gómez-Díaz, Álvaro González-Molina, Sofía Vidal-Serrano, Jesús Díez-Manglano, Fernando Salgado, María Soto-Martín, Manuel Ollero-Baturone and on behalf of the PROTEO RESEARCHERS
Oxidative Stress, Telomere Shortening, and Apoptosis Associated to Sarcopenia and Frailty in Patients with Multimorbidity
Reprinted from: *Journal of Clinical Medicine* 2020, 9, 2669, doi:10.3390/jcm9082669 47

Nathaniel R. Johnson, Christopher J. Kotarsky, Kyle J. Hackney, Kara A. Trautman, Nathan D. Dicks, Wonwoo Byun, Jill F. Keith, Shannon L. David and Sherri N. Stastny
Measures Derived from Panoramic Ultrasonography and Animal-Based Protein Intake Are Related to Muscular Performance in Middle-Aged Adults
Reprinted from: *Journal of Clinical Medicine* 2021, 10, 988, doi:10.3390/jcm10050988 59

Mariana Cevei, Roxana Ramona Onofrei, Felicia Cioara and Dorina Stoicanescu
Correlations between the Quality of Life Domains and Clinical Variables in Sarcopenic Osteoporotic Postmenopausal Women
Reprinted from: *Journal of Clinical Medicine* 2020, 9, 441, doi:10.3390/jcm9020441 79

Anna Arnal-Gómez, Maria A. Cebrià i Iranzo, Jose M. Tomas, Maria A. Tortosa-Chuliá, Mercè Balasch-Bernat, Trinidad Sentandreu-Mañó, Silvia Forcano and Natalia Cezón-Serrano
Using the Updated EWGSOP2 Definition in Diagnosing Sarcopenia in Spanish Older Adults: Clinical Approach
Reprinted from: *Journal of Clinical Medicine* 2021, 10, 1018, doi:10.3390/jcm10051018 91

Gianluca Testa, Andrea Vescio, Danilo Zuccalà, Vincenzo Petrantoni, Mirko Amico, Giorgio Ivan Russo, Giuseppe Sessa and Vito Pavone
Diagnosis, Treatment and Prevention of Sarcopenia in Hip Fractured Patients: Where We Are and Where We Are Going: A Systematic Review
Reprinted from: *Journal of Clinical Medicine* 2020, 9, 2997, doi:10.3390/jcm9092997 105

Marianna Avola, Giulia Rita Agata Mangano, Gianluca Testa, Sebastiano Mangano, Andrea Vescio, Vito Pavone and Michele Vecchio
Rehabilitation Strategies for Patients with Femoral Neck Fractures in Sarcopenia: A Narrative Review
Reprinted from: *Journal of Clinical Medicine* 2020, 9, 3115, doi:10.3390/jcm9103115 119

Nejc Šarabon, Žiga Kozinc, Stefan Löfler and Christian Hofer
Resistance Exercise, Electrical Muscle Stimulation, and Whole-Body Vibration in Older Adults: Systematic Review and Meta-Analysis of Randomized Controlled Trials
Reprinted from: *Journal of Clinical Medicine* 2020, 9, 2902, doi:10.3390/jcm9092902 135

Andreas Mæchel Fritzen, Søren Peter Andersen, Khaled Abdul Nasser Qadri, Frank D. Thøgersen, Thomas Krag, Mette C. Ørngreen, John Vissing and Tina D. Jeppesen
Effect of Aerobic Exercise Training and Deconditioning on Oxidative Capacity and Muscle Mitochondrial Enzyme Machinery in Young and Elderly Individuals
Reprinted from: *Journal of Clinical Medicine* 2020, 9, 3113, doi:10.3390/jcm9103113 157

Ilse J. M. Hagedoorn, Niala den Braber, Milou M. Oosterwijk, Christina M. Gant, Gerjan Navis, Miriam M. R. Vollenbroek-Hutten, Bert-Jan F. van Beijnum, Stephan J. L. Bakker and Gozewijn D. Laverman
Low Physical Activity in Patients with Complicated Type 2 Diabetes Mellitus Is Associated with Low Muscle Mass and Low Protein Intake
Reprinted from: *Journal of Clinical Medicine* 2020, 9, 3104, doi:10.3390/jcm9103104 173

Francisco Miguel Martínez-Arnau, Cristina Buigues, Rosa Fonfría-Vivas and Omar Cauli
Respiratory Muscle Strengths and Their Association with Lean Mass and Handgrip Strengths in Older Institutionalized Individuals
Reprinted from: *Journal of Clinical Medicine* 2020, 9, 2727, doi:10.3390/jcm9092727 185

Andreas Mæchel Fritzen, Frank D. Thøgersen, Khaled Abdul Nasser Qadri, Thomas Krag, Marie-Louise Sveen, John Vissing and Tina D. Jeppesen
Preserved Capacity for Adaptations in Strength and Muscle Regulatory Factors in Elderly in Response to Resistance Exercise Training and Deconditioning
Reprinted from: *Journal of Clinical Medicine* 2020, 9, 2188, doi:10.3390/jcm9072188 203

Francesco Bellanti, Aurelio Lo Buglio, Stefano Quiete, Giuseppe Pellegrino, Michał Dobrakowski, Aleksandra Kasperczyk, Sławomir Kasperczyk and Gianluigi Vendemiale
Comparison of Three Nutritional Screening Tools with the New Glim Criteria for Malnutrition and Association with Sarcopenia in Hospitalized Older Patients
Reprinted from: *Journal of Clinical Medicine* 2020, 9, 1898, doi:10.3390/jcm9061898 219

Agnieszka Wiśniowska-Szurlej, Agnieszka Ćwirlej-Sozańska, Natalia Wołoszyn, Bernard Sozański and Anna Wilmowska-Pietruszyńska
Effects of Physical Exercises and Verbal Stimulation on the Functional Efficiency and Use of Free Time in an Older Population under Institutional Care: A Randomized Controlled Trial
Reprinted from: *Journal of Clinical Medicine* 2020, 9, 477, doi:10.3390/jcm9020477 231

Hyuma Makizako, Yuki Nakai, Kazutoshi Tomioka, Yoshiaki Taniguchi, Nana Sato, Ayumi Wada, Ryoji Kiyama, Kota Tsutsumimoto, Mitsuru Ohishi, Yuto Kiuchi, Takuro Kubozono and Toshihiro Takenaka
Effects of a Multicomponent Exercise Program in Physical Function and Muscle Mass in Sarcopenic/Pre-Sarcopenic Adults
Reprinted from: *Journal of Clinical Medicine* **2020**, *9*, 1386, doi:10.3390/jcm9051386 . . . . **251**

Takumi Kawaguchi, Sachiyo Yoshio, Yuzuru Sakamoto, Ryuki Hashida, Shunji Koya, Keisuke Hirota, Dan Nakano, Sakura Yamamura, Takashi Niizeki, Hiroo Matsuse and Takuji Torimura
Impact of Decorin on the Physical Function and Prognosis of Patients with Hepatocellular Carcinoma
Reprinted from: *Journal of Clinical Medicine* **2020**, *9*, 936, doi:10.3390/jcm9040936 . . . . **263**

About the Editor

Gianluca Testa

Gianluca Testa is a researcher professor at University of Catania, Italy, since January 2018. He is one of the youngest nominated researchers in Italy, a medical doctor and surgeon, and an expert in the field of Orthopaedics and Traumatology. He practices at Universitary Hospital Policlinico Rodolico - San Marco, in Catania, treating both pediatric and older people. He is a delegate for the region Sicily of the Italian Pediatric Orthopaedics and Traumatology Society (S.I.T.O.P.) and for the Italian External Fixation Society (S.I.F.E.).

Preface to "Prevention and Treatment of Sarcopenia"

Sarcopenia represents the decline in skeletal muscle mass and function with age, characterized by the muscle fiber's quality, strength, muscle endurance, and metabolic ability decreasing, as well as the fat and connective tissue growing.

Reduction of muscle strength with aging leads to loss of functional capacity, causing disability, mortality, and other adverse health outcomes. Because of the increase of the proportion of elderly in the population, sarcopenia-related morbidity will become an increasing area of health care resource utilization.

Diagnostic screening consists of individuation of body composition, assessed by DEXA, anthropometry, bioelectrical impedance, MRI, or CT scan. Management is possible with resistance training exercise and vibration therapy, nutritional supplements, and pharmacological treatment.

The book includes articles from different nationalities, treating the experimental and medical applications of sarcopenia. The consequences of sarcopenia in frailty are treated in relation to other associated pathologies or lesions, as femoral neck fractures and hepatocellular carcinoma.

Gianluca Testa
Editor

Article

Prevalence of Sarcopenia Employing Population-Specific Cut-Points: Cross-Sectional Data from the Geelong Osteoporosis Study, Australia

Sophia X. Sui [1,*], Kara L. Holloway-Kew [1], Natalie K. Hyde [1], Lana J. Williams [1], Monica C. Tembo [1], Sarah Leach [2] and Julie A. Pasco [1,3,4,5]

1. Deakin University, IMPACT—Institute for Mental and Physical Health and Clinical Translation, Geelong, VIC 3220, Australia; k.holloway@deakin.edu.au (K.L.H.-K.); natalie.hyde@deakin.edu.au (N.K.H.); l.williams@deakin.edu.au (L.J.W.); mctembo@deakin.edu.au (M.C.T.); julie.pasco@deakin.edu.au (J.A.P.)
2. GMHBA, Geelong, VIC 3220, Australia; SarahLeach@GMHBA.COM.AU
3. Department of Medicine—Western Health, The University of Melbourne, St Albans, VIC 3021, Australia
4. Department of Epidemiology and Preventive Medicine, Monash University, Prahran, VIC 3181, Australia
5. University Hospital Geelong, Barwon Health, Geelong, VIC 3220, Australia
* Correspondence: ssui@deakin.edu.au; Tel.: +61-342-153-306; Fax: +61-342-153-491

Abstract: Background: Prevalence estimates for sarcopenia vary depending on the ascertainment criteria and thresholds applied. We aimed to estimate the prevalence of sarcopenia using two international definitions but employing Australian population-specific cut-points. Methods: Participants ($n = 665$; 323 women) aged 60–96 years old were from the Geelong Osteoporosis Study. Handgrip strength (HGS) was measured by dynamometers and appendicular lean mass (ALM) by whole-body dual-energy X-ray absorptiometry. Physical performance was assessed using gait speed (GS, men only) and/or the timed up-and-go (TUG) test. Using cut-points equivalent to two standard deviations (SDs) below the mean young reference range from the same population and recommendations from the European Working Group on Sarcopenia in Older People (EWGSOP), sarcopenia was identified by low ALM/height^2 (<5.30 kg for women; <6.94 kg for men) + low HGS (<16 kg women; <31 kg men); low ALM/height^2 + slow TUG (>9.3 s); low ALM/height^2 + slow GS (<0.8 m/s). For the Foundation for the National Institutes of Health (FNIH) equivalent, sarcopenia was identified as low ALM/BMI (<0.512 m^2 women, <0.827 m^2 men) + low HGS (<16 kg women; <31 kg men). Receiver Operating Characteristic curves were also applied to determine optimal cut-points for ALM/BMI (<0.579 m^2 women, <0.913 m^2 men) that discriminated poor physical performance. Prevalence estimates were standardized to the Australian population and compared to estimates using international thresholds. Results: Using population-specific cut-points and low ALM/height^2 + HGS, point-estimates for sarcopenia prevalence were 0.9% for women and 2.9% for men. Using ALM/height^2 + TUG, prevalence was 2.5% for women and 4.1% for men, and using ALM/height^2 + GS, sarcopenia was identified for 1.6% of men. Using ALM/BMI + HGS, prevalence estimates were 5.5–10.4% for women and 11.6–18.4% for men. Conclusions: This study highlights the range of prevalence estimates that result from employing different criteria for sarcopenia. While population-specific criteria could be pertinent for some populations, a consensus is needed to identify which deficits in skeletal muscle health are important for establishing an operational definition for sarcopenia.

Keywords: sarcopenia; skeletal muscle; prevalence; muscle strength; physical functional performance; epidemiologic studies; aging

1. Introduction

While sarcopenia is characterized by age-related declines in skeletal muscle mass, strength and function, currently, there is no unanimously agreed operational definition for sarcopenia [1–4]. Several operational definitions have been developed, notably by the

European Working Group on Sarcopenia in Older People (EWGSOP1 and EWGSOP2) [3,5] and the Foundation for the National Institutes of Health (FNIH) [4]. Sarcopenia parameters usually include low muscle mass and low muscle strength or performance to identify sarcopenia, but different algorithms have been proposed. For example, the EWGSOP suggests that muscle mass be expressed relative to height, while the FNIH recommends adjustment by BMI. Such disparities contribute to poor agreement in the literature between prevalence estimates for sarcopenia [6–8]. Furthermore, the EWGSOP1, EWGSOP2 and FNIH present different cut-points for identifying low muscle mass, strength and/or performance, which have been identified on the basis of different criteria [4,5,9,10], using data largely from European or American populations [3–5]. However, in the more recent EWGSOP2, reference data have been drawn from a range of populations [5], including Australia [11]. We have recently published prevalence estimates for sarcopenia using criteria recommended by the EWGSOP1, EWGSOP2 and FNIH [8], but there remains a lack of consensus about whether or not population-specific reference data should be used to identify low muscle mass and function [9,12]. The Australian and New Zealand Society for Sarcopenia and Frailty Research (ANZSSFR) recently recommended EWGSOP1 criteria but suggested employing population-specific cut-points [12].

The aim of this study was to calculate and compare prevalence estimates of sarcopenia in a sample of older women and men using the EWGSOP and FNIH ascertainment criteria but employing cut-points derived from the same population.

2. Methods

2.1. Study Design

The Geelong Osteoporosis Study (GOS) is a population-based, prospective study in Australia. Further detailed information about the GOS is published elsewhere [13]. Participants were randomly selected from the electoral roll for the Barwon Statistical Division until there were at least 100 women and 100 men in each 5-year age group from 20 to 69 years and 200 of each sex for age groups 70–79 years and ≥80 years [13]. Inclusion criterion was a listing on the electoral roll for the Barwon Statistical Division; participants were excluded if residency in the region was less than 6 months or if they were not able to provide written informed consent. At baseline (1993–1997), an age-stratified sample of 1494 women was enrolled, with 77% response; in 2005, this sample was supplemented with a further 246 women aged 20–29 years. Baseline data for 1540 men were collected during 2001–2006 (67% response). Participants were followed-up every few years. The study was approved by the Barwon Health Human Research Ethics Committee. Written informed consent was obtained from all participants.

2.2. Participants

Cross-sectional data from the 15-year assessment waves for women and men were used in this analysis. To determine prevalence estimates of sarcopenia in older adults, we included data from the 15-year assessment for 323 women (ages 60–95 years), collected during 2010–2014, and for 342 men (ages 60–96 years), collected during 2016–2019. The sample was almost entirely Caucasian (~98%).

2.3. Measures

Weight and height were measured to the nearest ±0.1 kg and ±0.1 cm and body mass index (BMI) calculated as weight/height^2 (kg/m^2). Appendicular lean mass (ALM) (kg) was obtained from whole-body dual-energy X-ray absorptiometry (DXA; Lunar Prodigy-Pro, Madison, WI, USA), which provided lean mass measures for the arms and legs. Short-term precision (calculated as the coefficient of variation on repeated whole body scans) was 0.9% for ALM. ALM was expressed relative to height^2 (ALM/height^2, kg/m^2) or relative to BMI (ALM/BMI, m^2).

Handgrip strength (HGS) was measured using a hand-held analog dynamometer (Jamar, Sammons Preston, Bolingbrook, IL, USA) for women and a digital dynamometer

(Vernier, LoggerPro3) for men. The testing procedure was demonstrated to participants before the measurement trials. With the participant seated in a comfortable position and the arm holding the dynamometer flexed at the elbow to 90 degrees, the participant was asked to squeeze the device as hard as possible for several seconds and the peak reading was recorded. This procedure was repeated for each hand. For women, the readings were performed in duplicate on each hand with no time interval between trials, and for men, trials were repeated in triplicate on each hand, holding the peak for 3 s with a 5-s interval between trials. The mean of the maximum value for each hand was used in further analyses. Measures from the Vernier device were transformed to Jamar equivalent values according to the following equation: HGS_{Jamar} (kg) = 9.50 + 0.818*$HGS_{Vernier}$ (kg) + 8.80*Sex, where sex = 1 for men, which was developed by measuring the maximum HGS on each device for 45 adults aged 21–67 years [8].

The timed up-and-go (TUG) test was used as a measure of mobility but also includes static and dynamic balance [14]. This involved timing the participant (in seconds) to rise from a chair (without armrests), walk to a marked line (3 m distance), turn around, return to the chair and sit down. For men only, usual gait speed (GS, m/s) was also determined by measuring the time taken (in seconds) to walk a distance of 4 m. All measures were collected by trained personnel.

2.4. Population-Specific Cut-Points

Table 1 presents the Australian population-specific and international cut-points for the components of sarcopenia. Population-specific cut-points were determined as equivalent to 2 standard deviations (SDs) below sex-specific mean values for young reference groups (age $\leq$ 49 years) generated from the same population, as previously described [11,15–17]. For women, the cut-point for low HGS was <16 kg [16]. Using the same approach, the mean $\pm$SD for HGS among 111 men (ages 33–49 years) was 44.8 $\pm$ 6.9 kg, and thus, the cut-point for low HGS was <31 kg. Low lean mass was identified as ALM/height^2 <5.30 kg/m^2 for women and 6.94 kg/m^2 for men [11], and low ALM/BMI as <0.512 m^2 for women and 0.827 m^2 for men [15], corresponding to T-scores < -2 [11,15].

Table 1. Applied threshold values for women and men used in different definitions.

Population-Specific Cut-Points	Women	Men
ALM/height^2 + HGS	<5.30 kg/m^2 + <16 kg	<6.94 kg/m^2 + <31 kg
ALM/height^2 + TUG	<5.30 kg/m^2 + >9.3 s	<6.94 kg/m^2 + >9.3 s
ALM/height^2 + GS	-	<6.94 kg/m^2 + <0.8 m/s
ALM/BMI + HGS	<0.512 m^2 + <16 kg	<0.827 m^2 + <31 kg
ALM/BMI$_{ROC}$ + HGS	<0.579 m^2 + <16 kg	0.913 m^2 + <31 kg
International Cut-Points		
ALM/height2EWGSOP1 + HGS (3)	<5.67 kg/m^2 + <20 kg	<7.23 kg/m^2 + <30 kg
ALM/height2EWGSOP1 + GS (3)	-	<7.23 kg/m^2 + <0.8 m/s
ALM/height2EWGSOP2 + HGS (5)	<5.5 kg/m^2 + <16 kg	<7.0 kg/m^2 + <27 kg
ALM/height2EWGSOP2 + TUG (5)	<5.5 kg/m^2 + >20 s	<7.0 kg/m^2 + >20 s
ALM/BMIFNIH + HGS (4)	<0.512 m^2 + <16 kg	<0.789 m^2 + <26 kg

ALM: appendicular lean mass; ALM/height^2: appendicular lean mass/height^2; ALM/BMI: appendicular lean mass/body mass index; HGS: handgrip strength; TUG: timed up-and-go; GS: gait speed; EWGSOP: European Working Group on Sarcopenia in Older People; FNIH: Foundation for the National Institutes of Health; ROC: receiver operating characteristic.

We used a cut-point of <0.8 m/s for GS to identify slowness (poor muscle performance) in line with extant literature [2,6,18]. The mean $\pm$SD for TUG among women was 6.98 $\pm$ 1.14 s, and thus, slow TUG was identified as >9.3 s. We also used TUG as a proxy for GS [2,14] for men, and since the cut-points for slow GS are the same for both sexes in the literature [3–5], we used the same threshold for TUG for both women and men.

Furthermore, as the FNIH cut-points for ALM/BMI were identified on the basis of discriminating clinically significant weakness [18], we estimated cut-points for low ALM/BMI that best discriminated the presence or absence of slow TUG (>9.3 s) [2,6,9,18]. The locations of optimal cut-points were determined by the principle that the sensitivity and specificity are closest to the value of the area under the receiver operating characteristic (ROC) curve, and the absolute value of the difference between the sensitivity and specificity is the smallest [19]. The ALM/BMI that best predicted slow TUG was <0.579 m^2 (sensitivity 0.63, specificity 0.60) for women and <0.913 m^2 (sensitivity 0.73, specificity 0.57) for men (Appendix A Figure A1). The area under the ROC curve was 0.64 (95% CI 0.58–0.70) for women and 0.68 (0.63–0.74) for men ($p < 0.001$).

2.5. Sarcopenia Ascertainment

Based on EWGSOP1 [3] and EWGSOP2 [5], sarcopenia corresponds to low ALM/height^2 and low HGS (ALM/height^2 + HGS); low ALM/height^2 and slow GS (ALM/height^2 + GS); or low ALM/height^2 and slow TUG (ALM/height^2 + TUG). According to FNIH [4], sarcopenia is defined as low ALM/BMI and low HGS (ALM/BMI + HGS) (Table 1). Furthermore, severe sarcopenia was determined using a combination involving low lean mass, muscle strength and physical performance, that is, ALM/height^2 + HGS + TUG for EWGSOP and ALM/BMI + HGS + TUG for FNIH.

2.6. Statistical Analysis

Data for women and men were analyzed separately. Histograms were used to check the distribution of data for normality. Means and SDs were presented for normally distributed data, and medians and interquartile ranges for skewed data. Prevalence for each age decade was calculated. Age-standardized prevalence estimates (mean and 95% confidence interval (CI)) were calculated according to 2011 census data from the Australian Bureau of Statistics [20]. Age-adjusted multivariable logistic regression models were developed to examine sex differences (pooled data) in the likelihood for sarcopenia. To compare prevalence estimates obtained with different cut-points, the kappa coefficient (κ) and 95% CIs were calculated and the strength of agreement was interpreted as small ($\kappa < 0.40$), medium ($\kappa = 0.40$–0.75) or high ($\kappa > 0.75$) [7]. Analyses were performed using SPSS (v24, IBM SPSS Statistics Inc., Chicago, IL, USA) and Minitab (v18, Minitab, State College, PA, USA).

3. Results

3.1. Participant Characteristics

Table 2 shows the participant characteristics. There were 12 women (3.7%) and 23 men (6.7%) with low ALM/height^2, 70 women (21.7%) and 110 men (32.2%) with low ALM/BMI and 50 women (15.5%) and 87 men (25.6%) with low HGS. A slow TUG was recorded for 143 women (44.7%) and 169 men (49.7%) and a slow GS for 102 men (30.4%). Using the cut-point values obtained from ROC curves, 162 (50.2%) women and 197 (57.6%) men were identified as having low ALM/BMI$_{ROC}$.

Table 2. Participant characteristics. Data are presented as mean (±SD) or median (IQR).

	Women (n = 323)	Men (n = 342)
Age (yr)	70 (64–75)	70 (66–78)
Weight (kg)	74.0 (±15.4)	83.9 (±13.8)
Height (m)	1.59 (±0.06)	1.73 (±0.07)
BMI (kg/m^2)	29.0 (±5.8)	28.0 (±4.1)
HGS (kg)	21 (±6)	36 (±6)
ALM/height^2 (kg/m^2)	6.60 (±0.79)	8.25 (±0.93)
ALM/BMI (m^2)	0.593 (±0.102)	0.888 (±0.124)
TUG (s)	9.1 (7.9–10.8)	9.2 (8.0–10.7)
Gait speed (m/s)	-	0.9 (±0.2)

BMI: body mass index; ALM: appendicular lean mass; HGS: handgrip strength; ALM/height^2: appendicular lean mass/height^2; ALM/BMI: appendicular lean mass/body mass index; TUG: timed up-and-go. Missing data: HGS $n = 1$ man; TUG $n = 3$ women, 2 men; GS $n = 323$ women, 7 men.

There was a pattern of increasing prevalence of sarcopenia with advancing age in both sexes across all the definitions (Table 3). The point estimates for men were higher than for women, especially for those aged ≥80 yr; however, 95% CIs for different age groups overlapped.

3.2. Sarcopenia Prevalence in Men Compared with Women

After adjusting for age, and according to FNIH-related definitions, men were more likely than women to have sarcopenia; for ALM/BMI + HGS, odds ratio (OR) 2.45 (95%CI 1.32–4.56; p = 0.005) and for ALM/BMI$_{ROC}$ + HGS, OR 2.27 (95%CI 1.39–3.72; p = 0.001). When EWGSOP-related definitions were used, men appeared to be more likely than women to have sarcopenia, but differences were not significant; for ALM/height^2 + HGS, OR 2.8 (95%CI 0.77–10.5; p = 0.11), and for ALM/height^2 + TUG, OR 1.5 (95%CI 0.6–3.7; p = 0.37).

3.3. Age-Standardized Estimates of Sarcopenia

The age-standardized estimates of sarcopenia according to different definitions and population-specific cut-points are shown in Table 3 and Figure 1. Using ALM/height^2 + low HGS, point estimates for sarcopenia prevalence were 0.9% for women and 2.9% for men. Using ALM/height^2 + TUG, estimates were 2.5% for women and 4.1% for men, and using ALM/height^2 + GS, the estimate for men was 1.6%. Using ALM/BMI + HGS, point estimates ranged from 5.5% to 10.4% for women and from 11.6% to 18.4% for men. The prevalence estimates based on population-specific cut-points are shown in Figure 1 together with estimates based on recommended international criteria. Prevalence estimates using international cut-points (shown in Figure 1) have been published elsewhere [8].

3.4. Agreement

Table 4 shows the levels of agreement between different definitions of sarcopenia using international and population-specific cut-points. Levels of agreement ranged from poor through to high (κ = 0.1–1 for women and 0–0.8 for men). Note that the 100% agreement for women using the FNIH definition occurred because the international and population-specific thresholds were the same, even though they were obtained using different methods.

Table 3. Age- and sex-specific prevalence estimates of sarcopenia according to different assessment criteria.

Criteria	60–69 yr		70–79 yr		≥80 yr		All	Standardized Prevalence
Women	n = 151		n = 124		n = 48		n = 323	
	n, %	95%CI	n, %	95%CI	n, %	95%CI	n, %	Mean (%, 95%CI)
ALM/height² + HGS	0 (0)	-	2 (1.6)	-	1 (2.1)	-	3 (0.9)	0.9 (0.2–1.6)
ALM/height² + TUG	3 (2.0)	0.6–5.6	3 (2.4)	0.7–6.7	2 (4.3)	0.9–13.9	8 (2.7)	2.5 (0.8–4.3)
ALM/BMI + HGS	3 (2.0)	0.6–5.5	5 (4.0)	1.6–8.9	8 (16.7)	8.2–29.3	16 (5.0)	5.5 (3.1–7.9)
ALM/BMI$_{ROC}$ + HGS	5 (3.3)	1.3–7.7	8 (6.5)	3.3–12.4	16 (33.3)	21.5–47.7	29 (9.0)	10.4 (7.2–13.6)
Severe sarcopenia								
ALM/height² + HGS + TUG	1 (0.8)	-	1 (2.1)	-	1 (2.1)	-	2 (0.6)	1.0 (0–2.1)
ALM/BMI + HGS + TUG	2 (1.3)	0.3–5.2	3 (2.4)	0.7–7.2	8 (17.0)	8.7–30.5	13 (4.1)	4.8 (2.6–6.9)
ALM/BMI$_{ROC}$ + HGS + TUG	4 (2.7)	1.0–6.9	5 (4.0)	1.7–9.3	15 (31.9)	20.2–46.4	24 (7.5)	8.9 (6.0–11.8)
Men	n = 152		n = 117		n = 73		n = 342	
ALM/height² + HGS	0 (0)	-	3 (2.6)	-	8 (11.1)	-	11 (3.2)	2.9 (1.8–4.0)
ALM/height² + TUG	2 (1.3)	0.3–4.6	1 (0.9)	0.09–4.8	12 (16.4)	9.3–26.3	15 (4.4)	4.1 (2.4–5.8)
ALM/height² + GS	0	-	0	-	6 (8.3)	-	6 (1.8)	1.6 (1.0–2.2)
ALM/BMI + HGS	4 (2.6)	0.9–6.4	13 (11.2)	6.4–18.0	26 (36.1)	25.7–47.6	43 (12.6)	11.6 (8.6–14.5)
ALM/BMI$_{ROC}$ + HGS	13 (8.6)	5.0–14.2	21 (18.1)	12.1–26.1	33 (45.8)	34.7–57.4	67 (19.7)	18.4 (14.3–22.4)
Severe sarcopenia								
ALM/height² + HGS + TUG	0	-	0	-	7 (9.7%)	-	7 (2.1)	1.9 (1.3–2.5)
ALM/BMI + HGS + TUG	2 (1.3)	0.3–5.2	9 (7.8)	4.1–14.2	25 (34.7)	24.7–46.4	36 (10.7)	9.5 (7.0–12.0)
ALM/BMI$_{ROC}$ + HGS + TUG	4 (2.7)	1.0–6.9	14 (12.1)	7.3–19.4	32 (44.4)	33.4–56.0	50 (14.8)	13.4 (10.3–16.6)

ALM: appendicular lean mass; GS: gait speed; HGS: handgrip strength; ALM/height²: appendicular lean mass/height²; ALM/BMI: appendicular lean mass/body mass index; TUG: timed up-and-go; ROC: receiver operating characteristics. Missing data: HGS n = 1 man; TUG n = 3 women, 2 men; GS n = 323 women, 7 men.

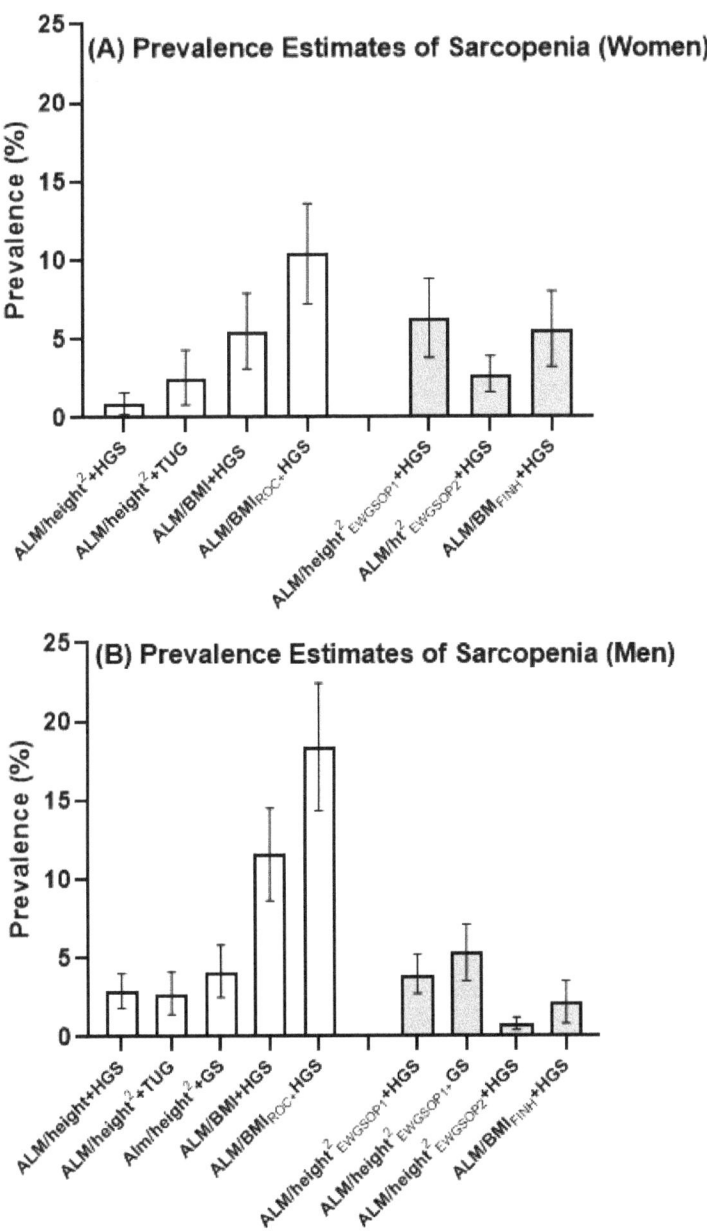

Figure 1. Prevalence estimates of sarcopenia for (**A**) women and (**B**) men aged 60 years and older. Error bars show 95% confidence intervals. Bars for estimates using population-specific cut-points are unshaded and those using international cut-points are shaded. EWGSOP: European Working Group on Sarcopenia in Older People; FNIH: Foundation for the National Institutes of Health; ALM: appendicular lean mass; GS: gait speed; HGS: handgrip strength; BMI: body mass index; TUG: timed up-and-go.

Table 4. Agreement between sarcopenia prevalence estimates according to different international and population-specific cut-points. Data are presented as κ, 95% confidence intervals and p-values.

Women	ALM/height² EWGSOP1 + HGS	ALM/height² EWGSOP2 + HGS	ALM/height² EWGSOP2 + GS	ALM/BMI FNIH + HGS	ALM/height² + HGS	ALM/height² + TUG	ALM/BMI + HGS
ALM/height² + HGS	0.2 (0.0–0.5)	0.4 (0.0–0.7)		0.1 (−0.1–0.2)	-		
p-value	<0.001	<0.001		0.02			
ALM/height² + TUG	0.3 (0.0–0.5)	0.2 (0.0–0.4)		0.1 (0.1–0.2)	0.4 (0–0.7)	0.1 (−0.1–0.2)	
p-value	<0.001	0.001		0.32	<0.001	0.3	
ALM/BMI + HGS	0.2 (0.0–0.4)	0.2 (0.0–0.4)		1	0.1 (0.0–0.3)	0.1 (0.0–0.2)	
p-value	0.001	0.001		<0.001	0.02	0.11	
ALM/BMI_{ROC} + HGS	0.3 (0.1–0.5)	0.3 (0.1–0.5)		0.7 (0.5–0.8)	0.1 (0.0–0.3)		0.7 (0.5–0.8)
p-value	<0.001	<0.001		<0.001	<0.001		<0.001

Men	ALM/height² EWGSOP1 + HGS	ALM/height² EWGSOP2 + GS	ALM/height² EWGSOP2 + HGS	ALM/BMI FNIH + HGS	ALM/height² + HGS	ALM/height² + TUG	ALM/height² + GS	ALM/BMI + HGS
ALM/height² + HGS	0.8 (0.6–1.0)	0.4 (0.2–0.7)	0.4 (0.1–0.7)	0.1 (−0.1–0.3)	-			
p-value	<0.001	<0.001	<0.001	0.13				
ALM/height² + TUG	0.4 (0.2–0.7)	0.5 (0.4–0.7)	0.3 (0.0–0.6)	0.1 (−0.1–0.2)	0.5 (0.3–0.8)	-		
p-value	<0.001	<0.001	<0.001	0.26	<0.001			
ALM/height² + GS	0.5 (0.3–0.8)	0.7 (0.4–0.9)	0.5 (0.1–0.8)	0.1 (−0.1–0.3)	0.7 (0.4–0.9)	0.8 (0.6–1.0)		
p-value	<0.001	<0.001	<0.001	0.11	<0.001	<0.001		
ALM/BMI + HGS	0.2 (0.0–0.3)	0.1 (0.0–0.3)	0.02 (0.0–0.1)	0.3 (0.1–0.4)	0.1 (0.0–0.3)	0.0, (−0.8–0.2)	0.07 (0–0.2)	
p-value	<0.001	0.02	0.30	<0.001	0.001	0.39	0.09	
ALM/BMI_{ROC} + HGS	0.2 (0.1–0.3)	0.2 (0.0–0.3)	0.0 (0.0–0.1)	0.2 (0.1–0.3)	0.1 (0.0–0.1)	0.0 (0.0–0.1)	0.1 (0.0–0.2)	0.7 (0.6–0.8)
p-value	<0.001	0.001	0.04	<0.001	0.172	0.182	0.02	<0.001

EWGSOP: European Working Group on Sarcopenia in Older People; FNIH: Foundation for the National Institutes of Health; ALM: appendicular lean mass; GS: gait speed; HGS: handgrip strength; ALM/height²: appendicular lean mass/height²; ALM/BMI: appendicular lean mass/body mass index; TUG: Timed-up-and-go. For population-specific cut-points, low values corresponded to T-score < −2, except where indicated as ROC (derived from receiver operating characteristic curves).

4. Discussion

We have reported sarcopenia prevalence in an Australian population using several cut-points for EWGSOP and FNIH definitions. Using these cut-points, we obtained substantial differences in prevalence estimates for sarcopenia, and the level of agreement between definitions varied widely. Using population-specific cut-points equivalent to T-scores <-2, the FNIH definition produced the greatest prevalence, while EWGSOP provided the lowest. As the cut-point for low ALM/BMI$_{ROC}$ that discriminated slow TUG was greater than ALM/BMI T-score <-2, the prevalence estimates for sarcopenia were correspondingly higher, and this was mainly a consequence of low ALM/BMI$_{ROC}$ among the elderly. Regardless, there was a pattern of increasing sarcopenia prevalence with advancing age across all definitions.

The higher prevalence estimates for sarcopenia for older ages was also found in a study in the Netherlands, where diagnostic criteria for sarcopenia influenced prevalence estimates in a middle-aged cohort (mean age 61.8 years for $n = 329$ women and 64.5 years for $n = 325$ men). The authors reported the prevalence of sarcopenia ranged from 0% to 15.6%, 0% to 21.8% and 0% to 25.8% in women aged <60, 60–69 and ≥70 years, respectively, and from 0% to 20.8%, 0% to 31.2% and 0% to 45.2% in men aged <60, 60–69 and ≥70 years, respectively. These results indicate an age-related increase in sarcopenia for all definitions reflecting a decline in muscle mass and performance with age [6,21–23].

For both women and men, when applying population-specific cut-points, we observed that for each age-decade, prevalence estimates were lower for EWGSOP than FNIH. The age-standardized estimates were lower according to EWGSOP than FNIH for both women and men. Dam et al. (2014) [7] of the FNIH research group reported that 2.3% of women and 1.3% of men (proportions outside the 95% CIs of our estimates) in their pooled samples from the USA were classified as having sarcopenia using FNIH, while the prevalence was 13.3% for women and 5.3% for men using EWGSOP1 (point estimates outside our 95% CIs for women, but not for men). Similarly, an Australian study by Sim et al. [2] found that FNIH diagnosed fewer women with sarcopenia than EWGSOP (9.4% vs. 24.1%). In addition, Sim et al. [2] applied Australian female population-specific definitions for FNIH (defined as ALM/BMI < 0.517 m^2 + HGS < 17 kg) and EWGSOP (defined as ALM/height^2 < 5.28 kg/m^2 + HGS < 17 kg). However, the percentage was similar after harmonizing the cut-points.

Our results showed that overall, the agreement between FNIH and EWGSOP was poor, regardless of the cut-points employed. The poor agreement between the original EWGSOP (EWGSOP1) and FNIH definitions is well documented in a number of studies [6–8,24]. For example, Dam et al. [7] examined the difference between FNIH definitions and EWGSOP1. The agreement between the FNIH criteria (low HGS and low lean mass) and EWGSOP was poor in women ($\kappa = 0.14$) and medium in men ($\kappa = 0.53$). However, to our knowledge, this is the first study to examine the agreement between the EWGSOP and FNIH definitions after applying population-specific cut-points in an Australian setting. Masanes et al. [25] found that small differences in cut-points for low lean mass produced substantial variations in prevalence estimates for sarcopenia, and our findings are consistent with their results.

Although the cut-points recommended by EWGSOP [3,5] were adopted from different studies, the method for identifying deficits differed; while some identified low muscle mass and poor performance using the lower portion of the population distribution, the FNIH used a Classification and Regression Tree analysis [10] to identify clinically relevant criteria [4]. In our study, the population-specific cut-points were consistently identified using the lower portion of the population distribution, with the exception of ALM/BMI, where we also used ROC curves to identify low ALM/BMI values that corresponded to poor physical performance. There is still a need to reach a consensus as to which deficits in skeletal muscle health, and the extent of these deficits, are important in defining sarcopenia. Our results highlight disparities in prevalence estimates arising from the thresholds employed, suggesting that population-specific cut-points might be useful in certain populations.

Our study has both strengths and weaknesses. The participants were selected at random from the electoral roll and represent a broad adulthood age range. Almost the entire sample was Caucasian, and this might limit the generalization of our results to other ethnic groups in Australia and beyond. Whereas in this study, we used the mean of the maximum HGS for each hand as being indicative of strength, in some other studies, the maximum irrespective of handedness has been used. In recognition that the methods reported in the literature to identify maximum HGS vary, our choice of one method over another is a potential limitation. Prevalence data for sarcopenia in this study may have been influenced by differential participation and retention bias related to muscle health. Data were also lacking for participants who had physical impairments that prevented them from performance testing. Although data for women and men were pooled to identify sex differences, prevalence estimates for women and men have otherwise been analyzed separately as they were collected at different times.

In conclusion, this study takes a step towards a response to ANZSSFR's call to investigate evidence-based cut-points for EWGSOP criteria for the populations of Australian and New Zealand [12]. We have provided population-based data which will help clinicians and researchers in the field establish new operational definitions for identifying individuals with sarcopenia in the Australian population. However, it is yet to be decided which deficits in skeletal muscle health are important in identifying sarcopenia. Until a universally agreed operational definition of sarcopenia exists internationally and in Australia, prevalence data should be reported with consideration of the ascertainment criteria used and, thus, interpreted in context.

Author Contributions: All authors have taken responsibility for the integrity of the data and the accuracy of the data analysis. Concept and design: S.X.S. and J.A.P. Drafting of the manuscript: S.X.S. Acquisition, analysis, and interpretation of data: all authors. Critical revision of the manuscript for intellectual content: all authors. Statistical analysis: S.X.S. Supervision: K.L.H.-K., N.K.H., L.J.W. and J.A.P. All authors have read and agreed to the published version of the manuscript.

Funding: The Geelong Osteoporosis Study was funded by the National Health and Medical Research Council (NHMRC), Australia (projects 251638 and 628582). S.X.S. was supported by a Deakin Postgraduate Scholarship in conjunction with the Geelong Medical and Health Benefits Association (GMHBA). K.L.H.-K. was supported by an Alfred Deakin Postdoctoral Research Fellowship, N.K.H. by a Dean's Research Postdoctoral Fellowship (Deakin University) and L.J.W. by an NHMRC Career Development Fellowship (1064272) and an NHMRC Investigator Grant (1174060). The funding organizations played no role in the design or conduct of the study, in the collection, management, analysis and interpretation of the data, nor in the preparation, review and approval of the manuscript.

Institutional Review Board Statement: The study was conducted according to the guidelines of the Declaration of Helsinki, and approved by the Human Research Ethics Committee at Barwon HealthInformed Consent Statement: Written informed consent was obtained from all participants in the study.

Data Availability Statement: The data presented in this study are available on request from the corresponding author.

Acknowledgments: The authors acknowledge the men and women who participated in the study, and the staff who contributed to the data collection.

Conflicts of Interest: All authors declare that no competing interests exist.

Ethical Approval: All procedures performed in the studies involving human participants were in accordance with the ethical standards of the institutional and national research committees and with the 1964 Helsinki declaration and its later amendments or comparable ethical standards. The study was approved by the Human Research Ethics Committee at Barwon Health.

Abbreviations

ALM	Appendicular lean mass
ANZSSFR	Australian and New Zealand Society for Sarcopenia and Frailty Research
BMI	Body mass index
CI	Confidence interval
DXA	Dual-energy X-ray absorptiometry
EWGSOP	European Working Group on Sarcopenia in Older People
FNIH	Foundation for the National Institutes of Health
GOS	Geelong Osteoporosis Study
GS	Gait speed
HGS	Handgrip strength
TUG	Timed up-and-go
ROC	Receiver operating characteristic

Appendix A

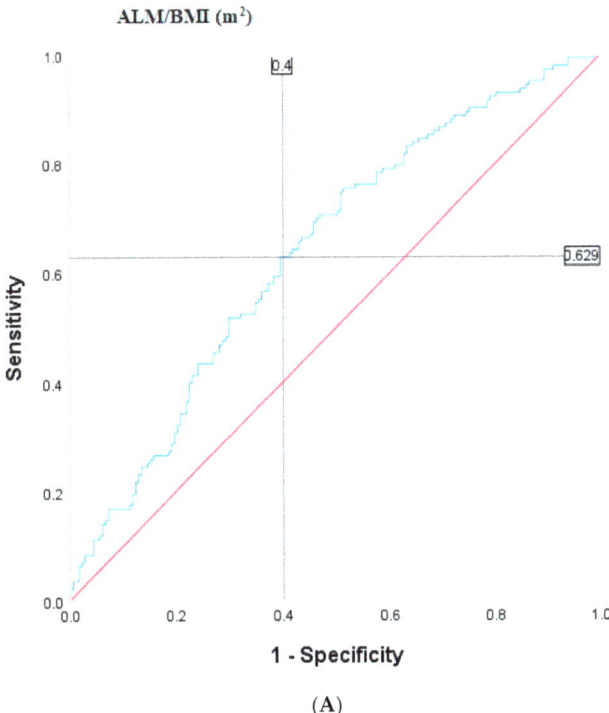

(A)

Figure A1. *Cont.*

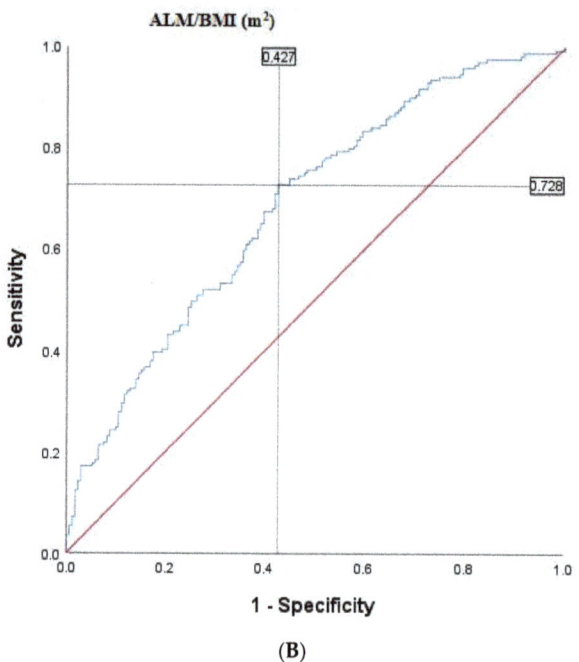

(B)

Figure A1. ROC analysis for optimal discrimination of slow timed up-and-go (TUG; slow TUG < 9.3 s) for ALM/BMI ((**A**,**B**) for women and men, respectively). (**A**) ALM/BMI that best predicted slow TUG (Women); (**B**) ALM/BMI that best predicted slow TUG (Men).

References

1. Fielding, R.A.; Vellas, B.; Evans, W.J.; Bhasin, S.; Morley, J.E.; Newman, A.B.; Van Kan, G.A.; Andrieu, S.; Bauer, J.; Breuille, D.; et al. Sarcopenia: An undiagnosed condition in older adults. Current consensus definition: Prevalence, etiology, and consequences. International Working Group on Sarcopenia. *J. Am. Med. Dir. Assoc.* **2011**, *12*, 249–256. [CrossRef] [PubMed]
2. Sim, M.; Prince, R.L.; Scott, D.; Daly, R.M.; Duque, G.; Inderjeeth, C.A.; Zhu, K.; Woodman, R.J.; Hodgson, J.M.; Lewis, J.R. Sarcopenia definitions and their associations with mortality in older Australian women. *J. Am. Med. Dir. Assoc.* **2019**, *20*, 76–82.e2. [CrossRef] [PubMed]
3. Cruz-Jentoft, A.J.; Baeyens, J.P.; Bauer, J.M.; Boirie, Y.; Cederholm, T.; Landi, F.; Martin, F.C.; Michel, J.-P.; Rolland, Y.; Schneider, S.M.; et al. Sarcopenia: European consensus on definition and diagnosis: Report of the European Working Group on Sarcopenia in Older People. *Age Ageing* **2010**, *39*, 412–423. [CrossRef] [PubMed]
4. Studenski, S.A.; Peters, K.W.; Alley, D.E.; Cawthon, P.M.; McLean, R.R.; Harris, T.B.; Ferrucci, L.; Guralnik, J.M.; Fragala, M.S.; Kenny, A.M.; et al. The FNIH Sarcopenia Project: Rationale, study description, conference recommendations, and final estimates. *J. Gerontol. Ser. A Boil. Sci. Med. Sci.* **2014**, *69*, 547–558. [CrossRef] [PubMed]
5. Cruz-Jentoft, A.J.; Bahat, G.; Bauer, J.; Boirie, Y.; Bruyère, O.; Cederholm, T.; Cooper, C.; Landi, F.; Rolland, Y.; Sayer, A.A.; et al. Sarcopenia: Revised European consensus on definition and diagnosis. *Age Ageing* **2019**, *48*, 16–31. [CrossRef] [PubMed]
6. Pagotto, V.; Silveira, E.A. Applicability and agreement of different diagnostic criteria for sarcopenia estimation in the elderly. *Arch. Gerontol. Geriatr.* **2014**, *59*, 288–294. [CrossRef]
7. Dam, T.-T.; Peters, K.W.; Fragala, M.; Cawthon, P.M.; Harris, T.B.; McLean, R.; Shardell, M.; Alley, D.E.; Kenny, A.; Ferrucci, L.; et al. An evidence-based comparison of operational criteria for the presence of sarcopenia. *J. Gerontol. Ser. A: Boil. Sci. Med. Sci.* **2014**, *69*, 584–590. [CrossRef]
8. Sui, S.X.; Holloway-Kew, K.L.; Hyde, N.K.; Williams, L.J.; Tembo, M.C.; Leach, S.; Pasco, J.A. Definition-specific prevalence estimates for sarcopenia in Australian population: The Geelong Osteoporosis Study. *JCSM Clin. Rep.* **2020**, *5*, 89–98.
9. Bahat, G.; Tufan, A.; Tufan, F.; Kilic, C.; Akpinar, T.S.; Kose, M.; Erten, N.; Karan, M.A.; Cruz-Jentoft, A.J. Cut-off points to identify sarcopenia according to European Working Group on Sarcopenia in Older People (EWGSOP) definition. *Clin. Nutr.* **2016**, *35*, 1557–1563. [CrossRef]
10. Breiman, L.; Friedman, J.H.; Olshen, R.A.; Stone, C.J. *Classification and Regression Trees*; Wadsworth International Group: Belmont, CA, USA, 1984.

11. Gould, H.; Brennan, S.L.; Kotowicz, M.A.; Nicholson, G.C.; Pasco, J.A. Total and appendicular lean mass reference ranges for Australian men and women: The Geelong Osteoporosis Study. *Calcif. Tissue Int.* **2014**, *94*, 363–372. [CrossRef]
12. Zanker, J.; Scott, D.; Reijnierse, E.M.; Brennan-Olsen, S.L.; Daly, R.M.; Girgis, C.M.; Grossmann, M.; Hayes, A.; Henwood, T.; Hirani, V.; et al. Establishing an operational definition of sarcopenia in Australia and New Zealand: Delphi method based consensus statement. *J. Nutr. Health Aging* **2019**, *23*, 105–110. [CrossRef] [PubMed]
13. Pasco, J.A.; Nicholson, G.C.; Kotowicz, M.A. Cohort profile: Geelong Osteoporosis Study. *Int. J. Epidemiol.* **2011**, *41*, 1565–1575. [CrossRef] [PubMed]
14. Bischoff, H.A.; Stähelin, H.B.; Monsch, A.U.; Iversen, M.D.; Weyh, A.; Von Dechend, M.; Akos, R.; Conzelmann, M.; Dick, W.; Theiler, R. Identifying a cut-off point for normal mobility: A comparison of the timed 'up and go' test in community-dwelling and institutionalised elderly women. *Age Ageing* **2003**, *32*, 315–320. [CrossRef] [PubMed]
15. Pasco, J.A.; Holloway-Kew, K.L.; Tembo, M.C.; Sui, S.X.; Anderson, K.B.; Rufus-Membere, P.; Hyde, N.K.; Williams, L.J.; Kotowicz, M.A. Normative data for lean mass using FNIH criteria in an Australian setting. *Calcif. Tissue Int.* **2018**, *104*, 475–479. [CrossRef] [PubMed]
16. Sui, S.X.; Holloway-Kew, K.L.; Hyde, N.K.; Williams, L.J.; Tembo, M.C.; Mohebbi, M.; Gojanovic, M.; Leach, S.; Pasco, J.A. Handgrip strength and muscle quality in Australian women: Cross-sectional data from the Geelong Osteoporosis Study. *J. Cachex Sarcopenia Muscle* **2020**, *11*, 690–697. [CrossRef] [PubMed]
17. Pasco, J.A.; Stuart, A.L.; Holloway-Kew, K.L.; Tembo, M.C.; Sui, S.X.; Anderson, K.B.; Hyde, N.K.; Williams, L.J.; Kotowicz, M.A. Lower-limb muscle strength: Normative data from an observational population-based study. *BMC Musculoskelet. Disord.* **2020**, *21*, 89. [CrossRef]
18. Cawthon, P.; Peters, K.W.; Shardell, M.D.; McLean, R.R.; Dam, T.-T.L.; Kenny, A.M.; Fragala, M.S.; Harris, T.B.; Kiel, D.P.; Guralnik, J.M.; et al. Cutpoints for low appendicular lean mass that identify older adults with clinically significant weakness. *J. Gerontol. Ser. A Boil. Sci. Med. Sci.* **2014**, *69*, 567–575. [CrossRef]
19. Unal, I. Defining an optimal cut-point value in ROC analysis: An alternative approach. *Comput. Math. Methods Med.* **2017**, *2017*, 1–14. [CrossRef]
20. Census of Population and Ageing: Age by Sex. Australian Bureau of Statistics. 2011. Available online: www.abs.gov.au (accessed on 19 November 2019).
21. Auyeung, T.W.; Lee, S.W.J.; Leung, J.; Kwok, T.; Woo, J. Age-associated decline of muscle mass, grip strength and gait speed: A 4-year longitudinal study of 3018 community-dwelling older Chinese. *Geriatr. Gerontol. Int.* **2014**, *14*, 76–84. [CrossRef]
22. Yoshida, D.; Suzuki, T.; Shimada, H.; Park, H.; Makizako, H.; Doi, T.; Anan, Y.; Tsutsumimoto, K.; Uemura, K.; Ito, T.; et al. Using two different algorithms to determine the prevalence of sarcopenia. *Geriatr. Gerontol. Int.* **2014**, *14*, 46–51. [CrossRef]
23. Lees, M.; Wilson, O.J.; Hind, K.; Ispoglou, T. Muscle quality as a complementary prognostic tool in conjunction with sarcopenia assessment in younger and older individuals. *Graefe's Arch. Clin. Exp. Ophthalmol.* **2019**, *119*, 1171–1181. [CrossRef]
24. Mayhew, A.J.; Amog, K.; Phillips, S.; Parise, G.; McNicholas, P.D.; De Souza, R.J.; Thabane, L.; Raina, P. The prevalence of sarcopenia in community-dwelling older adults, an exploration of differences between studies and within definitions: A systematic review and meta-analyses. *Age Ageing* **2019**, *48*, 48–56. [CrossRef] [PubMed]
25. Masanés, F.; Luque, X.R.I.; Salvà, A.; Serra-Rexach, J.A.; Artaza, I.; Formiga, F.; Cuesta, F.; Soto, A.L.; Ruiz, D.; Cruz-Jentoft, A.J. Cut-off points for muscle mass—not grip strength or gait speed—determine variations in sarcopenia prevalence. *J. Nutr. Heal. Aging* **2017**, *21*, 825–829. [CrossRef]

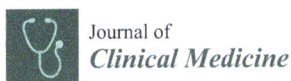

Review

Effect of Sleep Quality on the Prevalence of Sarcopenia in Older Adults: A Systematic Review with Meta-Analysis

Jacobo Á. Rubio-Arias [1,*], Raquel Rodríguez-Fernández [2], Luis Andreu [3,4], Luis M. Martínez-Aranda [4,5], Alejandro Martínez-Rodriguez [6] and Domingo J. Ramos-Campo [4]

1. LFE Research Group, Department of Health and Human Performance, Faculty of Physical Activity and Sport Science-INEF, Universidad Politécnica de Madrid, 28040 Madrid, Spain
2. Department of Methodology of Behavioral Sciences, Faculty of Psychology, Universidad Nacional de Educación a Distancia (UNED), 28040 Madrid, Spain; rrodriguez@psi.uned.es
3. International Chair of Sports Medicine, Universidad Católica San Antonio de Murcia (UCAM), 30107 Murcia, Spain; landreu@ucam.edu
4. Faculty of Sports, Universidad Católica San Antonio de Murcia (UCAM), 30107 Murcia, Spain; lmmartinez2@ucam.edu (L.M.M.-A.); Djramos@ucam.edu (D.J.R.-C.)
5. Neuroscience of Human Movement Research Group (Neuromove), Universidad Católica San Antonio de Murcia (UCAM), 30107 Murcia, Spain
6. Department of Analytical Chemistry, Nutrition and Food Science, Faculty of Science, Alicante University, 03690 Alicante, Spain; amartinezrodriguez@ua.es
* Correspondence: ja.rubio@upm.es or jacobo.rubio2@gmail.com

Received: 8 November 2019; Accepted: 3 December 2019; Published: 6 December 2019

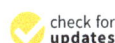

Abstract: Sarcopenia is an age-related condition. However, the prevalence of sarcopenia may increase due to a range of other factors, such as sleep quality/duration. Therefore, the aim of the study is to conduct a systematic review with meta-analysis to determine the prevalence of sarcopenia in older adults based on their self-reported sleep duration. Methods: Three electronic databases were used—PubMed-Medline, Web of Science, and Cochrane Library. We included studies that measured the prevalence of sarcopenia, divided according to sleep quality and excluded studies (a) involving populations with neuromuscular pathologies, (b) not showing prevalence values (cases/control) on sarcopenia, and (c) not including classificatory models to determine sleep quality. Results: high prevalence values in older adults with both long and short sleep duration were shown. However, prevalence values were higher in those with inadequate sleep (<6–8 h or low efficiency) (OR 0.76; 95% CI (0.70–0.83); Q = 1.446; p = 0.695; test for overall effect, Z = 6.01, p < 0.00001). Likewise, higher prevalence levels were shown in men (OR 1.61; 95% CI (0.82–3.16); Q = 11.80; p = 0.0189) compared to women (OR 0.77; 95% CI (0.29–2.03); Q = 21.35; p = 0.0003). Therefore, the prevalence of sarcopenia appears to be associated with sleep quality, with higher prevalence values in older adults who have inadequate sleep.

Keywords: muscle-mass; sleep efficiency; sleep duration; insomnia

1. Introduction

Together with the increment of the world population and life span over the years, a parallel increase in chronic diseases [1] has been observed, such as sarcopenia. This pathology has become a serious global public health problem [2] since it can lead to a considerable increase in costs due to the frequency and duration of hospitalization, as well as an increase in the number of falls as a consequence of muscle weakness [3,4]. In addition, people who suffer a high loss of muscle mass have an increased risk of other health problems, such as heart failure, chronic obstructive pulmonary diseases, kidney failure [5] or osteoporosis [6] and, therefore, a greater risk of bone fracture, turning sarcopenia into a major health problem that should be addressed in order to determine the possible factors associated with sarcopenia.

Sarcopenia has been defined as a decrease and deterioration of muscle mass associated with aging [7]. Thus, the skeletal muscle mass is progressively lost during aging and is partially replaced by fat and connective tissue due to a reduction and leakage of type II fibers generated by a slow degenerative neurological process [8]. This decrease in muscle mass due to aging also generates a decrease in muscle strength and, therefore, a physical disability generating a functional limitation (activities of the daily life) as well as a decrease in the life quality [9,10] with an associated increase in the risk of mortality [11,12]. In addition, this muscle mass loss has a greater impact on women during menopause as a consequence of the decrease in the estrogen levels after the fifth decade of life [13]. Sex differences in body composition are well known [14], with men having a higher cross-sectional area in skeletal muscle than women and greater muscle in the upper body [15]. Additionally, women are at higher risk of developing sarcopenic obesity due to increased fat and lower muscle mass [14]. Nevertheless, the results of prevalence related to sex are inconsistent [2]. In these circumstances, efforts are required to identify the factors associated with sarcopenia and to implement interventions for the prevention or the incidence reduction of this pathology among the elderly population [16], considering sex as a modifying variable.

However, the loss of muscle mass (sarcopenia) is not only related to age and sex but also depends on a number of endogenous and exogenous factors that influence the prevalence values of sarcopenia. The most studied and validated factors that can generate an effect on the sarcopenia are age (main moderating variable), genetic factors, birth weight, early growth, diet, physical activity, other chronic diseases, and hormonal changes (secondary variables) [17,18]. In line with this, a recent systematic review with meta-analysis on the general population [2] concludes that the prevalence of sarcopenia can be modified by other factors such as race, nutrition, quality of life, and sex among others.

Nonetheless, the scientific literature shows a gap between the role that sleep quality could play and the effects on the prevalence of sarcopenia. As Buchmann et al. (2016) [19] suggest, sleep is associated with a biological and mental regeneration process. Moreover, Vitale et al. (2019) [20] reported that the maintenance of circadian rhythms can be altered by aging and the development of many chronic diseases, including sarcopenia. The preservation of circadian rhythm is very important for the sustainment of cellular physiology, metabolism, and function in the skeletal muscle. Therefore, people who have an inadequate sleeping time could have an increased risk of mortality compared to those who sleep the recommended daily hours [21]. In addition, under low sleep conditions, the cognitive abilities might be affected and can be an increment in the risk of mortality and falling in older adults [22]. In this way, sex may also play a significant role in sleep quality, due to the fact that women have a greater predisposition of insomnia found among different criteria, frequencies, and duration [23]. Nevertheless, the association between muscle mass, sleep quality, and sex is not clear yet and no studies have been found to support such affirmation.

Certainly, the lack of sleep not only leads to a deterioration of cognitive abilities but can also have a negative effect at the cellular level on muscle physiology. It impairs muscle recovery due to increased stimulation of protein degradation, which is detrimental for protein synthesis and promotes muscle atrophy [24]. In addition to the negative effect on muscle mass, it has been associated with cardiovascular disease [25], type II diabetes [26], hypertension [25], obesity [27], and colorectal cancer [28]. In this regard, public health should include sleep duration/quality as one of the risk factors associated with a large number of diseases.

Some correlational studies have determined the effect of sleep duration on muscle mass, showing that less sleep duration or quality leads to a loss of muscle mass [29]. However, no meta-analyses addressing the effect of sleep duration or quality on the prevalence of sarcopenia have been found. Therefore, the objectives of this systematic review with meta-analysis are (1) to analyze the overall prevalence of sarcopenia in people with optimal sleep duration/quality compared to those with inadequate sleep quality, (2) to analyze whether the prevalence of sarcopenia is correlated to the sex of the participants. Our starting hypothesis is that people with poor rest show a higher prevalence of sarcopenia than those who rest in better conditions and, in addition, men will have a lower prevalence compared to women.

2. Experimental Section

2.1. Study Design

A systematic review with meta-analysis was performed following the recommendations of PRISMA (preferred reporting items for systematic review and meta-analysis) [30]. All the analyses were performed in duplicate (J.A.R.A. and L.A.), all disagreements on inclusion/exclusion were discussed and resolved by consensus. The extrinsic characteristics of the publications and the substantive characteristics—population, sex, associated pathology, habits of alcohol, tobacco, physical activity, age, and BMI—were extracted from the studies that were finally included in the quantitative analysis. Finally, the methodological characteristics—duration of sleep, quality of sleep, muscular mass and presence or not of sarcopenia—were also considered. All subjects included in the analysis were classified as cases or control differentiating sleep and sex.

2.2. Search and Data Sources

Three electronic databases were used: PubMed-Medline, Web of Science, and Cochrane Library. The search was conducted without search date restriction and ended on 28 July 2019. The key search words and strategy were "Sleep Disorders" OR "Sleep Deprivation" OR "Sleep Hygiene" OR "Sleep duration" OR insomnia OR sleep* and "muscle mass" OR "muscular atrophy" OR sarcopenia.

2.3. Data extraction and Inclusion/Exclusion Criteria

The following inclusion criteria were considered: prevalence studies analyzing the effect of sleep on sarcopenia and conducted in adults (>40). Studies were excluded if they included (a) populations with neuromuscular pathologies, (b) studies that did not show prevalence values (cases/control) on sarcopenia, and (c) studies that did not include classificatory models that allowed sleep quality to be determined.

2.4. Outcomes

The variables to determine the prevalence of sarcopenia as a function of sleep were (1) the presence or absence of sarcopenia, and (2) sleep quality. Sleep can be assessed to estimate adequate or inadequate sleep in terms of quality or duration in different ways. For the questionnaires, adequate-sleep (sleep well) for those who obtained between very good or quite good in the percentage of quality and not-adequate-sleep (sleep bad), rather bad or very bad were considered [19]. Regarding the hours of sleep, they were considered inadequate (<6–8) and adequate (≥8), following the recommendations of the National Sleep Foundation [21].

2.5. Assessment of Risk of Bias

The Q-index was used to assess the methodological quality, a scale that allows us to quantify the bias, obtaining a final score between 0 (minimum quality) and 1 (maximum quality). This rescaled quality range (called Qi in MetaXL) has a monotonic relationship to ICC bias, defined as the variance of the study bias divided by the sum of the variance of bias within and between studies [31,32]. Quality analysis was performed on each study based on the method of assessing sleep quality and sarcopenia, giving higher preference to the studies that measured the sleep with instruments previously validated for this purpose, as well as sarcopenia with DXA or BIA. Therefore, the studies using both DXA and a validated questionnaire to analyze sleep quality were scored with 1. The following criteria were conducted:

(Q1) Were the target population and the observation period well defined?: yes = 1 and no = 0;

(Q2) Diagnostic criteria, use of diagnostic system reported: sarcopenia = DXA or BIA and sleep quality = instruments validated = 1 and own system/symptoms described/no system/not specified = 0;

(Q3) Method of case ascertainment: community survey/multiple institutions = 2, inpatient/inpatients and outpatients/case registers = 1, and not specified = 0;

(Q4) Administration of measurement protocol: administered interview = 3, systematic case-note review = 2, chart diagnosis/case records = 1 and not specified = 0;

(Q5) Catchment area: broadly representative (national or multi-site survey) = 2, small area/not representative (single community, single university) = 1, and convenience sampling/other (primary care sample/treatment group) = 0; and

(Q6) Prevalence measure: point prevalence (e.g., one month) = 2, 12-month prevalence = 1 and lifetime prevalence = 0.

In addition, the overall publication bias of the studies was analyzed using the funnel plot, dividing between older adults who slept well and those who had inadequate sleep.

2.6. Data Synthesis and Statistical Analysis

Meta-analysis and statistical analysis were performed using MetaXL software version 2.0 (Sunrise Beach, Queensland, Australia). The prevalence of sarcopenia (cases vs. control) was initially calculated in the included studies for random-effects model analysis (no transformation methods) and then recalculated under a rescaled quality of bias effects model. For the analysis, the sleep category was considered (sleep well and sleep poorly) for the calculation of the overall prevalence of sarcopenia, and this method was applied under the random-effects model and effects in quality of the rescaled bias using three possible transformations (None, Logit, and Arcsine) [31,32] to contrast the effects of the prevalence of sarcopenia. In all cases, pooled prevalence values were shown, 95% CI, heterogeneity I^2, Cochran's Q, chi^2, p, tau^2. On the other hand, the grouped odds ratios (OR) and their IC95% were also calculated following a model of "quality effects" [31,33] to analyze the association between those who sleep well (control) and those who sleep poorly (effect). In addition, OR and sleep category analysis were estimated, excluding studies that did not report participants' total hours of sleep and only showed sleep quality [19,34]. Heterogeneity between studies was conducted using the I^2 statistic, and the variation between studies was calculated using the tau^2 statistic (τ^2) [35]. I^2 values between 30–60% were considered as moderate levels of heterogeneity, while a value of $\tau^2 > 1$ suggested the presence of substantial statistical heterogeneity. The minimum level of significance was set as $p \leq 0.05$.

3. Results

3.1. General Characteristics of the Studies

A total of 551 items were identified from the selected databases, and 0/0 items were included from other sources. After the removal of duplicated articles from the different databases, 361 titles and abstracts, as well as 106 articles, were reviewed, and 255 were removed. Finally, statistical analysis was performed on a total of 6 studies [19,34,36–39] (5 were performed in Asia and only 1 in Europe; Figure 1), with a mean age of 68.7 years (range = 44–80 years). Table 1 shows the descriptive characteristics of the studies included in our analysis. The selected studies included 6405 (990 cases and 5415 controls) older adults with adequate sleep and 12,708 (1762 cases and 10,946 controls) adults with inadequate sleep. However, only four studies contained data divided by sex (1232 men) including 142 cases with adequate sleep and 95 cases with inadequate sleep. In addition, 1381 women were enrolled in the four studies, with 109 cases in the adequate sleep group and 118 cases in the inadequate sleep group.

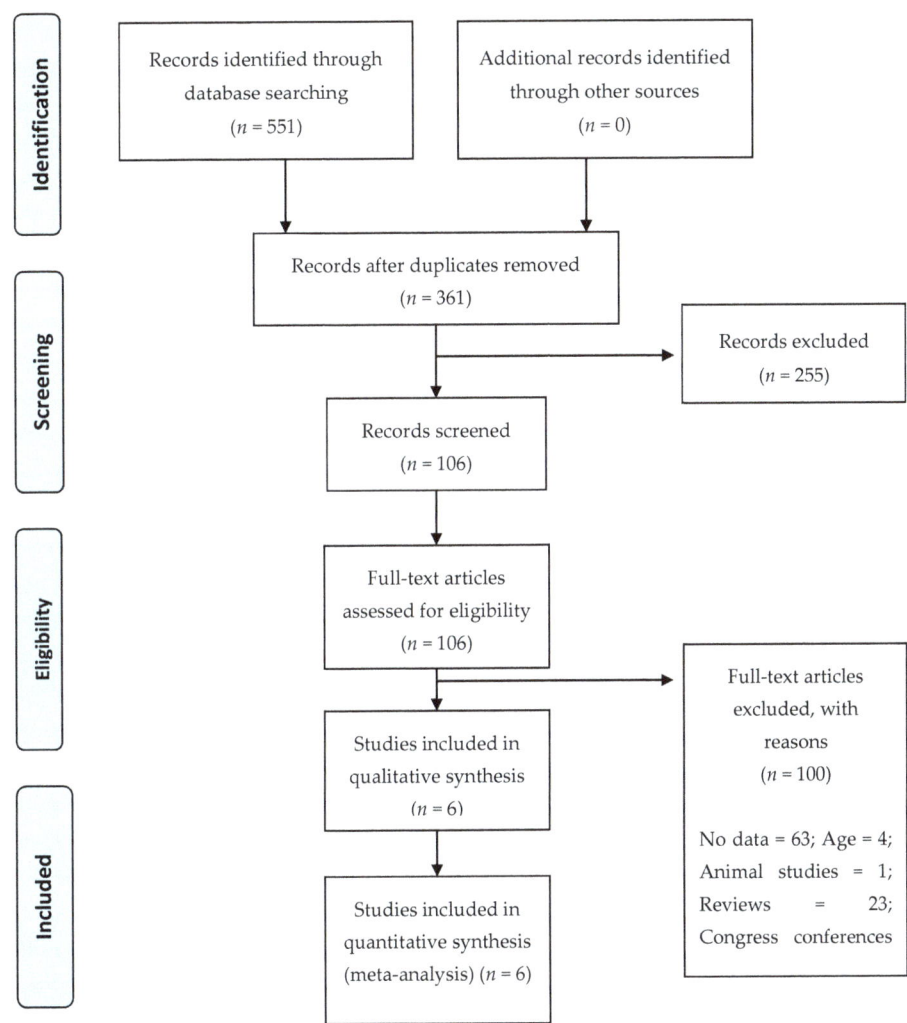

Figure 1. Flow diagram of the process of study selection.

Table 1. Characteristics of the included studies in the meta-analysis.

	Extrinsic Variables	Substantive Characteristics												Methodological Characteristics								
																Sleep Well			Sleep Poorly		
Study	Country of the Study	Sex	Alcohol	Tobacco	Level of Physical Activity	Muscle Mass	Sleep Quality	Age	Weight	Height	BMI	Type	Sex	Total	N	Cases	Control	N2	Cases	Control
Buchmann et al.	Berlin	Women	494	46	Moderate	DXA	PSQI	68			25.7	Cross-sectional	M	568	492	79	413	76	27	49
		Women	66	4	Moderate			69			31.2		W	628	508	64	444	120	13	107
		Men	424	59	Moderate			69			26.4		T	1196	1000	143	857	196	40	156
		Men	99	7	Moderate			69			30.2									
Chien et al.	Taiwan	Men			Regular	BIA	PSQI and Self-report	78.7	63.9	162.1	24.3	Cross-sectional	M	224	112	25	87	112	29	83
		Men			Regular			77.8	64.1	163.7	23.9		W	264	76	20	56	188	18	170
		Men			Regular			80	66.8	164.4	24.7		T	488	188	45	143	300	47	253
		Women			Regular			74.4	58.3	151.9	25.3									
		Women			Regular			74.5	57.9	153	24.8									
		Women			Regular			76.2	56.6	152.2	24.3									
Fu et al.	China	48.7% Men	No = 61.1%	No = 37.2%	Moderate	BIA	Self-report	68.24	70.24	163.38	25.9	Cohort study	T	920	468	52	416	452	43	409
		40.5% Men	No = 62.2%	No = 38.9%	Moderate			66.3	67.96	163.91	25.3									
		37.9% Men	No = 59.5%	No = 33.7%	Moderate			67.38	67.16	163.39	25.1									
		54% Men	No = 64.6%	No = 28.8%	Moderate			68.93	68.1	163.37	25.4									
Hu et al.	China	Men	57	62	Moderate	DXA	Self-report	70.8			23.6	Cross-Sectional Study	M	251	63	13	50	188	28	160
		Men	19	19	Moderate			72.6			18.7		W	356	63	14	49	293	57	236
		Women	16	1	Moderate			69.1			23.6		T	607	126	27	99	481	85	396
		Women	5	2	Moderate			72.3			20.3									
Ida et al.	Japan	Men	60%	72.1%		Self-report	PSQI	71.8			24.3	Cross-sectional study	M	189	105	14	91	84	22	62
		Women	17.2%	4.9%				72.8			23.9		W	129	71	11	60	58	24	34
													T	318	176	25	151	142	46	96
Kwon et al.	Korea	Men = 5819; Women = 8118	4.209	3.579	Regular	DXA	Self-report	44				Cross-sectional study	M							
		Men = 1339; Women = 872	635	797	Regular			45.2					W							
													T	16148	4938	819	4119	11210	1486	9724

M, men; W, women; T, total; DXA, densitometry; BIA, bioelectrical impedance analysis and PSQI, pittsburgh sleep quality index.

3.2. Quality of the Studies

The assessment of the methodological quality of the studies included in the quantitative analysis is summarised in Table 2.

Table 2. The score obtained by the studies on the quality scale.

		Q1	Q2	Q3	Q4	Q5	Q6	M.S.	Qi
Buchmann et al. 2016	[19]	1	1	2	3	1	2	10	1
Chien et al. 2015	[36]	1	1	2	3	1	2	9	1
Fu et al. 2019	[37]	1	1	0	3	1	2	7	0.8
Hu et al. 2017	[38]	1	1	2	3	1	2	10	1
Ida et al. 2019	[34]	1	0	0	3	0	2	7	0.6
Kwon et al. 2017	[39]	1	1	2	3	1	2	10	1

TS, Total score; Q1, Were the target population and the observation period well defined?; Q2, Diagnostic criteria; Q3, Method of case ascertainment; Q4, Administration of measurement protocol; Q5, Catchment Area; Q6, Prevalence measure. M.S. mean score; Qi stands for a quality rank.

When estimating a study quality, the mean score was 0.833 (range: 0.7–1). Three studies used bioelectrical impedance analysis (BIA) [33,36], three DXA [19,38,39] and only one study used a self-administered questionnaire [34]. Furthermore, three studies used the Pittsburg Sleep Quality Index (PSQI) [19,34,36], and the other three assessed the sleep duration/quality with self-reports. In addition, two studies [34,37] did not specify the case measurement system. The funnel plots suggest the presence of significant publication bias (Figure 2).

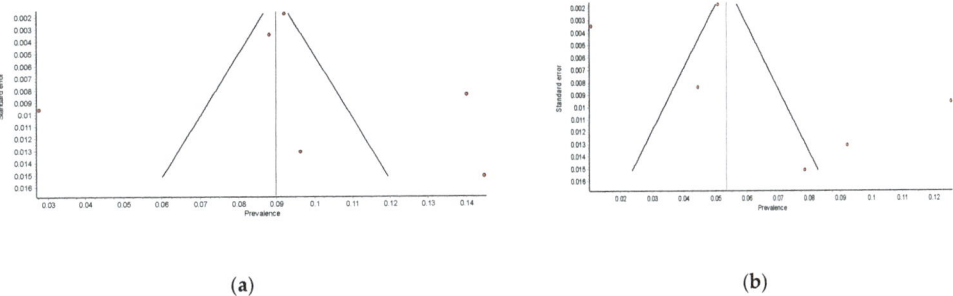

(a)   (b)

Figure 2. Funnel plot of the meta-analysis of the published studies. Each plotted point represents the standard error (SE) and the prevalence. (**a**) Sleep well, (**b**) sleep poorly.

3.3. Meta-Analysis

The overall results of the prevalence of sarcopenia in the studies included in our meta-analysis revealed a high prevalence (Figure 3). When the methodological quality of the studies was considered in the results (Table 2), the prevalence was decreased (Total = 19,677 participants, 2858 cases; 0.144, 95% CI (0.100–0.189); Q = 41.90, p = 0.0000) but maintaining a high heterogeneity (I^2 = 88).

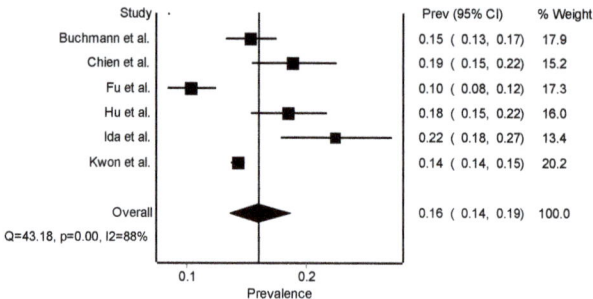

Figure 3. Overall prevalence of studies included in the analysis (method: random effects).

Results by Sleep Categories

The effects of the prevalence of sarcopenia sorted by categories are shown in Table 3. The prevalence values are grouped by sleep quality categories (sleep well and sleep poorly).

Table 3. Prevalence. Pooled results and CIs for three categories by transformation method and model.

Model	Transf.	Category	Sarcopenia and Self-Report or PSQI							Sarcopenia and Self-Report						
			Pooled	LCI	HCI	I² (%)	Cochran's Q	χ² (p)	tau2/ Q-Index	Pooled	LCI	HCI	I²	Cochran's Q	χ² (p)	tau2/ Q-Index
Inverse Variance	None	SW	0.056	0.053	0.059	95.786	118.642	0.000		0.052	0.049	0.055	94.549	55.035	0.000	
		SP	0.088	0.084	0.091	95.786	118.642	0.000		0.090	0.086	0.094	94.549	55.035	0.000	
	Logit	SW	0.384	0.052	0.058	95.241	105.072	0.000		0.363	0.049	0.055	90.653	32.094	0.000	
		SP	0.616	0.084	0.092	95.241	105.072	0.000		0.637	0.087	0.095	90.653	32.094	0.000	
	Double arcsine	SW	0.388	0.052	0.059	95.847	120.389	0.000		0.363	0.049	0.055	93.072	43.300	0.000	
		SP	0.612	0.084	0.092	95.847	120.389	0.000		0.637	0.087	0.095	93.072	43.300	0.000	
Random effects	None	SW	0.073	0.044	0.102	95.786	118.642	0.000	0.001	0.060	0.030	0.091	94.549	55.035	0.000	0.001
		SP	0.090	0.061	0.119	95.786	118.642	0.000	0.001	0.093	0.062	0.124	94.549	55.035	0.000	0.001
	Logit	SW	0.460	0.046	0.103	95.241	105.072	0.000	0.264	0.399	0.041	0.083	90.653	32.094	0.000	0.126
		SP	0.540	0.055	0.119	95.241	105.072	0.000	0.264	0.601	0.062	0.122	90.653	32.094	0.000	0.126
	Double arcsine	SW	0.453	0.044	0.102	95.847	120.389	0.000	0.018	0.395	0.036	0.086	93.072	43.300	0.000	0.011
		SP	0.547	0.056	0.120	95.847	120.389	0.000	0.018	0.605	0.061	0.123	93.072	43.300	0.000	0.011
Quality effects	None	SW	0.056	-0.001	0.113	95.786	118.642	0.000	1.698	0.052	0.000	0.104	94.549	55.035	0.000	1.356
		SP	0.088	0.031	0.145	95.786	118.642	0.000	1.698	0.091	0.039	0.143	94.549	55.035	0.000	1.356
	Logit	SW	0.384	0.024	0.118	95.241	105.072	0.000	1.714	0.362	0.028	0.093	90.653	32.094	0.000	0.804
		SP	0.616	0.040	0.182	95.241	105.072	0.000	1.714	0.638	0.051	0.158	90.653	32.094	0.000	0.804
	Double arcsine	SW	0.379	0.011	0.112	95.847	120.389	0.000	1.583	0.353	0.015	0.096	93.072	43.300	0.000	1.013
		SP	0.621	0.030	0.155	95.847	120.389	0.000	1.583	0.647	0.042	0.148	93.072	43.300	0.000	1.013

Transf., transformation; HCI, higher CI; LCI, lower CI; SW, sleep well; SP, sleep poorly.

People who sleep well had lower values than those who sleep poorly and the prevalence in all the sub-analyses was high, suggesting a prevalence of sarcopenia independently of the category. However, the OR value was not significant (OR 0.81; 95% CI (0.41–1.60); Q = 34.04; $p = 0.0000$; test for overall effect, Z = 0.12, $p = 0.91$) when analysing the relationship between sarcopenia and sleep quality. Nonetheless, when the relationship between sleep quality and sarcopenia was analyzed after excluding the Buchmann et al. [19] and Ida et al. [34] studies from the analysis due to high heterogeneity, the sleep quality was associated with sarcopenia (OR 0.76; 95% CI (0.70–0.83); Q = 1.446; $p = 0.695$; test for overall effect, Z = 6.01, $p < 0.00001$). Likewise, the subjects who self-reported fewer sleeping hours showed a higher prevalence of sarcopenia.

Due to the high heterogeneity of the studies included in the meta-analysis, a gender analysis of prevalence was performed (Figure 4). Only four studies provided sex-dependent data. Non-significant associations for men (OR 1.61; 95% CI (0.82–3.16); Q = 11.80; $p = 0.0189$) or women (OR 0.77; 95% CI (0.29–2.03); Q = 21.35; $p = 0.0003$) were observed. However, the heterogeneity still showed high value in all the sub-analyses that were performed (including the quality of the studies and without any transformation), due to the heterogeneity of the methodologies, the types of studies and other parameters that were not taken into consideration for the analysis of the prevalence of sarcopenia.

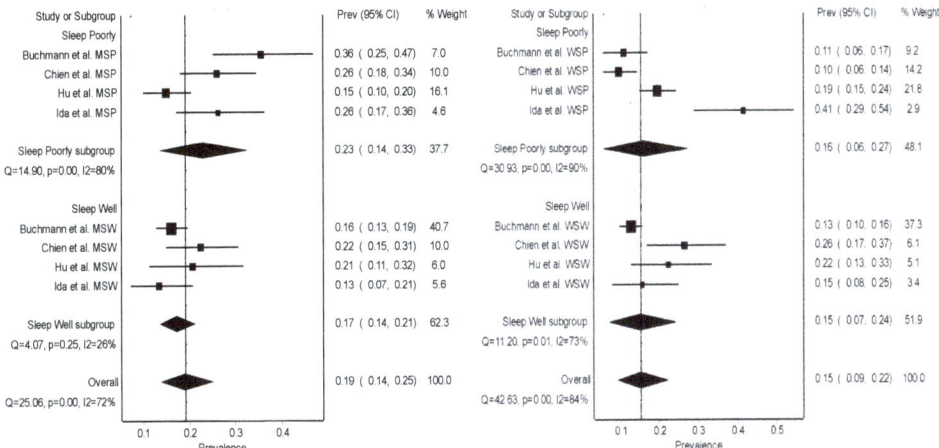

Figure 4. Prevalence of sarcopenia according to the sex of the participants. MSP, men sleep poorly; MSW, men sleep well; SWP, women sleep poorly; and WSW, women sleep well.

4. Discussion

The main finding of this research is that those subjects having inadequate sleep show a higher prevalence of sarcopenia values than those who reported adequate sleep. In addition, our results revealed a high prevalence of sarcopenia in older adults.

The results showed that a higher prevalence of sarcopenia values from those who do not sleep adequately were almost twice the value of the grouped prevalence, according to the model and the transformation that were used in the analysis. In line with our findings, Chien et al. [36], observed a significant association between sleep duration and the prevalence of sarcopenia on a sample of 488 adults (224 men and 264 women) from Taiwan, even though the assessment of sarcopenia was performed by electrical bioimpedance (BIA). Moreover, in the only study carried out in Europe, focused on the German subjects [19], similar results to those described above were observed, with the addition of the association between the sleep length and the quantity of muscle mass and recommending longitudinal studies to better understand the potential association. Similarly, Hu et al. [38] observed a relationship between sleep hours and sarcopenia in a Chinese cohort (n = 920, 95 cases). However, in this case, a U-shaped association in the prevalence of sarcopenia was obtained, in which older adults with short or long sleep length obtained higher values compared to those with normal sleep duration.

One plausible explanation to this findings is that the participants with an inefficient sleep may have differences in hormonal regulation (anabolic and catabolic balance), with elevated levels of cortisol (catabolic hormone promoting protein degradation), and low levels of IGF-1 (anabolic hormones promoting protein synthesis), developing a positive balance towards muscle degradation and, therefore, favoring the loss of muscle mass [19,40]. Likewise, Buchmann et al. [19] also observed elevated c-reactive protein (CRP) values. CRP is a pro-inflammatory cytokine and has been proposed as a possible cause of muscular atrophy [41] and also associated with sleep deprivation in high concentrations [42]. The sleep restriction generates hormonal imbalances and pro-inflammatory effects, favoring the loss of muscle mass with age. This could be one reason for the higher prevalence of sarcopenia values of sarcopenia in people with inadequate sleep. We must consider that the losses of muscle strength and muscle mass are associated and, therefore, related to a decrease in the functional capacity and quality of life [43]. Further studies to determine the effects of sleep deprivation in patients diagnosed with sarcopenia are necessary.

Interestingly, our results suggest a higher prevalence of sarcopenia in men compared to women (men = 0.19, 95% CI (0.14–0.25); women = 0.15, 95% CI (0.09–0.22)). These results are in line with previous studies in which the prevalence of sarcopenia can occur at earlier ages, as shown by Kwon et al. [39]. They observed a prevalence of sarcopenia of 14.3% in a group of 16,148 Koreans (44.1 ± 0.2 years), being higher in men (18.7%) than in women (9.7%). This can be explained by the fact that men had a higher muscle mass compared to women, but also a larger magnitude in muscle decrease was observed in men versus women as age increased [14]. On the contrary, in previous studies where the prevalence of sarcopenia was identified at different age intervals, a lower prevalence in men compared to women was observed [44]. Although age is the main causal effect of sarcopenia, the prediction ratio of increased sarcopenia based on age is difficult to verify, due to the multitude of factors that could have an influence in the prevalence values [45]. Nonetheless, it is estimated that the prevalence of clinically significant sarcopenia ranges from 8.8% in elderly women to 17.5% in elderly men, but it should be noted that these values may be higher or lower depending on the environmental factors [46]. In our study, only four articles considered gender as a sarcopenia-modifying variable, with very different methodologies and difficult interpretation. Therefore, the effect of sex on the prevalence of sarcopenia is unclear and more studies are needed to determine this interaction.

In summary, a direct association between sleep duration and prevalence of sarcopenia were confirmed in all the studies included in the quantitative data analysis. However, the interaction of gender and sleep duration/quality is not entirely clear. Hu et al. [38] observed that the prevalence of sarcopenia due to sleep deprivation was more pronounced in women. Similar results were described by Chien et al. [36] and Ida et al. [34]. However, Buchmann et al. [19] reported poor associations between sleep deprivation and the prevalence of sarcopenia in women. This discrepancy could be justified based on the ethnicity of the participants [2] or the age range difference between the studies. This higher and more evident prevalence in women could be associated with the negative effects of menopause. Thus, a decrease in the estrogen levels during menopause could play a potential role in decreasing the muscle mass after the fifth decade of life [13]. In addition, muscle mass seems to play an important role in osteoporosis in women, since muscle contractions involve a mechanical load on the bone that could promote the rate of bone regeneration [47]. Therefore, it could be stated that there is a close link between muscle strength, muscle mass, and bone tissue [48]; and that menopausal women are a sensitive population for the prevalence of sarcopenia, although to determine the gender role of this prevalence more studies would be needed. In addition, physical activity and programmed exercise should be considered, as it could play a relevant role in the prevalence of sarcopenia by improving sleep quality [49].

Finally, the results of this review should be interpreted with caution, since several limitations could be influencing them. For example, the high heterogeneity shown in the analyses could not be corrected by means of the rescaled bias scale. Another point to consider is the origin of the studied population. In five of the analyzed studies, the subjects cohort was from Asia, while only one single study was performed using a European population and the way of measuring the cut-off point and the provenance could be biasing the results [2], resulting in different tendencies between men and women. Other limitations are the way in which the sarcopenia [6] is conceptualized, resulting in prevalence variations due to the different techniques developed to measure sarcopenia, as well as the classification of the pathologic incidence [50] and that sleep quality was only self-reported throughout questionnaires and not objectively monitored; and the low number of articles included for the data for quantitative analysis (low security measure).

5. Conclusions

The main conclusion is the observed association between sleep duration/quality and the prevalence of sarcopenia. In addition, this prevalence seems to be higher in men than in women. These results could have a practical application for the public health since it can help us to consider sleep quality as a risk factor, as well as the need to incorporate therapies in order to improve the sleep quality and to reduce the negative effects of age-associated sarcopenia.

Author Contributions: Conceptualization, J.Á.R.-A., L.A. and R.R.-F.; methodology, R.R.-F.; software, J.Á.R.-A., A.M.-R. and L.M.M.-A.; formal analysis, J.Á.R.-A. and D.J.R.-C.; investigation, J.Á.R.-A., R.R.-F., L.A., L.M.M.-A., A.M.-R. and D.J.R.-C.; writing—original draft preparation, J.Á.R.-A.; writing—review and editing, R.R.-F., L.A., L.M.M.-A., A.M.-R. and D.J.R.-C.; supervision, J.Á.R.-A., R.R.-F., L.A., L.M.M.-A., A.M.-R. and D.J.R.-C.

Funding: This research received no external funding.

Acknowledgments: The authors thank to G. Sanz for proofreading in English writing. No sources of funding were used in the preparation of this article.

Conflicts of Interest: The authors declare no conflict of interest.

References

1. Tobergte, D.R.; Curtis, S. Informe Mundial sobre el Envejecimiento y la Salud. *OMS* **2015**.
2. Shafiee, G.; Keshtkar, A.; Soltani, A.; Ahadi, Z.; Larijani, B.; Heshmat, R. Prevalence of sarcopenia in the world: A systematic review and meta-Analysis of general population studies. *J. Diabetes Metab. Disord.* **2017**, *16*, 1–10. [CrossRef] [PubMed]
3. Antunes, A.C.; Araujo, D.A.; Verissimo, M.T.; Amaral, T.F. Sarcopenia and hospitalisation costs in older adults: A cross-Sectional study. *Nutr. Diet.* **2017**, *74*, 46–50. [CrossRef] [PubMed]
4. Beaudart, C.; Zaaria, M.; Pasleau, F.; Reginster, J.Y.; Bruyere, O. Health outcomes of sarcopenia: A systematic review and meta-Analysis. *PLoS ONE* **2017**, *12*, e0169548. [CrossRef] [PubMed]
5. Morley, J.E.; Anker, S.D.; Von Haehling, S. Prevalence, incidence, and clinical impact of sarcopenia: Facts, numbers, and epidemiology—Update 2014. *J. Cachexia Sarcopenia Muscle* **2014**, *5*, 253–259. [CrossRef]
6. Cruz-Jentoft, A.J.; Bahat, G.; Bauer, J.; Boirie, Y.; Bruyere, O.; Cederholm, T.; Cooper, C.; Landi, F.; Rolland, Y.; Sayer, A.A.; et al. Sarcopenia: Revised European consensus on definition and diagnosis. *Age Ageing* **2019**, *48*, 16–31. [CrossRef]
7. Rosenberg, I.H. Sarcopenia: Origins and clinical relevance. *J. Nutr.* **1997**, *127*, 990S–991S. [CrossRef]
8. Lexell, J. Human aging, muscle mass, and fiber type composition. *J. Gerontol. Ser. A Biol. Sci. Med. Sci.* **1995**, *50*, 11–16.
9. Hairi, N.N.; Cumming, R.G.; Naganathan, V.; Handelsman, D.J.; Le Couteur, D.G.; Creasey, H.; Waite, L.M.; Seibel, M.J.; Sambrook, P.N. Loss of muscle strength, mass (sarcopenia), and quality (specific force) and its relationship with functional limitation and physical disability: The concord health and ageing in men project. *J. Am. Geriatr. Soc.* **2010**, *58*, 2055–2062. [CrossRef]
10. Rizzoli, R.; Reginster, J.Y.; Arnal, J.F.; Bautmans, I.; Beaudart, C.; Bischoff-Ferrari, H.; Biver, E.; Boonen, S.; Brandi, M.L.; Chines, A.; et al. Quality of life in sarcopenia and frailty. *Calcif. Tissue Int.* **2013**, *93*, 101–120. [CrossRef]
11. Rantanen, T. Muscle strength, disability and mortality. *Scand. J. Med. Sci. Sports* **2003**, *13*, 3–8. [CrossRef] [PubMed]
12. Arango-Lopera, V.E.; Arroyo, P.; Gutierrez-Robledo, L.M.; Perez-Zepeda, M.U.; Cesari, M. Mortality as an adverse outcome of sarcopenia. *J. Nutr. Health Aging* **2013**, *17*, 259–262. [CrossRef] [PubMed]
13. Messier, V.; Rabasa-Lhoret, R.; Barbat-Artigas, S.; Elisha, B.; Karelis, A.D.; Aubertin-Leheudre, M. Menopause and sarcopenia: A potential role for sex hormones. *Maturitas* **2011**, *68*, 331–336. [CrossRef] [PubMed]
14. Bredella, M.A. *Sex Differences in Body Composition BT-Sex and Gender Factors Affecting Metabolic Homeostasis, Diabetes and Obesity*; Mauvais-Jarvis, F., Ed.; Springer International Publishing: Cham, Germany, 2017; pp. 9–27. ISBN 978-3-319-70178-3.
15. Janssen, I.; Heymsfield, S.B.; Wang, Z.M.; Ross, R. Skeletal muscle mass and distribution in 468 men and women aged 18–88 yr. *J. Appl. Physiol.* **2000**, *89*, 81–88. [CrossRef] [PubMed]
16. Melton, L.J.; Khosla, S.; Riggs, B.L. Epidemiology of sarcopenia. *Mayo Clin. Proc.* **2000**, *48*, 625–630. [CrossRef]
17. Shimokata, H.; Shimada, H.; Satake, S.; Endo, N.; Shibasaki, K.; Ogawa, S.; Arai, H. Chapter 2 Epidemiology of sarcopenia. *Geriatr. Gerontol. Int.* **2018**, *18*, 13–22. [CrossRef]

18. Dodds, R.M.; Roberts, H.C.; Cooper, C.; Sayer, A.A. The Epidemiology of Sarcopenia. *J. Clin. Densitom.* **2015**, *27*, 355–363. [CrossRef]
19. Buchmann, N.; Spira, D.; Norman, K.; Demuth, I.; Eckardt, R.; Steinhagen-Thiessen, E. Sleep, Muscle Mass and Muscle Function in Older People. *Dtsch. Aerzteblatt Int.* **2016**, *113*, 253.
20. Vitale, J.; Bonato, M.; La Torre, A.; Banfi, G. The Role of the Molecular Clock in Promoting Skeletal Muscle Growth and Protecting against Sarcopenia. *Int. J. Mol. Sci.* **2019**, *20*, 4318. [CrossRef]
21. Hirshkowitz, M.; Whiton, K.; Albert, S.M.; Alessi, C.; Bruni, O.; DonCarlos, L.; Hazen, N.; Herman, J.; Katz, E.S.; Kheirandish-Gozal, L.; et al. National Sleep Foundation's sleep time duration recommendations: Methodology and results summary. *Sleep Health* **2015**, *1*, 233–243. [CrossRef]
22. Ancoli-Israel, S.; Cooke, J.R. Prevalence and comorbidity of insomnia and effect on functioning in elderly populations. *J. Am. Geriatr. Soc.* **2005**, *53*, S264–S271. [CrossRef] [PubMed]
23. Zhang, B.; Wing, Y.K. Sex differences in insomnia: A meta-Analysis. *Sleep* **2006**, *29*, 85–93. [CrossRef] [PubMed]
24. Dattilo, M.; Antunes, H.K.M.; Medeiros, A.; Monico Neto, M.; Souza, H.S.; Tufik, S.; De Mello, M.T. Sleep and muscle recovery: Endocrinological and molecular basis for a new and promising hypothesis. *Med. Hypotheses* **2011**, *77*, 220–222. [CrossRef] [PubMed]
25. Cappuccio, F.P.; Cooper, D.; Delia, L.; Strazzullo, P.; Miller, M.A. Sleep duration predicts cardiovascular outcomes: A systematic review and meta-Analysis of prospective studies. *Eur. Heart J.* **2011**, *32*, 1484–1492. [CrossRef]
26. Tuomilehto, H.; Peltonen, M.; Partinen, M.; Lavigne, G.; Eriksson, J.G.; Herder, C.; Aunola, S.; Keinanen-Kiukaanniemi, S.; Ilanne-Parikka, P.; Uusitupa, M.; et al. Sleep duration, lifestyle intervention, and incidence of type 2 diabetes in impaired glucose tolerance: The finnish diabetes prevention study. *Diabetes Care* **2009**, *32*, 1965–1971. [CrossRef]
27. Cappuccio, F.P.; Taggart, F.M.; Kandala, N.B.; Currie, A.; Peile, E.; Stranges, S.; Miller, M.A. Meta-Analysis of short sleep duration and obesity in children and adults. *Sleep* **2008**, *31*, 619–626. [CrossRef]
28. Zhao, H.; Yin, J.Y.; Yang, W.S.; Qin, Q.; Li, T.T.; Shi, Y.; Deng, Q.; Wei, S.; Liu, L.; Wang, X.; et al. Sleep duration and cancer risk: A systematic review and meta-Analysis of prospective studies. *Asian Pac. J. Cancer Prev.* **2013**, *14*, 7509–7515. [CrossRef]
29. Chen, H.C.; Hsu, N.W.; Chou, P. The association between sleep duration and hand grip strength in community-Dwelling older adults: The yilan study, Taiwan. *Sleep* **2017**, *40*, zsx021. [CrossRef]
30. Liberati, A.; Altman, D.G.; Tetzlaff, J.; Mulrow, C.; Gotzsche, P.C.; Ioannidis, J.P.A.; Clarke, M.; Devereaux, P.J.; Kleijnen, J.; Moher, D. The PRISMA statement for reporting systematic reviews and meta-analyses of studies that evaluate health care interventions: Explanation and elaboration. *J. Clin. Epidemiol.* **2009**, *6*, e1000100.
31. Barendregt, J.J.; Doi, S.A. *MetaXL User Guide: Version 5.3*; EpiGear International Pty Ltd.: Queensland, Australia, 2016.
32. Barendregt, J.J.; Doi, S.A.; Lee, Y.Y.; Norman, R.E.; Vos, T. Meta-Analysis of prevalence. *J. Epidemiol. Community Health* **2013**, *67*, 974–978. [CrossRef]
33. Colimon, K.M. *Fundamentos De Epidemiologia*; Diaz de Santos: Madrid, Spain, 1990; ISBN 9788578110796.
34. Ida, S.; Kaneko, R.; Nagata, H.; Noguchi, Y.; Araki, Y.; Nakai, M.; Ito, S.; Ishihara, Y.; Imataka, K.; Murata, K. Association between sarcopenia and sleep disorder in older patients with diabetes. *Geriatr. Gerontol. Int.* **2019**, *19*, 399–403. [CrossRef] [PubMed]
35. Higgins, J.P.T. Measuring inconsistency in meta-Analyses. *BMJ* **2003**, *327*, 557–560. [CrossRef] [PubMed]
36. Chien, M.Y.; Wang, L.Y.; Chen, H.C. The Relationship of Sleep Duration with Obesity and Sarcopenia in Community-Dwelling Older Adults. *Gerontology* **2015**, *61*, 399–406. [CrossRef] [PubMed]
37. Fu, L.; Yu, X.; Zhang, W.; Han, P.; Kang, L.; Ma, Y.; Jia, L.; Yu, H.; Chen, X.; Hou, L.; et al. The Relationship Between Sleep Duration, Falls, and Muscle Mass: A Cohort Study in an Elderly Chinese Population. *Rejuvenation Res.* **2018**. [CrossRef]
38. Hu, X.; Jiang, J.; Wang, H.; Zhang, L.; Dong, B.; Yang, M. Association between sleep duration and sarcopenia among community-Dwelling older adults: A cross-Sectional study. *Medicine* **2017**, *96*, e6268. [CrossRef]
39. Kwon, Y.J.; Jang, S.Y.; Park, E.C.; Cho, A.R.; Shim, J.Y.; Linton, J.A. Long sleep duration is associated with sarcopenia in Korean adults based on data from the 2008–2011 KNHANES. *J. Clin. Sleep Med.* **2017**, *13*, 1097–1104. [CrossRef]

40. Stitt, T.N.; Drujan, D.; Clarke, B.A.; Panaro, F.; Timofeyva, Y.; Kline, W.O.; Gonzalez, M.; Yancopoulos, G.D.; Glass, D.J. The IGF-1/PI3K/Akt pathway prevents expression of muscle atrophy-Induced ubiquitin ligases by inhibiting FOXO transcription factors. *Mol. Cell* **2004**, *14*, 395–403. [CrossRef]
41. Schaap, L.A.; Pluijm, S.M.F.; Deeg, D.J.H.; Visser, M. Inflammatory Markers and Loss of Muscle Mass (Sarcopenia) and Strength. *Am. J. Med.* **2006**, *119*, e9–e526. [CrossRef]
42. Van Leeuwen, W.M.A.; Lehto, M.; Karisola, P.; Lindholm, H.; Luukkonen, R.; Sallinen, M.; Harma, M.; Porkka-Heiskanen, T.; Alenius, H. Sleep restriction increases the risk of developing cardiovascular diseases by augmenting proinflammatory responses through IL-17 and CRP. *PLoS ONE* **2009**, *4*, e4589. [CrossRef]
43. Verlaan, S.; Aspray, T.J.; Bauer, J.M.; Cederholm, T.; Hemsworth, J.; Hill, T.R.; McPhee, J.S.; Piasecki, M.; Seal, C.; Sieber, C.C.; et al. Nutritional status, body composition, and quality of life in community-Dwelling sarcopenic and non-Sarcopenic older adults: A case-Control study. *Clin. Nutr.* **2017**, *36*, 267–274. [CrossRef]
44. Salva, A.; Serra-Rexach, J.A.; Artaza, I.; Formiga, F.; Rojano, I.; Luque, X.; Cuesta, F.; Lopez-Soto, A.; Masanes, F.; Ruiz, D.; et al. La prevalencia de sarcopenia en residencias de Espana: Comparacion de los resultados del estudio multicentrico ELLI con otras poblaciones. *Rev. Esp. Geriatr. Gerontol.* **2016**, *51*, 260–264. [CrossRef] [PubMed]
45. Piovezan, R.D.; Abucham, J.; Dos Santos, R.V.T.; Mello, M.T.; Tufik, S.; Poyares, D. The impact of sleep on age-Related sarcopenia: Possible connections and clinical implications. *Ageing Res. Rev.* **2015**, *23*, 210–220. [CrossRef] [PubMed]
46. Morley, J.E.; Baumgartner, R.; Roubenoff, R.; Mayer, J.; Nair, K.S. Sarcopenia. *J. Lab. Clin. Med.* **2001**, *137*, 231–243. [CrossRef] [PubMed]
47. Schoenau, E. From mechanostat theory to development of the "functional muscle-Bone-Unit". *J. Musculoskelet. Neuronal Interact.* **2005**, *5*, 232.
48. Gregg, E.W.; Kriska, A.M.; Salamone, L.M.; Roberts, M.M.; Anderson, S.J.; Ferrell, R.E.; Kuller, L.H.; Cauley, J.A. The epidemiology of quantitative ultrasound: A review of the relationships with bone mass, osteoporosis and fracture risk. *Osteoporos. Int.* **1997**, *7*, 89–99. [CrossRef]
49. Rubio-Arias, J.; Marin-Cascales, E.; Ramos-Campo, D.J.; Hernandez, A.V.; Perez-Lopez, F.R. Effect of exercise on sleep quality and insomnia in middle-Aged women: A systematic review and meta-Analysis of randomized controlled trials. *Maturitas* **2017**, *100*, 49–56. [CrossRef]
50. Pagotto, V.; Silveira, E.A. Methods, diagnostic criteria, cutoff points, and prevalence of sarcopenia among older people. *Sci. World J.* **2014**, *2014*, 231312. [CrossRef]

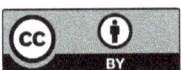 © 2019 by the authors. Licensee MDPI, Basel, Switzerland. This article is an open access article distributed under the terms and conditions of the Creative Commons Attribution (CC BY) license (http://creativecommons.org/licenses/by/4.0/).

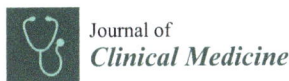
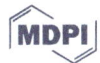

Article

Impact of Psychological Distress and Sleep Quality on Balance Confidence, Muscle Strength, and Functional Balance in Community-Dwelling Middle-Aged and Older People

Raquel Fábrega-Cuadros, Agustín Aibar-Almazán *, Antonio Martínez-Amat and Fidel Hita-Contreras

Department of Health Sciences, Faculty of Health Sciences, University of Jaén, 23071 Jaén, Spain; rfabrega@ujaen.es (R.F.-C.); amamat@ujaen.es (A.M.-A.); fhita@ujaen.es (F.H.-C.)
* Correspondence: aaibar@ujaen.es; Tel.: +34-953-213-408

Received: 19 August 2020; Accepted: 21 September 2020; Published: 22 September 2020

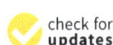

Abstract: The objective was to evaluate the associations of psychological distress and sleep quality with balance confidence, muscle strength, and functional balance among community-dwelling middle-aged and older people. An analytical cross-sectional study was conducted ($n = 304$). Balance confidence (Activities-specific Balance Confidence scale, ABC), muscle strength (hand grip dynamometer), and functional balance (Timed Up-and-Go test) were assessed. Psychological distress and sleep quality were evaluated by the Hospital Anxiety and Depression Scale and the Pittsburgh Sleep Quality Index, respectively. Age, sex, physical activity level, nutritional status, and fatigue were included as possible confounders. Multivariate linear and logistic regressions were performed. Higher values of anxiety (OR = 1.10), fatigue (OR = 1.04), and older age (OR = 1.08) were associated with an increased risk of falling (ABC < 67%). Greater muscle strength was associated with male sex and improved nutritional status (adjusted $R^2 = 0.39$). On the other hand, being older and using sleeping medication were linked to poorer functional balance (adjusted $R^2 = 0.115$). In conclusion, greater anxiety levels and the use of sleep medication were linked to a high risk of falling and poorer functional balance, respectively. No associations were found between muscle strength and sleep quality, anxiety, or depression.

Keywords: fall risk; balance; muscle strength; anxiety; depression; sleep quality

1. Introduction

Aging brings with it a series of changes that can affect the mobility and independence of people [1]. These changes affect the mood and attitude towards their environment, and this depends largely on the degree of acceptance of aging since it contributes to the feeling of happiness and satisfaction with life, whose lack can cause feelings of loneliness and sadness [2].

Certain disorders associated with this process, such as anxiety and/or depression, are psychological indicators of a decrease in quality of life [3]. Specifically, the prevalence of depression in the geriatric population worldwide is 7%, and its incidence increases with age [4]. Conversely, the prevalence of anxiety in people over 60 years old ranges between 0.7% and 18.6%, values far below those of younger adults [5].

Sleep quality is a key contributor to good health, and its importance among the older population cannot be overstated, given that sleep disorders and the difficulty to fall asleep become more common with age [6]. It has been shown that although the need to sleep remains the same throughout an individual's life, the ability to get enough sleep does in fact decrease with age. This brings about several adverse health outcomes such as reduced physical function, depression, increased risk of falls, and mortality [7].

Falls represent a major health care problem among older people and are linked to increased morbidity, mortality, and health costs [8]. Around 30% of older people living in the community experience a fall each year [9]. Fall risk factors have been studied in detail and include demographic, environmental, and health-related factors [10]. Balance confidence is one of the most important psychological factors linked to falls and the deterioration of balance, and its decrease can lead to diminished independence and participation in activities of daily living, thus creating a vicious circle that affects the quality of life and creates more isolated and dependent people [11]. On the other hand, the impaired functional balance has been shown to be one of the most important predictors of falls [12].

Muscle strength also declines with age more sharply than muscle mass [13]. It has been reported that muscle loss in older women decreases 3.7% per decade, however, strength decreases 15% per decade until age 70 when the loss accelerates considerably [14]. Moreover, in 2018 the European Working Group on Sarcopenia (EWGSOP2) listed low strength as a primary indicator of probable sarcopenia [15]. A decrease in muscle strength contributes to an elevated prevalence of falls and the loss of functional capacity and is a major cause of disability, mortality, and other adverse health outcomes [16].

Not many studies have examined the impact of psychological distress and sleep quality on balance confidence and function, and muscle strength in older people, which, in many cases, have shown inconclusive results and have focused on sleep duration or insomnia. Based on all of the above, the objective of this study was to evaluate the associations of psychological distress and sleep quality with the risk of falling according to balance confidence, functional balance, and muscle strength among community-dwelling middle-aged and older individuals.

2. Experimental Section

2.1. Study Design and Participants

An analytical cross-sectional study was conducted, to which end 315 community-dwelling middle-aged and older people were initially contacted and 304 finally took part. Recruitment was performed by contacting several senior centers from the Eastern Andalusia region. Prior to the beginning of the study, all participants provided their written informed consent. The research was approved by the Research Ethics Committee of the University of Jaén, Spain (NOV.18/2.TES), and was conducted in accordance with the Declaration of Helsinki, good clinical practices, and all applicable laws and regulations.

Community-dwelling ambulatory adults aged 50 years and older, able to understand and complete the required questionnaires and willing to give written informed consent to participate in the study were included in the protocol. Exclusion criteria were: conditions that limit physical activity, chronic and/or severe medical disease or any neuropsychiatric disorder that could influence their responses to the questionnaires.

2.2. Study Parameters

2.2.1. Balance Confidence

The Activities-specific Balance Confidence scale (ABC) was used to assess balance confidence in the performance of activities of daily living [17]. This is a 16-item questionnaire that quantifies the level of confidence in performing a specific task without losing balance or becoming unsteady [18]. Each item score ranges from 0–100%, and the total score is obtained by summing the ratings (0–1600) and then dividing by 16. A higher percentage indicates a greater level of balance confidence. A score of <67% has been identified as a reliable means of predicting a future fall [19]. This cut-off was used to identify which participants were at high risk of falling.

2.2.2. Muscle Strength

Muscle strength was assessed with an analog dynamometer (TKK 5001, Grip-A, Takei, Tokyo, Japan). Participants were required to apply their maximum handgrip strength three times with the dominant hand, each separated by 30 s. The maximal measured effort was regarded as their handgrip strength [20].

2.2.3. Functional Balance

The Timed Up-and-Go (TUG) test [21] is a simple and valid method for predicting changes in functional balance in older adults [22]. It is a sensitive and specific measure for identifying community-dwelling adults who are at risk of falls [23]. In the TUG test, individuals rise from a seated position on a chair, walk three meters, turn around, return, and sit down again. The time required to complete this task was recorded.

2.2.4. Sleep Quality

Sleep quality was assessed using the Pittsburgh Sleep Quality Index (PSQI) [24,25]. It comprises 19 self-rated questions and 5 more (only used for clinical purposes) to be completed by bedmates or roommates. The 19 items (ranged from 0–3) generate a total score and seven different domains or subscales (subjective sleep quality, sleep latency, sleep duration, habitual sleep efficiency, sleep disturbance, use of sleeping medication, and daytime dysfunction). Higher scores indicate poorer subjective sleep quality.

2.2.5. Psychological Distress

The Hospital Anxiety and Depression Scale (HADS) is a self-administered questionnaire widely used to assess psychological distress in the general population [26,27]. This questionnaire contains 14 items, 7 related to anxiety symptoms, and 7 to depressive symptoms. Each item ranges from 0–3, and the total scores for both anxiety and depression range from 0 to 21, with higher scores indicating more severe symptoms.

2.2.6. Fatigue Severity

In order to assess fatigue severity during the last 7 days, the Fatigue Severity Scale was used [28]. This questionnaire consists of 9 items (rated from 1–7) and produces a total score where larger values imply greater fatigue.

2.2.7. Nutritional Status

The Mini Nutritional Assessment survey (MNA) was used to evaluate nutritional status [29,30]. It has 18 questions that include anthropometric measures, health status, dietary patterns, and subjective assessments of nutritional and health status. Higher scores indicate better nutritional status.

2.2.8. Physical Activity Level

Physical activity level was assessed with the International Physical Activity Questionnaire-Short Form (IPAQ-SF) [31]. It consists of seven items that measure physical activity within three intensity levels (walking, moderate, and vigorous) during an average week. Physical activity was evaluated by combining the activity score of both moderate and vigorous-intensity activity (min/day) for each work and recreational activity domain. Responses were converted to Metabolic Equivalent Task minutes per week (MET-min / week) according to the scoring protocol.

2.3. Sample Size Calculation

For sample size calculation, at least 20 subjects per variable are required in the linear regression model [32], while a minimum of 10 subjects per variable was needed in the logistic regression model [33].

Since 15 possible predicting variables were considered (7 domains plus the total score of the PSQI, anxiety, depression, as well as physical activity level, nutritional status, fatigue, sex, and age as possible confounders), over 300 subjects were required for the purposes of our analysis. The final number of participants was 304.

2.4. Statistical Analysis

Continuous variables were described using means and standard deviations, and for categorical variables frequencies and percentages were used. The Kolmogorov–Smirnov test was performed to evaluate the normal distribution of the data. To analyze the differences between participants with and without risk of falling (ABC), Student's t test (continuous independent variables), and the Chi-squared test (sex) were used. In order to analyze the independent associations, a multivariate logistic regression was performed. Those variables with significant individual associations ($p < 0.05$) were selected for the stepwise logistic regression model. The odds ratio (OR) can be considered as significant when the 95% confidence interval (CI) does not include 1.00. The Chi-squared and Hosmer–Lemeshow tests were conducted to assess the overall goodness-of-fit for each of the steps of the model, as well as for the final model. To explore the possible individual associations of muscle strength and functional balance with PSQI, HADS, FSS, MNA, and IPAQ-SF scores, as well as with age (independent variables), Pearson's correlation was used. As for the analysis of the independent associations, the same procedure was applied, but using a stepwise multivariate linear regression. Functional balance and muscle strength were individually introduced as dependent variables in separate models. We first looked into the bivariate correlation coefficients, and any independent variables with significant associations ($p < 0.05$) were included in the multivariate linear regression. Adjusted R^2 was used to calculate the effect size coefficient of multiple determination in the linear models. R^2 can be considered insignificant when <0.02, small if between 0.02 and 0.15, medium if between 0.15 and 0.35, and large if >0.35 [34]. A 95% confidence level was used ($p < 0.05$). Data management and analysis were performed using the SPSS statistical package for the social sciences for Windows (SPSS Inc., Chicago, IL, USA).

3. Results

A total of 304 participants (72.04 ± 7.88 years) took part in this study. When studying the ABC score (23.42 ± 7.25), 24.01% of participants were at risk of falling. The analysis revealed (Table 1) that participants with an ABC score < 67 were individually associated with the largest values of anxiety ($p = 0.002$), depression ($p = 0.001$), fatigue ($p = < 0.001$), increased age ($p < 0.001$), and worse nutritional status ($p = 0.002$).

Table 1. Individual differences according to the risk of falling.

		All Participants ($n = 304$)		Risk of Falling (ABC)				p-Value
				No ($n = 231$)		Yes ($n = 73$)		
		Mean	SD	Mean	SD	Mean	SD	
PSQI	Sleep quality	1.01	0.82	1.00	0.80	1.04	0.87	0.738
	Sleep latency	1.18	1.09	1.16	1.08	1.26	1.11	0.475
	Sleep duration	1.00	0.97	1.00	0.98	1.01	0.94	0.890
	Sleep efficiency	0.95	1.10	0.97	1.11	0.90	1.08	0.658
	Sleep disturbances	1.23	0.58	1.22	0.57	1.27	0.61	0.461
	Use of sleeping medication	1.01	1.34	1.02	1.34	0.97	1.34	0.804
	Daytime dysfunction	0.49	0.63	0.46	0.61	0.59	0.68	0.130
	Total score	6.87	4.70	6.82	4.58	7.04	5.11	0.725

Table 1. Cont.

		All Participants (n = 304)		Risk of Falling (ABC)				p-Value
				No (n = 231)		Yes (n = 73)		
Anxiety		5.74	4.02	5.34	4.07	7.01	3.58	0.002
Depression		4.99	3.44	4.62	3.38	6.14	3.39	0.001
Physical activity level, MET-min/week		1367.96	2213.43	1310.16	1817.89	1549.29	3157.97	0.422
Nutritional status		26.31	2.08	26.52	1.99	25.64	2.22	0.002
Fatigue		21.33	15.25	18.87	13.96	29.14	16.58	<0.001
Age, years		72.04	7.88	70.99	7.27	75.38	8.82	<0.001
		n	%	n	%	n	%	
Sex	Male	255	83.88	37	16.02	12	16.44	0.932
	Female	49	16.12	194	83.98	61	83.56	

ABC: Activities-Specific Balance Confidence Scale. MET: Metabolic Equivalent of Task. PSQI: Pittsburgh Sleep Quality Index. SD: Standard Deviation.

The multivariate logistic regression that looked into the risk of falls as assessed with the ABC score revealed several significant results. Higher values of anxiety (OR = 1.10, 95% CI = 1.02–1.18), fatigue (OR = 1.04, 95% CI = 1.02–1.06), and older age (OR = 1.08, 95% CI = 1.04–1.12) were independently associated with ABC scores < 67%. The Hosmer–Lemeshow test showed a good fit of the model (Chi-squared = 2.403, p = 0.966), which was able to classify correctly 78.29% of all participants at high risk of suffering a future fall, according to the ABC score (Table 2).

Table 2. Multivariate logistic regression analyses for factors associated with the risk of falling (determined through the ABC score).

		OR	95% CI	p-Value
	Anxiety	1.10	1.02–1.18	0.012
Risk of falling (ABC)	Fatigue	1.04	1.02–1.06	0.000
	Age	1.08	1.04–1.12	0.000

ABC: Activities-Specific Balance Confidence Scale. CI: Confidence Interval. OR: Odds Ratio.

As for functional balance (9.86 ± 2.91 s) and muscle strength (19.43 ± 6.42 kg), the individual associations are shown in Table 3. Muscle strength was only associated with anxiety (p = 0.001), fatigue (p = 0.020), and nutritional status (p = 0.038), whereas poor functional balance was related to greater age (p < 0.001) and physical activity level (p = 0.035), as well as with the use-of-sleeping-medication domain in PSQI (p = 0.028). Regarding sex differences, men displayed greater muscle strength (both p < 0.001), but worse functional balance (p = 0.005).

Table 3. Pearson's correlations of functional balance and muscle strength, with PSQI scores and possible confounders.

		Muscle Strength		Functional Balance	
		r	p-Value	r	p-Value
PSQI	Sleep quality	0.06	0.264	0.03	0.654
	Sleep latency	0.07	0.231	0.00	0.950
	Sleep duration	0.05	0.427	0.02	0.790
	Sleep efficiency	−0.00	0.963	−0.02	0.747
	Sleep disturbances	0.01	0.808	−0.02	0.665
	Use of sleeping medication	0.03	0.602	0.13	0.028
	Daytime dysfunction	0.01	0.854	0.04	0.474
	Total score	0.05	0.416	0.04	0.464

Table 3. Cont.

	Muscle Strength		Functional Balance	
	r	p-Value	r	p-Value
Anxiety	−0.18	0.001	0.05	0.355
Depression	−0.08	0.191	0.08	0.174
Nutritional status	−0.12	0.038	−0.05	0.401
Fatigue	−0.14	0.017	0.06	0.281
Age, years	−0.104	0.070	0.33	0.000
Physical activity level (MET-min / week)	0.103	0.075	−0.12	0.035

MET: Metabolic Equivalent of Task. PSQI: Pittsburgh Sleep Quality Index. r: Pearson's Correlation Coefficient.

Lastly, the linear regression analysis (Table 4) revealed that greater muscle strength was independently associated with the male sex ($p < 0.001$) and a better nutritional status ($p = 0.001$), and the effect size was large (adjusted $R^2 = 0.392$). On the other hand, being older ($p < 0.001$) and the use of sleeping medication ($p = 0.033$) were linked to poorer functional balance, although the effect size was small (adjusted $R^2 = 0.115$).

Table 4. Multivariate linear regression analyses for functional balance and muscle strength.

		B	β	95% CI		p-Value
Muscle strength	Sex	−10.74	−0.62	−12.28	−9.21	<0.001
	Nutritional status	0.44	0.14	00.17	0.71	0.002
Functional balance	Age	0.12	0.34	−0.09	−0.16	<0.001
	Use of sleeping medication	0.27	0.12	0.04	0.50	0.023

B: Unstandardized Coefficient. β: Standardized Coefficient. CI: Confidence Interval. MET: Metabolic Equivalent of Task. PSQI: Pittsburgh Sleep Quality Index.

4. Discussion

The objective of this study was to evaluate the associations of psychological distress and sleep quality with balance confidence, functional balance, and muscle strength among community-dwelling middle-aged and older individuals. In our study, anxiety, fatigue, older age, and the use of sleeping medication were shown to be associated with the risk of falling and poorer functional balance. Muscle strength was associated with being male and nutritional status.

In general, balance confidence scores are able to predict perceived physical function and even mobility in older adults [35]. Similar to our own study, a previously published paper also employed regression models to find a significant association of anxiety with confidence in balance, while depression was shown to be associated with avoidance of activity [36]. A systematic review with meta-analysis found an association between balance confidence and anxiety [37], and a similar link was established between depression and level of physical activity [38]. Regarding the association of age with balance confidence, Medley et al. [39] reported that participants with low balance confidence were older than those who reported high balance confidence. In our study, only anxiety, age, and fatigue were independently associated with the balance confidence. To our knowledge, this is the first study to observe an association between confidence in balance and fatigue in healthy middle-aged and older people, although there are studies that demonstrate this association, but in people with some pathology [40,41].

Muscle strength plays an important role in the execution of many activities of daily living and is considered an indicator of functional decline among community-dwelling older adults [42]. Low grip strength is predictive of poor outcomes and indicative of prolonged hospital stays, increased functional limitations, poor quality of life, and death [43]. For example, it has been shown that people who have a high level of grip strength have a significantly lower fear of falling than those who show lower levels [44,45]. In addition, it has been observed that the strength of the abductor muscles can identify older adults at risk of falling [46]. A recent study looking into the association between falls and lower-limb strength failed to find any link at a one-year follow-up [47]. Our study found no associations whatsoever between muscle strength and sleep quality, and increased muscle strength was independently associated only with being male (as in previous studies by Buchman et al. [48]) and with improved nutritional status. Other authors have agreed before that a poor diet is significantly associated with lower muscle strength, but they also linked it to lower physical function, longer TUG test time, depression, and risk of falling [49], although the results of the present study should be interpreted with caution since they are correlations and a cause-effect relationship cannot be established. Some recent studies even recommend the intake of supplementary proteins given their significant effect in increasing muscle mass and strength among elderly people with sarcopenia [50]. We must consider, however, that disparities in the literature may be due to a variety of population ages, measurement methods, and educational and cultural levels, which may have a confounding effect.

Balance confidence contributes to functional mobility performance [39], and there seems to be a strong link between balance self-efficacy and function capabilities [51]. A study by Brandão et al. [52] identified an association between excessive daytime sleepiness and quality of life, and also characterized the profile of older adults with poor sleep quality. Sleep duration is associated with inflammation markers (serum interleukin-6, tumor necrosis factor α, and C-reactive protein) in older adults, and in turn with mortality [53]. Loss of functional balance, as measured by the TUG test, is known to be one of the first signs of aging and is considered a marker for general health that is strongly associated with the risk of mortality [54]. In our results, and as far as individual associations are concerned, higher age, poorer sleep quality (use of sleep medication), and decreased levels of physical activity were linked to lower TUG scores. However, in the multivariate analysis model, such associations only held for the first two variables (age and poor sleep quality). The results of a study conducted among women indicate that a shorter sleep duration increased wakefulness after sleep onset, and decreased sleep efficiency are risk factors for functional or physical impairment in older women [55].

There are some limitations to our study that must be acknowledged. Firstly, its cross-sectional design did not allow for the evaluation of causal relationships. Secondly, sleep quality was assessed using self-report methods, and therefore the influence of recall bias must be considered. Thirdly, our study was conducted among people from a specific geographic area, and any generalization of its results should be limited to individuals with characteristics similar to those of our population sample. Future studies should consider exploring prospective designs, employing objective sleep quality assessment methods (polysomnography or actigraphy), and applying them to a general population of older adults.

5. Conclusions

Among middle-aged and older Spanish people, greater levels of anxiety and fatigue, as well as older age were associated with an increased risk of falling (assessed with the Activities-specific Balance Confidence scale). No associations were found with sleep quality and depression. Greater muscle strength was associated with being male and having a better nutritional status. Finally, increased age and the use of sleeping medication were linked to poorer functional balance.

Author Contributions: Conceptualization: R.F.-C. and F.H.-C.; methodology: R.F.-C. and A.A.-A.; formal analysis: F.H.-C. and R.F.-C.; supervision: A.M.-A. and A.A.-A.; writing—original draft preparation: R.F.-C. and F.H.-C.; writing—review and editing: A.M.-A. and A.A.-A.; funding acquisition: A.M.-A. and F.H.-C. All authors have read and agreed to the published version of the manuscript.

Funding: This research was supported by the project 1260735, integrated into the 2014–2020 Operational Programme FEDER in Andalusia.

Conflicts of Interest: The authors declare no conflict of interest.

References

1. Sulbrandt, C.J.; Pino, Z.P.; Oyarzún, G.M. Active and healthy aging. Research and policies for population aging. *Rev. Chil. Enferm. Respir.* **2012**, *28*, 269–271.
2. Dziechciaż, M.; Filip, R. Biological psychological and social determinants of old age: Bio-psycho-social aspects of human aging. *Ann. Agric. Environ. Med.* **2014**, *21*, 835–838. [CrossRef] [PubMed]
3. Alvarado, A.M.; Salazar, A.M. Aging concept analysis. *Gerokomos* **2014**, *25*, 57–62.
4. Wen, Y.; Liu, C.; Liao, J.; Yin, Y.; Wu, D. Incidence and risk factors of depressive symptoms in 4 years of follow-up among mid-aged and elderly community-dwelling Chinese adults: Findings from the China Health and Retirement Longitudinal Study. *BMJ Open* **2019**, *9*, e029529. [CrossRef] [PubMed]
5. Hohls, J.K.; Köning, H.H.; Raynik, Y.I.; Hajek, A. A systematic review of the association of anxiety with health care utilization and costs in people aged 65 years and older. *J. Affec. Disord.* **2018**, *232*, 163–176. [CrossRef]
6. Cybulski, M.; Cybulski, L.; Krajewska-Kulak, E.; Orzechowska, M.; Cwalina, U.; Kowalczuk, K. Sleep disorders among educationally active elderly people in Bialystok, Poland: A cross-sectional study. *BMC Geriatr.* **2019**, *19*, 225. [CrossRef] [PubMed]
7. Neikrug, A.B.; Ancoli-Israel, S. Sleep disorders in the older adult—A mini-review. *Gerontology* **2010**, *56*, 181–189. [CrossRef]
8. Tinetti, M.E. Clinical practice. Preventing falls in elderly persons. *N. Engl. J. Med.* **2003**, *348*, 42–49. [CrossRef]
9. Sun, D.Q.; Huang, J.; Varadhan, R.; Agrawal, Y. Race and fall risk: Data from the National Health and Aging Trends Study (NHATS). *Age Ageing* **2016**, *45*, 120–127. [CrossRef]
10. Deandrea, S.; Lucenteforte, E.; Bravi, F.; Foschi, R.; La Vecchia, C.; Negri, E. Risk Factors for Falls in Community-Dwelling Older People: A Systematic Review and Meta-Analysis. *Epidemiology* **2010**, *21*, 658–668. [CrossRef]
11. Scheffer, A.C.; Schuurmans, M.J.; Van Dijk, N.; Van der Hooft, T.; De Rooij, S.E. Fear of falling: Measurement strategy, prevalence, risk factors and consequences among older persons. *Age Ageing* **2008**, *37*, 19–24. [CrossRef] [PubMed]
12. Jácome, C.; Cruz, J.; Gabriel, R.; Figueiredo, D.; Marques, A. Functional Balance in Older Adults with Chronic Obstructive Pulmonary Disease. *J. Aging Phys. Act.* **2014**, *22*, 357–363. [CrossRef]
13. Cruz-Jentoft, A.J.; Bahat, G.; Bauer, J.; Boirie, Y.; Bruyère, O.; Cederholm, T.; Cooper, C.; Landi, F.; Rolland, Y.; Sayer, A.A.; et al. Sarcopenia: Revised European consensus on definition and diagnosis. *Age Ageing* **2019**, *48*, 16–31. [CrossRef]
14. Siparsky, P.N.; Kirkendall, D.T.; Garrett, W.E., Jr. Muscle changes in aging: Understanding sarcopenia. *Sports Health* **2014**, *6*, 36–40. [CrossRef] [PubMed]
15. Mitchell, W.K.; Williams, J.; Atherton, P.; Larvin, M.; Lund, J.; Narici, M. Sarcopenia, dynapenia, and the impact of advancing age on human skeletal muscle size and strength; a quantitative review. *Front. Physiol.* **2012**, *3*, 260. [CrossRef] [PubMed]
16. Dhillon, R.J.; Hasni, S. Pathogenesis and Management of Sarcopenia. *Clin. Geriatr. Med.* **2017**, *33*, 17–26. [CrossRef] [PubMed]
17. Powell, L.E.; Myers, A.M. The Activities-specific Balance Confidence (ABC) Scale. *J. Gerontol. A Biol. Sci. Med. Sci.* **1995**, *50A*, M28–M34. [CrossRef]
18. Montilla-Ibáñez, A.; Martínez-Amat, A.; Lomas-Vega, R.; Cruz-Díaz, D.; Torre-Cruz, M.J.; Casuso-Pérez, R.; Hita-Contreras, F. The Activities-specific Balance Confidence scale: Reliability and validity in Spanish patients with vestibular disorders. *Disabil. Rehabil.* **2017**, *39*, 697–703. [CrossRef]
19. Lajoie, Y.; Gallagher, S.P. Predicting falls within the elderly community: Comparison of postural sway, reaction time, the Berg balance scale and the Activities-specific Balance Confidence (ABC) scale for comparing fallers and non-fallers. *Arch. Gerontol. Geriatr.* **2004**, *38*, 11–26. [CrossRef]
20. Beaudart, C.; Rolland, Y.; Cruz-Jentoft, A.J.; Bauer, J.M.; Sieber, C.; Cooper, C.; Al-Daghri, N.; Araujo de Carvalho, I.; Bautmans, I.; Bernabei, R.; et al. Assessment of Muscle Function and Physical Performance in Daily Clinical Practice: A position paper endorsed by the European Society for Clinical and Economic Aspects of Osteoporosis, Osteoarthritis and Musculoskeletal Diseases (ESCEO). *Calcif. Tissue Int.* **2019**, *105*, 1–14. [CrossRef]
21. Podsiadlo, D.; Richardson, S. The timed "Up & Go": A test of basic functional mobility for frail elderly persons. *J. Am. Geriatr. Soc.* **1991**, *39*, 142–148. [PubMed]

22. Benavent-Caballer, V.; Sendín-Magdalena, A.; Lisón, J.F.; Rosado-Calatayud, P.; Amer-Cuenca, J.J.; Salvador-Coloma, P.; Segura-Ortí, E. Physical factors underlying the Timed "Up and Go" test in older adults. *Geriatr. Nurs.* **2016**, *37*, 122–127. [CrossRef] [PubMed]
23. Shumway-Cook, A.; Brauer, S.; Woollacott, M. Predicting the probability for falls in community-dwelling older adults using the Timed Up & Go Test. *Phys. Ther.* **2000**, *80*, 896–903. [PubMed]
24. Buysse, D.J.; Reynolds, C.F., 3rd; Monk, T.H.; Berman, S.R.; Kupfer, D.J. The Pittsburgh Sleep Quality Index: A new instrument for psychiatric practice and research. *Psychiatry Res.* **1989**, *28*, 193–213. [CrossRef]
25. Hita-Contreras, F.; Martínez-López, E.; Latorre-Román, P.A.; Garrido, F.; Santos, M.A.; Martínez-Amat, A. Reliability and validity of the Spanish version of the Pittsburgh Sleep Quality Index (PSQI) in patients with fibromyalgia. *Rheumatol. Int.* **2014**, *34*, 929–936. [CrossRef]
26. Zigmond, A.S.; Snaith, P.R. The hospital anxiety and depression scale. *Acta Psychiatr. Scand.* **1983**, *67*, 361–370. [CrossRef]
27. Herrero, M.J.; Blanch, J.; Peri, J.M.; De Pablo, J.; Pintor, L.; Bulbena, A. A validation study of the hospital anxiety and depression scale (HADS) in a Spanish population. *Gen. Hosp. Psychiatry* **2003**, *25*, 277–283. [CrossRef]
28. Krupp, L.B.; LaRocca, N.G.; Muir-Nash, J.; Steinberg, A.D. The fatigue severity scale. Application to patients with multiple sclerosis and systemic lupus erythematosus. *Arch. Neurol.* **1989**, *46*, 1121–1123. [CrossRef] [PubMed]
29. Vellas, B.; Guigoz, Y.; Garry, P.J.; Nourhashemi, F.; Bennahum, D.; Lauque, S.; Albarede, J.L. The Mini Nutritional Assessment (MNA) and its use in grading the nutritional state of elderly patients. *Nutrition* **1999**, *15*, 116–122. [CrossRef]
30. Muñoz Díaz, B.; Molina-Recio, G.; Romero-Saldaña, M.; Redondo Sánchez, J.; Aguado Taberné, C.; Arias Blanco, C.; Molina-Luque, R.; Martínez De La Iglesia, J. Validation (in Spanish) of the Mini Nutritional Assessment survey to assess the nutritional status of patients over 65 years of age. *Fam. Pract.* **2019**, *36*, 172–178. [CrossRef]
31. Craig, C.L.; Marshall, A.L.; Sjöström, M.; Bauman, A.E.; Booth, M.L.; Ainsworth, B.E.; Pratt, M.; Ekelund, U.; Yngve, A.; Sallis, J.F.; et al. International physical activity questionnaire: 12-country reliability and validity. *Med. Sci. Sports Exerc.* **2003**, *35*, 1381–1395. [CrossRef]
32. Concato, J.; Peduzzi, P.; Holford, T.R.; Feinstein, A.R. Importance of events per independent variable in proportional hazards analysis. I. Background, goals, and general strategy. *J. Clin. Epidemiol.* **1995**, *48*, 1495–1501. [CrossRef]
33. Ortega Calvo, M.; Cayuela Domínguez, A. Unconditioned logistic regression and sample size: A bibliographic review. *Rev. Esp. Salud Publica* **2002**, *76*, 85–93. [CrossRef] [PubMed]
34. Cohen, J. A power primer. *Psychol. Bull.* **1992**, *112*, 155–159. [CrossRef] [PubMed]
35. Torkia, C.; Best, K.L.; Miller, W.C.; Eng, J.J. Balance Confidence: A Predictor of Perceived Physical Function, Perceived Mobility, and Perceived Recovery 1 Year After Inpatient Stroke Rehabilitation. *Arch. Phys. Med. Rehabil.* **2016**, *97*, 1064–1071. [CrossRef] [PubMed]
36. Hull, S.L.; Kneebone, I.I.; Farquharson, L. Anxiety, Depression, and Fall-Related Psychological Concerns in Community-Dwelling Older People. *Am. J. Geriatr. Psychiatry* **2013**, *21*, 1287–1291. [CrossRef] [PubMed]
37. Payette, M.C.; Bélanger, C.; Léveille, V.; Grenier, S. Fall-Related Psychological Concerns and Anxiety among Community-Dwelling Older Adults: Systematic Review and Meta-Analysis. *PLoS ONE* **2016**, *11*, e0152848. [CrossRef]
38. Hughes, C.C.; Kneebone, I.I.; Jones, F.; Brady, B.A. Theoretical and Empirical Review of Psychological Factors Associated with Falls-Related Psychological Concerns in Community-Dwelling Older People. *Int. Psychogeriatr.* **2015**, *27*, 1071–1087. [CrossRef]
39. Medley, A.; Thompson, M. Contribution of age and balance confidence to functional mobility test performance: Diagnostic accuracy of L test and normal-paced timed up and go. *J. Geriatr. Phys. Ther.* **2015**, *38*, 8–16. [CrossRef]
40. Miller, K.K.; Combs, S.A.; Puymbroeck, M.V.; Altenburger, P.A.; Kean, J.; Dierks, T.A.; Schmid, A.A. Fatigue and Pain: Relationships with Physical Performance and Patient Beliefs after Stroke. *Top. Stroke Rehabil.* **2013**, *20*, 347–355. [CrossRef]

41. Abasiyanik, Z.; Özdoğar, A.T.; Sağıcı, Ö.; Baba, C.; Ertekin, Ö.; Özakbaş, S. Explanatory factors of balance confidence in persons with multiple sclerosis: Beyond the physical functions. *Mult. Scler. Relat. Disord.* **2020**, *43*, 102239. [CrossRef] [PubMed]
42. Hicks, G.E.; Shardell, M.; Alley, D.E.; Miller, R.R.; Bandinelli, S.; Guralnik, J.; Lauretani, F.; Simonsick, E.M.; Ferruci, L. Absolute strength and loss of strength as predictors of mobility decline in older adults: The InCHIANTI study. *J. Gerontol. A Biol. Sci. Med. Sci.* **2012**, *67*, 66–73. [CrossRef] [PubMed]
43. Ibrahim, K.; May, C.; Patel, H.P.; Baxter, M.; Sayer, A.A.; Roberts, H. A feasibility study of implementing grip strength measurement into routine hospital practice (GRImP): Study protocol. *Pilot Feasibility Stud.* **2016**, *2*, 27. [CrossRef] [PubMed]
44. Kim, Y.S.; Lee, O.; Lee, J.H.; Kim, J.H.; Choi, B.Y.; Kim, M.J.; Kim, T.G. The Association between Levels of Muscle Strength and Fear of Falling in Korean Olders. *Korean J. Sports Med.* **2013**, *31*, 13–19. [CrossRef]
45. Silveira, T.; Pegorari, M.; Castro, S.; Ruas, G.; Novais-Shimano, S.; Patrizzi, L. Association of falls, fear of falling, handgrip strength and gait speed with frailty levels in the community elderly. *Medicina (Ribeirao Preto)* **2015**, *48*, 549–556. [CrossRef]
46. Gafner, S.C.; Germaine Bastiaenen, C.H.; Ferrari, S.; Gold, G.; Trombetti, A.; Terrier, P.; Hikfiker, R.; Allet, L. The Role of Hip Abductor Strength in Identifying Older Persons at Risk of Falls: A Diagnostic Accuracy Study. *Clin. Interv. Aging* **2020**, *15*, 645–654. [CrossRef]
47. Mello, J.P.; Cangussu-Oliveira, L.M.; Campos, R.C.; Tavares, F.V.; Capato, L.L.; García, B.M.; Carvalho de Abreu, D.C. Relationship Between Lower Limb Muscle Strength and Future Falls Among Community-Dwelling Older Adults with No History of Falls: A Prospective 1-Year Study. *J. Appl. Gerontol.* **2020**. online ahead of print. [CrossRef]
48. Buchmann, N.; Spira, D.; Norman, K.; Demuth, I.; Eckardt, R.; Steinhagen-Thiessen, E. Sleep, Muscle Mass and Muscle Function in Older People. *Dtsch. Arztebl. Int.* **2016**, *113*, 253–260.
49. Van Rijssen, N.M.; Rojer, A.G.M.; Trappenburg, M.C.; Reijnierse, E.M.; Meskers, C.G.M.; Maier, A.B.; van der Schueren, M.A.E. Is being malnourished according to the ESPEN definition for malnutrition associated with clinically relevant outcome measures in geriatric outpatients? *Eur. Geriatr. Med.* **2018**, *9*, 389–394. [CrossRef]
50. Gielen, E.; Beckwée, D.; Delaere, A.; De Breucker, S.; Vandewoude, M.; Bautmans, I. Sarcopenia Guidelines Development Group of the Belgian Society of Gerontology and Geriatrics (BSGG). Nutritional interventions to improve muscle mass, muscle strength, and physical performance in older people: An umbrella review of systematic reviews and meta-analyses. *Nutr. Rev.* **2020**, nuaa011. [CrossRef]
51. Kafri, M.; Hutzler, Y.; Korsensky, O.; Laufer, Y. Functional Performance and Balance in the Oldest-Old. *J. Geriatr. Phys. Ther.* **2019**, *42*, 183–188. [CrossRef] [PubMed]
52. Brandão, G.S.; Camelier, F.W.R.; Callou Sampaio, A.A.; Brandão, G.A.; Silva, A.S.; Freitas Gomes, G.S.B.; Donner, C.F.; Franco Oliveira, L.V.; Camelier, A.A. Association of sleep quality with excessive daytime somnolence and quality of life of elderlies of community. *Multidiscip. Respir. Med.* **2018**, *13*, 8. [CrossRef] [PubMed]
53. Hall, M.H.; Smagula, S.F.; Boudreau, R.M.; Ayonayon, H.N.; Goldman, S.E.; Harris, T.B.; Naydeck, B.L.; Rubin, S.M.; Samuelsson, L.; Satterfield, S.; et al. Association between Sleep Duration and Mortality Is Mediated by Markers of Inflammation and Health in Older Adults: The Health, Aging and Body Composition Study. *Sleep* **2015**, *38*, 189–195. [CrossRef] [PubMed]
54. Dommershuijsen, L.J.; Isik, B.M.; Darweesh, S.K.L.; van der Geest, J.N.; Ikram, M.K.; Ikram, M.A. Unravelling the association between gait and mortality—One step at a time. *J. Gerontol. A Biol. Sci. Med. Sci.* **2020**, *75*, 1184–1190. [CrossRef] [PubMed]
55. Spira, A.P.; Covinsky, K.; Rebok, G.W.; Punjabi, N.M.; Stone, K.L.; Hillier, T.A.; Ensrud, K.E.; Yaffe, K. Poor sleep quality and functional decline in older women. *J. Am. Geriatr. Soc.* **2012**, *60*, 1092–1098. [CrossRef]

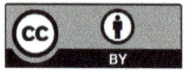

© 2020 by the authors. Licensee MDPI, Basel, Switzerland. This article is an open access article distributed under the terms and conditions of the Creative Commons Attribution (CC BY) license (http://creativecommons.org/licenses/by/4.0/).

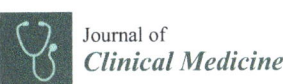

Brief Report

Dynapenia and Low Cognition: A Cross-Sectional Association in Postmenopausal Women

Julie A. Pasco [1,2,3,4,*], Amanda L. Stuart [1], Sophia X. Sui [1], Kara L. Holloway-Kew [1], Natalie K. Hyde [1], Monica C. Tembo [1], Pamela Rufus-Membere [1], Mark A. Kotowicz [1,2,3] and Lana J. Williams [1]

1. IMPACT—The Institute for Mental and Physical Health and Clinical Translation, School of Medicine, Deakin University, Geelong, VIC 3220, Australia; a.stuart@deakin.edu.au (A.L.S.); ssui@deakin.edu.au (S.X.S.); k.holloway@deakin.edu.au (K.L.H.-K.); natalie.hyde@deakin.edu.au (N.K.H.); mctembo@deakin.edu.au (M.C.T.); pamela.r@deakin.edu.au (P.R.-M.); mark.kotowicz@deakin.edu.au (M.A.K.); l.williams@deakin.edu.au (L.J.W.)
2. Department of Medicine-Western Health, The University of Melbourne, St Albans, VIC 3021, Australia
3. Barwon Health, Geelong, VIC 3220, Australia
4. Department of Epidemiology and Preventive Medicine, Monash University, Melbourne, VIC 3004, Australia
* Correspondence: julie.pasco@deakin.edu.au; Tel.: +61-3-421-53331

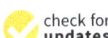

Citation: Pasco, J.A.; Stuart, A.L.; Sui, S.X.; Holloway-Kew, K.L.; Hyde, N.K.; Tembo, M.C.; Rufus-Membere, P.; Kotowicz, M.A.; Williams, L.J. Dynapenia and Low Cognition: A Cross-Sectional Association in Postmenopausal Women. *J. Clin. Med.* **2021**, *10*, 173. https://doi.org/10.3390/jcm10020173

Received: 8 December 2020
Accepted: 4 January 2021
Published: 6 January 2021

Publisher's Note: MDPI stays neutral with regard to jurisdictional claims in published maps and institutional affiliations.

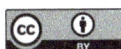

Copyright: © 2021 by the authors. Licensee MDPI, Basel, Switzerland. This article is an open access article distributed under the terms and conditions of the Creative Commons Attribution (CC BY) license (https://creativecommons.org/licenses/by/4.0/).

Abstract: Dynapenia is a key contributor to physical frailty. Cognitive impairment and dementia accompany frailty, yet links between skeletal muscle and neurocognition are poorly understood. We examined the cross-sectional relationship between lower limb muscle strength and global cognitive function. Participants were 127 women aged 51–87 years, from the Geelong Osteoporosis Study. Peak eccentric strength of the hip-flexors and hip abductors was determined using a hand-held dynamometer, and dynapenia identified as muscle strength t-scores < -1. Cognition was assessed using the Mini-Mental State Examination (MMSE), and MMSE scores below the median were rated as low. Associations between dynapenia and low cognition were examined using logistic regression models. Hip-flexor dynapenia was detected in 38 (71.7%) women with low cognition and 36 (48.7%) with good cognition ($p = 0.009$); for hip abductor dynapenia, the pattern was similar (21 (39.6%) vs. 9 (12.2%); $p < 0.001$). While the observed difference for hip-flexor strength was attenuated after adjusting for age and height (adjusted Odds Ratio (OR) 1.95, 95%CI 0.86–4.41), low cognition was nearly 4-fold more likely in association with hip abductor dynapenia (adjusted OR 3.76, 95%CI 1.44–9.83). No other confounders were identified. Our data suggest that low strength of the hip abductors and low cognition are associated and this could be a consequence of poor muscle function contributing to cognitive decline or vice versa. As muscle weakness is responsive to physical interventions, this warrants further investigation.

Keywords: cognition; brain-body cross-talk; muscle strength; older persons; sarcopenia

1. Introduction

Dynapenia refers to age-associated loss of skeletal muscle strength [1]. From about age 50 years, muscle strength declines by 10–15% per decade up to age 70 years, reaching losses of 25–40% per decade thereafter [2,3]. The rate of decline in muscle strength surpasses age-related loss of skeletal muscle mass and is a key contributor to physical frailty; physical frailty is known to accompany cognitive impairment and dementia [4].

Low muscle strength is also a key characteristic of sarcopenia. This is evident in the revised operational definition from the European Working Group on Sarcopenia in Older People (EWGSOP2), which focuses on low muscle strength as the primary parameter of sarcopenia; low muscle mass (or quality) confirms the diagnosis, and poor physical performance identifies severe sarcopenia [5]. Sarcopenia has been associated with cognitive impairment and Alzheimer's disease [6].

Muscle deterioration during ageing is a consequence of decreases in the number and cross-sectional area of muscle fibres [7] and reductions in the number of motoneurons [8].

Thus, loss of muscle strength in older people is attributable, at least in part, to neurologic mechanisms that alter the number of functioning motor units [9]. However, links between dynapenia and cognitive function are poorly understood. As handgrip strength is easily measured, predicts adverse health outcomes, and is considered to indicate global skeletal muscle strength [10], EWGSOP2 recommends handgrip strength for assessing muscle strength in the diagnosis for sarcopenia. However, not all studies support good agreement between handgrip and lower limb muscle strength [11]. Several reviews have described associations between upper body strength measures and cognition by assessing handgrip strength [12–14], but links between lower body strength measures (e.g., hip flexor or hip abductor strength) have not been well investigated. The main goal of this study was to examine the relationship between lower limb skeletal muscle strength and global cognitive function in older women (>50 years), as older ages are at highest risk for age-related physical and mental decline. We hypothesise that dynapenia will be associated with low cognition.

2. Materials and Methods

An age-stratified, population-based cohort of 1494 women (age 20–94 years) was recruited for the Geelong Osteoporosis Study between 1994 and 1997, with 77.1% response, using a random-selection process from electoral rolls [15]; the cohort was predominantly Caucasian (~98%). A listing on the electoral roll for the Barwon Statistical Division fulfilled inclusion criteria; residence in the region for less than 6 months and inability to provide informed consent necessitated exclusion. Six years later (2000–2003), 638 of 1048 women who were re-assessed at follow-up were aged over 50 years. Among these, 127 (ages 51–87 years) provided measures of cognitive function in combination with muscle strength, weight, height, and information about their lifestyle behaviours, meeting criteria for inclusion in this analysis. There were no further exclusion criteria for the analysis. Written informed consent was obtained from all participants. The Barwon Health Human Research Ethics Committee approved the study (project 92/01).

Global cognitive function was assessed using the Mini-Mental State Examination (MMSE) [16]; scores below the median were rated as low cognition and scores above the median were rated as good cognition. Peak eccentric muscle strength of the hip flexors and abductors were measured using a hand-held dynamometer (HHD; Nicholas Manual Muscle Tester, Lafayette Instrument Company, Lafayette, IN, USA) [17]. HHD provides good to excellent reliability and validity when compared with fixed dynamometry for most measures of isometric lower limb strength [18]. To measure hip flexion strength, the seated participant raised the test thigh 10 cm above the bench; with the HHD positioned 5 cm proximal to the patella, the examiner applied a downward force while the participant resisted, until resistance could no longer be sustained. For hip abduction strength, the side-lying participant raised the outstretched test leg 20 cm above the bench; the HHD was positioned 10 cm proximal to the lateral malleolus. Measurements were repeated bilaterally, and the maximum of triplicate measures for each muscle group was used in analyses. Multiplying the maximal registered force (kg) by 9.81 converted the force to Newtons (N). Dynapenia refers to muscle strength t-scores < 1 for hip flexors and hip abductors [19]. All MMSE tests were conducted by one of the authors (A.L.S.), and HHD assessments were performed by other trained research personnel.

Data on current smoking, alcohol use, and mobility were collected by self-report. The usual consumption of different alcoholic beverages was recorded as glasses per week, and the average daily total was categorised as <1 or ≥1 glass/day. Participants with mobility described as someone who 'moves, walks, and works energetically and participates in vigorous exercise' were classified as being physically active.

Descriptive characteristics of participants were presented as mean (±SD), median (IQR), or n (%). Intergroup differences were identified by Student's t-test for parametric data, Mann–Whitney test for non-parametric data, and chi-square test for categorical data. Associations between dynapenia (exposure) and low cognitive performance (outcome) were examined using binary logistic regression models before and after adjusting for potential confounders and effect modifiers. Statistical analyses were performed using Minitab (version 16, Minitab, State College, PA, USA).

3. Results

Participant characteristics are listed in Table 1. The median MMSE score was 29 (range 22–30). Mean muscle strength measures for hip flexors and abductors were lower for women with low cognition in comparison with those with good cognition. The group with low cognition was older, had shorter stature, and was less likely to consume, on average, one or more alcoholic drinks each day; otherwise no other differences were detected.

Table 1. Participant characteristics for the whole group and according to categories of cognition. Data are shown as mean (±SD), median (interquartile range, IQR), or number (%).

	All	Cognition		
		Low (MMSE * < 29)	Good (MMSE * ≥ 29)	p
n	127	53	74	
MMSE * score	29.0 (28.0–30.0)	28.0 (27.0–28.0)	29.5 (29.0–30.0)	<0.001
Age (year)	68.1 (59.0–75.9)	70.4 (64.7–78.3)	62.1 (56.5–73.3)	<0.001
Weight (kg)	70.7 (±14.7)	68.8 (±13.9)	72.0 (±15.1)	0.216
Height (cm)	1.59 (±0.06)	1.57 (±0.06)	1.60 (±0.06)	0.001
BMI ** (kg/m^2)	28.0 (±5.2)	28.0 (±4.9)	28.0 (±5.5)	0.959
Current smokers	11 (8.7%)	4 (7.6%)	7 (9.5%)	0.761
Alcohol ≥1 glass/d	20 (15.8%)	4 (7.6%)	16 (21.6%)	0.032
Physically active	6 (4.7%)	2 (3.8%)	4 (5.4%)	0.999
Muscle strength (N)				
Hip flexors	144 (±0.48)	127 (±41)	156 (±49)	<0.001
Hip abductors	127 (±40)	116 (±40)	135 (±38)	0.007

* MMSE Mini-Mental State Examination. ** BMI: Body Mass Index.

While hip flexor dynapenia was detected in 38 (71.7%) women with low cognition and 36 (48.7%) with good cognition (p = 0.009), this difference was attenuated after adjustments were made for age and height (adjusted Odds Ratio (OR) 1.95, 95%CI 0.86–4.41, p = 0.110).

For hip abductors, dynapenia was detected for 21 (39.6%) women with low cognition and 9 (12.2%) of those with good cognition (p < 0.001). This association was sustained after adjustment for age and height; those with hip abductor dynapenia were nearly four-fold more likely to have low cognition (adjusted OR 3.76, 95%CI 1.44–9.83, p = 0.007). Body Mass Index (BMI), smoking, alcohol consumption, and mobility did not contribute to the model. No effect modifiers were identified.

4. Discussion

Here we present data that describe a cross-sectional association between lower limb muscle strength and global cognitive function in postmenopausal women. These findings are concordant with cross-sectional data from the I-Lan Longitudinal Aging Study (ILAS) involving 731 elderly men and women (mean age 73.4 years) for whom MMSE-derived global cognitive impairment was associated with low handgrip strength (adjusted OR 2.23, 95%CI 1.29–3.86) [20]. Similarly, cross-sectional data for 292 men (ages 60–96 years) from the Geelong Osteoporosis Study revealed that handgrip strength was associated with psychomotor function and overall cognitive performance assessed by the CogState Brief Battery [21], and another cross-sectional study of 39 men (ages 61–79 years) reported that knee extensor strength was positively associated with global cognitive function also assessed by MMSE [22]. Moreover, there are longitudinal data that describe increases in muscle strength [23] and torque [24] in association with improvements in cognitive performance following loading of skeletal muscle through progressive resistance training regimens. Conclusions from a recent systematic review were that resistance training elicited functional changes in the brain, including improvements in executive function [25].

Previous work in animal models suggest that restriction of skeletal muscle activity in the hind legs of mice affect neurogenic areas of the brain [26] and produce changes in memory and spatial learning [27]. These findings align with observations in the literature that physical inactivity is a common risk factor for Alzheimer's disease and, conversely, that voluntary exercise improves cognitive function [28,29].

Cognitive changes following skeletal muscle loading may operate through the release from contracting muscle of chemical messengers, such as brain-derived neurotrophic factor (BDNF), which trigger neurobiological changes [29,30]. Age-related declines in skeletal muscle and cognitive capabilities have common pathophysiological pathways, including chronic inflammation, oxidative stress, and endocrine imbalances; they also share risk factors associated with adverse lifestyle behaviours, such as physical inactivity, smoking, and excessive use of alcohol, that might contribute to brain–body cross-talk by mediating these pathophysiological pathways [31–34]. While we accounted for differences in body habitus and lifestyle behaviours, biomarker data that indicate biological imbalances were not available.

However, an important forte of our study design is that assessment of muscle strength and cognitive function were obtained independently, thereby minimising potential differential measurement bias. We also recognise as weaknesses that the data are cross-sectional, and there is the possibility that low cognitive function might have impacted on the ability to perform the muscle strength tests. Although several variables, including lifestyle behaviours, were considered as confounders, residual confounding is likely. It is noted that our results should be interpreted with caution because of the small numbers of participants in some sub-groups (such as nine women with hip abductor dynapenia and good cognition), and we recognise that the findings may not be generalisable beyond our sample of white postmenopausal women. Moreover, while we have investigated only lower limb muscle strength in association with global cognition, there is scope to explore this further using other indices of muscle performance and cognitive function in specific domains.

5. Conclusions

Our cross-sectional analyses suggest that low muscle strength and low cognition are associated, and this could be related to muscle function deficits contributing to cognitive decline or vice versa. Longitudinal studies are needed to address temporal changes in skeletal muscle performance and cognitive function. We propose that future cross-sectional studies use different neuroimaging methods (e.g., functional near-infrared spectroscopy, electroencephalography, functional magnetic resonance imaging) and/or assess neurochemical substances (e.g., neurotransmitters, neurotrophic factors) in order to further elucidate the underlying neurobiological mechanisms of the relationship between skeletal muscle strength and cognitive performance. Emerging pharmacological therapies for preventing muscle loss, such as antibodies against myostatin and activin receptor types IIA and IIB [35,36], might provide potential novel agents for the management of cognitive decline. Similarly, pharmacological therapies for preventing cognitive decline might provide potential novel agents for the management of muscle decay. There is evidence to support life course approaches for preventing and managing physical and cognitive performance [29,37–40]. Thus, there may be potential for future clinical trials involving such novel therapies, together with interventions focused on specific modes of exercise, diet, and health behaviours that could be championed as public health strategies for both physical and mental health benefits.

Author Contributions: Conceptualization: J.A.P.; methodology: J.A.P. and L.J.W.; formal analysis: J.A.P.; investigation: A.L.S., K.L.H.-K., N.K.H., M.C.T., and P.R.-M.; resources: J.A.P., M.A.K., and L.J.W.; data curation: J.A.P.; writing—original draft preparation: J.A.P.; writing—review and editing, J.A.P., A.L.S., S.X.S., K.L.H.-K., N.K.H., M.C.T., P.R.-M., M.A.K., and L.J.W.; project administration: J.A.P. and M.A.K.; funding acquisition: J.A.P., M.A.K., and L.J.W. All authors have read and agreed to the published version of the manuscript.

Funding: The Geelong Osteoporosis Study was funded by the National Health and Medical Research Council (NHMRC), Australia (projects 251638, 628582). S.X.S., M.C.T., and P.R.M. were supported by Deakin Postgraduate Scholarships; K.L.H.-K. was supported by an Alfred Deakin Postdoctoral Research Fellowship; N.K.H. was supported by a Deakin Postdoctoral Research Fellowship; and L.J.W. was supported by a NHMRC Career Development Fellowship (1064272) and a NHMRC Investigator grant (1174060). However, these funding organisations played no role in the design and conduct of the study, in the collection, management, analysis and interpretation of the data, or in the preparation, review, and approval of the manuscript.

Institutional Review Board Statement: The study was conducted according to the guidelines of the Declaration of Helsinki, and approved by the Human Research Ethics Committee at Barwon Health (project 92/01).

Informed Consent Statement: Informed consent was obtained from all participants involved in the study.

Data Availability Statement: The data presented in this study are available on request from the corresponding author. The data are not publicly available due to ethical restrictions.

Acknowledgments: The authors acknowledge the study participants.

Conflicts of Interest: The authors declare no conflict of interest. J.A.P. has received grants from the National Health and Medical Research Council (NHMRC) Australia, the BUPA Foundation, Amgen-GSK OA-ANZBMS, Amgen Australia, Deakin University, the Western Alliance, and the Beischer Foundation; K.L.H.-K. has received grants from Deakin University, Amgen-GSK OA-ANZBMS and Amgen Australia; N.K.H. has received grants from Deakin University and the Beischer Foundation; M.A.K. has received grants from the NHMRC, Amgen-GSK OA-ANZBMS, Amgen Australia, and the Western Alliance; L.J.W. has received grants from Deakin University and the NHMRC.

References

1. Clark, B.C.; Manini, T.M. Sarcopenia =/= dynapenia. *J. Gerontol. A Biol. Sci. Med. Sci.* **2008**, *63*, 829–834. [CrossRef] [PubMed]
2. Goodpaster, B.H.; Park, S.W.; Harris, T.B.; Kritchevsky, S.B.; Nevitt, M.; Schwartz, A.V.; Simonsick, E.M.; Tylavsky, F.A.; Visser, M.; Newman, A.B.; et al. The loss of skeletal muscle strength, mass, and quality in older adults: The Health, Aging and Body Composition study. *J. Gerontol. Ser. A Boil. Sci. Med. Sci.* **2006**, *61*, 1059–1064. [CrossRef]
3. Hughes, V.A.; Frontera, W.R.; Wood, M.; Evans, W.J.; Dallal, G.E.; Roubenoff, R.; Singh, M.A.F. Longitudinal muscle strength changes in older adults: Influence of muscle mass, physical activity, and health. *J. Gerontol. Ser. A Boil. Sci. Med. Sci.* **2001**, *56*, B209–B217. [CrossRef] [PubMed]
4. Robertson, D.A.; Savva, G.M.; Kenny, R.A. Frailty and cognitive impairment—A review of the evidence and causal mecha-nisms. *Ageing Res. Rev.* **2013**, *12*, 840–851. [CrossRef] [PubMed]
5. Cruz-Jentoft, A.J.; Bahat, G.; Bauer, J.; Boirie, Y.; Bruyère, O.; Cederholm, T.; Cooper, C.; Landi, F.; Rolland, Y.; Sayer, A.A.; et al. Sarcopenia: Revised European consensus on definition and diagnosis. *Age Ageing* **2019**, *48*, 16–31. [CrossRef]
6. Sugimoto, T.; Ono, R.; Murata, S.; Saji, N.; Matsui, Y.; Niida, S.; Toba, K.; Sakurai, T.; Niida, S. Prevalence and associated factors of sarcopenia in elderly subjects with amnestic mild cognitive impairment or Alzheimer disease. *Curr. Alzheimer Res.* **2016**, *13*, 718–726. [CrossRef]
7. Faulkner, J.A.; Larkin, L.M.; Claflin, D.R.; Brooks, S.V. Age-related changes in the structure and function of skeletal muscles. *Clin. Exp. Pharmacol. Physiol.* **2007**, *34*, 1091–1096. [CrossRef]
8. Drey, M.; Krieger, B.; Sieber, C.C.; Bauer, J.M.; Hettwer, S.; Bertsch, T.; Dahinden, P.; Mäder, A.; Vrijbloed, J.W.; Schuster, G.; et al. Motoneuron loss is associated with sarcopenia. *J. Am. Med. Dir. Assoc.* **2014**, *15*, 435–439. [CrossRef]
9. Kaya, R.D.; Nakazawa, M.; Hoffman, R.L.; Clark, B.C. Interrelationship between muscle strength, motor units, and aging. *Exp. Gerontol.* **2013**, *48*, 920–925. [CrossRef]
10. Rantanen, T.; Era, P.; Heikkinen, E. Maximal isometric strength and mobility among 75-year-old men and women. *Age Ageing* **1994**, *23*, 132–137. [CrossRef]
11. Yeung, S.S.; Reijnierse, E.M.; Trappenburg, M.C.; Hogrel, J.-Y.; McPhee, J.S.; Piasecki, M.; Sipilä, S.; Salpakoski, A.; Butler-Browne, G.; Pääsuke, M.; et al. Handgrip strength cannot be assumed a proxy for overall muscle strength. *J. Am. Med. Dir. Assoc.* **2018**, *19*, 703–709. [CrossRef] [PubMed]

12. Carson, R.G. Get a grip: Individual variations in grip strength are a marker of brain health. *Neurobiol. Aging* **2018**, *71*, 189–222. [CrossRef] [PubMed]
13. Fritz, N.E.; McCarthy, C.J.; Adamo, D.E. Handgrip strength as a means of monitoring progression of cognitive decline—A scoping review. *Ageing Res. Rev.* **2017**, *35*, 112–123. [CrossRef] [PubMed]
14. Shaughnessy, K.A.; Hackney, K.J.; Clark, B.C.; Kraemer, W.J.; Terbizan, D.J.; Bailey, R.R.; McGrath, R. A narrative review of handgrip strength and cognitive functioning: Bringing a new characteristic to muscle memory. *J. Alzheimer's Dis.* **2020**, *73*, 1265–1278. [CrossRef] [PubMed]
15. Pasco, J.A.; Nicholson, G.C.; Kotowicz, M.A. Cohort profile: Geelong Osteoporosis Study. *Int. J. Epidemiol.* **2011**, *41*, 1565–1575. [CrossRef] [PubMed]
16. Bossers, W.J.R.; Van Der Woude, L.H.; Boersma, F.; Scherder, E.J.; Van Heuvelen, M.J. Recommended measures for the assessment of cognitive and physical performance in older patients with dementia: A systematic review. *Dement. Geriatr. Cogn. Disord. Extra* **2012**, *2*, 589–609. [CrossRef]
17. Marino, M.; Nicholas, J.A.; Gleim, G.W.; Rosenthal, P.; Nicholas, S.J. The efficacy of manual assessment of muscle strength us-ing a new device. *Am. J. Sports Med.* **1982**, *10*, 360–364. [CrossRef]
18. Mentiplay, B.F.; Perraton, L.G.; Bower, K.J.; Adair, B.; Pua, Y.-H.; Williams, G.P.; McGaw, R.; Clark, R.A. Assessment of lower limb muscle strength and power using hand-held and fixed dynamometry: A reliability and validity study. *PLoS ONE* **2015**, *10*, e0140822. [CrossRef]
19. Pasco, J.A.; Stuart, A.L.; Holloway-Kew, K.L.; Tembo, M.C.; Sui, S.X.; Anderson, K.B.; Hyde, N.K.; Williams, L.J.; Kotowicz, M.A. Lower-limb muscle strength: Normative data from an observational population-based study. *BMC Musculoskelet. Disord.* **2020**, *21*, 1–8. [CrossRef]
20. Huang, C.-Y.; Hwang, A.-C.; Liu, L.-K.; Lee, W.-J.; Chen, L.-K.; Peng, L.; Lin, M.-H. Association of dynapenia, sarcopenia, and cognitive impairment among community-dwelling older Taiwanese. *Rejuvenation Res.* **2016**, *19*, 71–78. [CrossRef]
21. Sui, S.X.; Holloway-Kew, K.L.; Hyde, N.K.; Williams, L.J.; Leach, S.; Pasco, J.A. Muscle strength and gait speed rather than lean mass are better indicators for poor cognitive function in older men. *Sci. Rep.* **2020**, *10*, 1–9. [CrossRef] [PubMed]
22. Nakamoto, H.; Yoshitake, Y.; Takai, Y.; Kanehisa, H.; Kitamura, T.; Kawanishi, M.; Mori, S. Knee extensor strength is associated with Mini-Mental State Examination scores in elderly men. *Eur. J. Appl. Physiol.* **2012**, *112*, 1945–1953. [CrossRef] [PubMed]
23. Mavros, Y.; Gates, N.; Wilson, G.C.; Jain, N.; Meiklejohn, J.; Brodaty, H.; Wen, W.; Singh, N.; Baune, B.T.; Suo, C.; et al. Mediation of cognitive function improvements by strength gains after resistance training in older adults with mild cognitive impairment: Outcomes of the Study of Mental and Resistance Training. *J. Am. Geriatr. Soc.* **2017**, *65*, 550–559. [CrossRef] [PubMed]
24. Forte, R.; Boreham, C.A.; Leite, J.C.; De Vito, G.; Brennan, L.; Gibney, E.R.; Pesce, C. Enhancing cognitive functioning in the el-derly: Multicomponent vs resistance training. *Clin. Interv. Aging* **2013**, *8*, 19–27. [CrossRef]
25. Herold, F.; Törpel, A.; Schega, L.; Müller, N.G. Functional and/or structural brain changes in response to resistance exercises and resistance training lead to cognitive improvements—A systematic review. *Eur. Rev. Aging Phys. Act.* **2019**, *16*, 1–33. [CrossRef]
26. Adami, R.; Pagano, J.; Colombo, M.; Platonova, N.; Recchia, D.; Chiaramonte, R.; Bottinelli, R.; Canepari, M.; Bottai, D. Reduction of movement in neurological diseases: Effects on neural stem cells characteristics. *Front. Neurosci.* **2018**, *12*, 336. [CrossRef]
27. Wang, T.; Chen, H.; Lv, K.; Ji, G.; Zhang, Y.; Wang, Y.; Li, Y.; Qu, L. iTRAQ-based proteomics analysis of hippocampus in spatial memory deficiency rats induced by simulated microgravity. *J. Proteom.* **2017**, *160*, 64–73. [CrossRef]
28. Cass, S.P. Alzheimer's Disease and exercise: A literature review. *Curr. Sports Med. Rep.* **2017**, *16*, 19–22. [CrossRef]
29. Marston, K.J.; Brown, B.M.; Rainey-Smith, S.R.; Peiffer, J.J. Resistance exercise-induced responses in physiological factors linked with cognitive health. *J. Alzheimer's Dis.* **2019**, *68*, 39–64. [CrossRef]
30. Binder, D.K.; Scharfman, H.E. Brain-derived neurotrophic factor. *Growth Factors* **2004**, *22*, 123–131. [CrossRef]
31. Chang, K.V.; Hsu, T.H.; Wu, W.T.; Huang, K.C.; Han, D.S. Association between sarcopenia and cognitive impairment: A systematic review and meta-analysis. *J. Am. Med. Dir. Assoc.* **2016**, *17*, 1164.e7–1164.e15. [CrossRef] [PubMed]
32. Sui, S.X.; Pasco, J.A. Obesity and brain function: The brain–body crosstalk. *Medicina* **2020**, *56*, 499. [CrossRef] [PubMed]
33. Pasco, J.A. Age-related changes in muscle and bone. In *Osteosarcopenia: Bone, Muscle and Fat Interactions*; Duque, G., Ed.; Springer: New York, NY, USA, 2019; ISBN 978-3-030-25889-4.
34. Pasco, J.A.; Williams, L.J.; Jacka, F.; Stupka, N.; Brennan-Olsen, S.L.; Holloway-Kew, K.L.; Berk, M. Sarcopenia and the common mental disorders: A potential regulatory role of skeletal muscle on brain function? *Curr. Osteoporos. Rep.* **2015**, *13*, 351–357. [CrossRef] [PubMed]
35. Becker, C.; Lord, S.R.; Studenski, S.A.; Warden, S.J.; Fielding, R.A.; Recknor, C.P.; Hochberg, M.C.; Ferrari, S.L.; Blain, H.; Binder, E.F.; et al. Myostatin antibody (LY2495655) in older weak fallers: A proof-of-concept, randomised, phase 2 trial. *Lancet Diabetes Endocrinol.* **2015**, *3*, 948–957. [CrossRef]
36. Rooks, D.; Praestgaard, J.; Hariry, S.; Laurent, D.; Petricoul, O.; Perry, R.G.; Lach-Trifilieff, E.; Roubenoff, R. Treatment of sarcopenia with bimagrumab: Results from a phase II, randomized, controlled, proof-of-concept study. *J. Am. Geriatr. Soc.* **2017**, *65*, 1988–1995. [CrossRef]
37. Williams, D.P. Strength training for the prevention and treatment of dynapenia. *J. Bone Muscles Stud.* **2017**, *2017*, 13–21.
38. Audiffren, M.; André, N. The exercise–cognition relationship: A virtuous circle. *J. Sport Heal. Sci.* **2019**, *8*, 339–347. [CrossRef]

39. Cuesta, F.; Verdejo-Bravo, C.; Fernandez-Perez, C.; Martín-Sánchez, F.J. Effect of milk and other dairy products on the risk of frailty, sarcopenia, and cognitive performance decline in the elderly: A systematic review. *Adv. Nutr.* **2019**, *10* (suppl. 2), S105–S119. [CrossRef]
40. Scarmeas, N.; Anastasiou, C.A.; Yannakoulia, M. Nutrition and prevention of cognitive impairment. *Lancet Neurol.* **2018**, *17*, 1006–1015. [CrossRef]

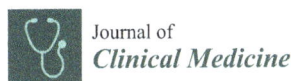

Article

Oxidative Stress, Telomere Shortening, and Apoptosis Associated to Sarcopenia and Frailty in Patients with Multimorbidity

Máximo Bernabeu-Wittel [1,*], Raquel Gómez-Díaz [2], Álvaro González-Molina [1], Sofía Vidal-Serrano [3], Jesús Díez-Manglano [4], Fernando Salgado [5], María Soto-Martín [6], Manuel Ollero-Baturone [1] and on behalf of the PROTEO RESEARCHERS [†]

1. Internal Medicine Department, Hospital Universitario Virgen del Rocío, 41013 Sevilla, Spain; aglezmolina@gmail.com (Á.G.-M.); m.ollero.baturone@gmail.com (M.O.-B.)
2. General and Multiple Use Laboratory, Instituto de Biomedicina de Sevilla, 41013 Sevilla, Spain; rgomez-ibis@us.es
3. Internal Medicine Department, Hospital San Juan de Dios del Aljarafe, 41930 Sevilla, Spain; sofiavidalserrano@gmail.com
4. Internal Medicine Department, Hospital Royo Villanova, 50015 Zaragoza, Spain; jdiez@aragon.es
5. Internal Medicine Department, Hospital Regional, 29010 Málaga, Spain; fersalord@gmail.com
6. Internal Medicine Department, Hospital Juan Ramón Jiménez, 21005 Huelva, Spain; msoto@hotmail.com
* Correspondence: wittel@cica.es; Tel./Fax: +34-(95)5012270
† All researchers from the PROTEO project listed at Acknowledgments.

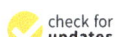

Received: 6 August 2020; Accepted: 14 August 2020; Published: 18 August 2020

Abstract: Background: The presence of oxidative stress, telomere shortening, and apoptosis in polypathological patients (PP) with sarcopenia and frailty remains unknown. Methods: Multicentric prospective observational study in order to assess oxidative stress markers (catalase, glutathione reductase (GR), total antioxidant capacity to reactive oxygen species (TAC-ROS), and superoxide dismutase (SOD)), absolute telomere length (aTL), and apoptosis (DNA fragmentation) in peripheral blood samples of a hospital-based population of PP. Associations of these biomarkers to sarcopenia, frailty, functional status, and 12-month mortality were analyzed. Results: Of the 444 recruited patients, 97 (21.8%), 278 (62.6%), and 80 (18%) were sarcopenic, frail, or both, respectively. Oxidative stress markers (lower TAC-ROS and higher SOD) were significantly enhanced and aTL significantly shortened in patients with sarcopenia, frailty or both syndromes. No evidence of apoptosis was detected in blood leukocytes of any of the patients. Both oxidative stress markers (GR, $p = 0.04$) and telomere shortening ($p = 0.001$) were associated to death risk and to less survival days. Conclusions: Oxidative stress markers and telomere length were enhanced and shortened, respectively, in blood samples of polypathological patients with sarcopenia and/or frailty. Both were associated to decreased survival. They could be useful in the clinical practice to assess vulnerable populations with multimorbidity and of potential interest as therapeutic targets.

Keywords: multimorbidity; polypathological patients; sarcopenia; frailty; oxidative stress; telomere length; apoptosis

1. Introduction

As a result of populations' aging throughout the world, the prevalence of chronic conditions has drastically increased; these coexist frequently in the same patient, conditioning deleterious relationships, faster clinical and functional deterioration, poorer quality of life, and higher mortality. Taking multimorbidity seriously is of nuclear importance for the sustainability of all healthcare systems [1–3]. Multimorbidity is narrowly correlated to aging. As a matter of fact, there is a direct and strong correlation between the development of different chronic conditions and longevity. The easy explanation of this correlation is the longer exposure to different risk factors (environmental agents, unhealthy lifestyles, inherited risk factors, overuse deterioration), which impact in the development of diseases and failures of multiple organs and systems [3,4].

Sarcopenia and frailty are two major geriatric syndromes closely related to the aging process [5,6]. The development of one or both of them is linked to progressive functional disability, loss of quality of life and death. Their prevalence in elderly populations approximates 10% and 15%, respectively; however, in the presence of chronic conditions and multimorbidity, these prevalences can raise to 20% and 60%, respectively [7]. Both syndromes are narrowly interrelated; as a matter of fact, they have currently an identical therapeutic approach based on physical activity and optimal nutrition. In a recent study, both sarcopenia and frailty were present in the same patient in 18% of the studied cases; that is to say that most sarcopenic patients were frail, and about one third of frail patients were sarcopenic [7]. Nevertheless, these percentages are different in other studies, probably due to sample selection criteria [8].

Both syndromes have commonalities sharing a nuclear issue, which is the physical function impairment, usually assessed by different tools like walking speed and hand grip strength. Such impairment may be responsible for the concurrent existence of a disability in both phenotypes, but they also express differences; as a matter of fact, sarcopenia rather tends to assume the lineaments of cachexia and "muscle wasting", whereas frailty status is largely dominated by a low physical performance, homeostasis disruption to stressors, and disabling condition.

The deep and intimal relation between sarcopenia and frailty probably reflects that they share similar or identical pathophysiological routes and molecular mechanisms. In this field, many metabolic imbalances and other molecular factors have been studied and correlated in some ways to both geriatric syndromes. Sarcopenia has been associated to genetic expression of apoptosis and muscular autophagy, muscle androgenic and vitamin D receptors, chronic inflammation, oxidative stress, and telomere shortening [9–11]. On the other hand, frailty has been associated to inflammation pathways (demonstrated in the case of C-reactive protein, interleukin-1β, the IL-1 receptor antagonist, IL-18, and tumor necrosis factor alpha), unspecific immunological alterations linked to immunosenescence (mainly thymus involution and the corresponding decrease of T and B lymphocyte precursors and the reduction in the proliferative capacity of the T and B lymphocytes), and oxidative stress [12–14].

From these data, the narrow relation between frailty and sarcopenia can be extracted. This is more so in patients with multimorbidity, in which aging and chronic conditions may trigger more oxidative stress, telomere shortening, and apoptosis. In these patients, sarcopenia and frailty could be the results of a multisite "rusting" produced by chronic inflammation processes and their consequent imbalance between the production of reactive oxygen species (ROS) and cellular antioxidant defenses, present in chronic neurological, pulmonary, and cardiovascular diseases, along with atherosclerosis, diabetes, obesity, and arthritis. Nevertheless, the role and weight of any of these molecular alterations in sarcopenic and/or frail populations with multimorbidity remain unknown.

For all these reasons, we have explored the main oxidative stress markers, telomere length, and apoptosis parameters in a hospital-based multicenter cohort of multimorbidity patients. We hypothesized that all these biological markers have a deep impact and association to sarcopenia and frailty.

2. Patients and Methods

2.1. Development of the Study

This was a prospective observational, multi-institutional (6 centers) study carried out by researchers from the Polypathological Patient and Advanced Age Study Group of the Spanish Society of Internal Medicine (all participant centers are listed on the PROTEO Researchers list). The study was approved by the ethics committee of all participant centers. The study inclusion period ranged from January 2012 to March 2016.

All patients treated in the Internal Medicine and Geriatric areas who accomplished inclusion criteria (≥18 years old and fulfilling criteria of polypathological patient (PP)) were included, after providing their written informed consent. The patient's sample was collected by performing prevalence surveys every 14 days during the study period. A total of 155 surveys were performed (29 ± 19 surveys per hospital).

After receiving informed consent, a complete set of demographical, socio-familial, clinical, functional, biological, and pharmacological data were collected from all included patients.

Sarcopenia was defined following EWGSOP criteria [15]. This was established by the presence of a gait speed ≤ 0.8 m/seg, plus a skeletal muscle mass <6.76 Kg/m^2 in women, and <10.76 Kg/m^2 in men (for those patients able to walk) or a hand grip strength lower than 50 percentile of his/her age group and gender, and a skeletal muscle mass <6.76 Kg/m^2 in women and <10.76 Kg/m^2 in men (for those patents unable to walk). Frailty was defined when fulfilling 3 or more of Fried's criteria (slowness, weakness, weight loss, exhaustion, and low physical activity) [16].

All patients were clinically followed during a 12-month period in order to assess mortality, as previously described [7]. Time survival was assessed, and in case of death, chronology of the demise was incorporated. Therefore, we looked at mortality as a time-dependent outcome. For the dichotomous outcome, subjects were categorized depending on whether or not they survived 12 months from their initial interview date. For the continuous outcome, survival time was defined as the number of days between the baseline interview and the date of death. All these data were collected by clinicians in charge who were active members of the investigation team.

Ethics Committee Approval: The present study has been approved by the ethics committee of all participant centers (ethical approval code: CEI2012/PI242). Ethical Guidelines for Authorship and Publishing: The authors certify that they comply with the ethical guidelines for publishing in the Journal Clinical Medicine.

2.2. Biological Parameters Determination

We determined blood or plasma biological parameters of all included patients, including oxidative stress markers, apoptosis expression, and telomere length.

Oxidative stress markers: We determined activity/levels of catalase, glutathione reductase (GR), total antioxidant capacity to reactive oxygen species (TAC-ROS), and superoxide dismutase (SOD). Colorimetric studies were performed using a monochromator-based UV–VIS spectrophotometer (Multiskan® GO; Thermo Fisher Scientific Corporation, Carlsbad, CA, USA).

Catalase activity (nmol/min/mL) was measured in patients' plasma using the colorimetrical procedure provided by Cayman's Catalase Assay Kit, Item No. 707002 (Cayman Chemical, Ann Arbor, MI, USA). The method is based on the reaction of the enzyme wit methanol in the presence of an optimal concentration of H_2O_2. The formaldehyde produced is measured colorimetrically with Purpald as the chromogen. Purpald specifically forms a bicyclic heterocycle with aldehydes, which upon oxidation changes from colorless to purple color [17,18].

Glutathione reductase activity (U/mL; 1 Unit = the amount of enzyme that will cause the oxidation of 1.0 nmol of NADP to NADP+ per minute at 25 °C) was analyzed in patients' plasma by measuring the rate of NADPH oxidation, using for this purpose the Cayman's Glutathione reductase Assay Kit, Item No. 703202 (Cayman Chemical, Ann Arbor, MI, USA). The oxidation of NADPH is accompanied by a decrease in absorbance at 340 nm and is directly proportional to the GR activity in the sample [18,19].

Total antioxidant capacity to reactive oxygen species (mM Trolox equivalents) was analyzed measuring the ability of patients' plasma antioxidants to inhibit the oxidation of ABTS® (2,2′-Azino-di-3-ethylbenzthiazoline sulphonatel) to ABTS®+ by metmyoglobin. For this purpose, the Cayman's Antioxidant Assay Kit, Item No. 709001 (Cayman Chemical, Ann Arbor, MI, USA) was used. The antioxidants cause suppression of the absorbance at 750 nm or 405 nm to a degree that is proportional to their concentration. This capacity of the antioxidants is compared to that of Trolox, a water-soluble tocopherol analogue, and is quantified as millimolar Trolox equivalents [20,21].

Superoxide dismutase activity (U/mL) was measured in patients' plasma using the colorimetrical absorbance procedure provided by Cayman's Superoxide Dismutase Assay Kit, Item No. 706002 (Cayman Chemical, Ann Arbor, MI, USA). The method utilizes a tetrazolium salt for detection of superoxide radicals generated by xanthine oxidase and hypoxanthine. One unit of SOD is defined as the amount of enzyme needed to exhibit 50% dismutation of the superoxide radical. This assay measures all types of SOD (Cu/Zn-SOD, Mn-SOD, and Fe-SOD) [18].

Telomere length: We assessed telomere length following the procedure described by O'Callaghan and Fenech, in which the absolute telomere length (aTL) was measured [22]. For this purpose, we used Telomere standard Human/rodent (teloF and teloR) as primers for telomere length (TL) analysis and 36B4 standard human primers for single copy gene (SCG) determinations. All these were supplied by TaqMan™ Array Human Telomere Extension by Telomerase (Thermofisher Scientific, Waltham, MA, USA).

First standard curves were constructed for both experiments (TL and SCG). Then, all patients' samples were analyzed, and aTL was calculated dividing the absolute result of TL by the result of SCG. This result was again divided by 92 (each somatic human cell has 46 chromosomes, and each chromosome has 2 telomeres) in order to obtain the mean aTL per single telomere [22].

Apoptosis: In order to detect apoptosis, we evaluated possible DNA fragmentation in patients' leucocytes. For this purpose, we performed a DNA conventional constant field gel electrophoresis loading in a 0.8% agarose gel panel a total or 300 ng from a normalized purified DNA mixture with a DNA concentration of 30 ng/uL. DNA was purified by means of standard techniques already established [22]. When apoptosis is present, the result is fragmentation of DNA into multiples of 180 base-pair lengths; a characteristic "ladder" effect is obtained when these fragments are resolved in the agarose gel electrophoresis [23].

Statistical analysis: The dichotomous variables were described as whole numbers and percentages, and the continuous variables as mean and standard deviation (or median and interquartile rank (IQR) in those with no criteria of normal distribution). The distribution of all variables was analyzed with the Kolmorogov–Smirnov test. Possible biological parameters associated to the presence of sarcopenia and death were investigated performing the Student's t for normally distributed quantitative variables, and Mann–Whitney U test.

Finally, we also evaluated the association of these biological parameters with functional status (by means of basal Barthel index), death risk (by means of PROFUND index), and survival (considering death as a time-dependent variable), using linear regression models. Statistical significance was considered when obtained p values were ≤0.05. Statistics were performed using the SPSS 22.0 software (IBM, Armonk, NY, USA).

3. Results

We included 444 patients with a mean age of 77.3 ± 8.4 years. Fifty-five percent were male. The main clinical features and biological parameters of the recruited patients are detailed in Table 1. Sarcopenia was present in 97 (21.8%), frailty in 278 (62.6%), and the remaining 69 (15.6%) were robust. Eighty patients (18% of the whole cohort) out of those with sarcopenia or frailty had simultaneously both phenotypes.

And combined sarcopenia and frailty were present in 80 (18%) patients. Mortality in the 12-months follow-up period was 40% (N = 178). A detailed clinical description of the included patients has already been published [7]; briefly, sarcopenia was more frequent in men, and associated to chronic lung diseases, cancer, lower BMI, and previous hospital admissions, whereas frailty was more frequent in women and associated to a higher number of polypathology categories, chronic pain, anxiety, and pressure ulcers; both phenotypes shared association with age, asthenia, and lower BI scores.

Table 1. Main clinical and biological features of a multicenter sample of 444 polypathological patients recruited for sarcopenia and frailty assessment.

Clinical Features	Mean (SD)/Median -IQR-/N (%)
Number of defining categories (major diseases) per patient	2.5 (0.5)
Prevalence of defining categories (major diseases)	
Heart diseases	374 (84.6%)
Kidney/autoimmune diseases	202 (45.7%)
Lung diseases	183 (41.4%)
Neurological diseases	133 (30.1%)
Peripheral arterial disease/diabetes with neuropathy	80 (18.1%)
Neoplasia/chronic anemia	70 (15.8%)
Degenerative osteoarticular disease	43 (9.7%)
Liver disease	28 (6.3%)
Number of other comorbidities per patient	5.9 (2.3)
Most frequent comorbidities	
Hypertension	380 (86%)
Dyslipemia	232 (52.5%)
Diabetes with no visceral involvement	216 (49%)
Atrial fibrillation	178 (40%)
Obesity	159 (36%)
Anxiety and depressive disorders	74 (17%)
Benign prostate hyperplasia	64 (14.5%)
Frequent symptoms	
Fatigue	304 (70%)
Anorexia	212 (48%)
Insomnia	194 (44%)
Chronic pain	178 (40%)
Cough	158 (36%)
Patients with basal III-IV class of NYHA//III-IV class of mMRC	128 (29%)
PROFUND index	6 -6-
Basal Barthel's Index	66 (30)
BMI (Kg/m^2)	30 (6.6%)
Main biological parameters	
Hemoglobin (d/dL)	11.3 (2)
Creatinin (mg/dL)	1.26 (1)
Albumin (g/dL)	3.2 (0.9)
Cholesterol (mg/dL)	151 (42)
Triglicerydes (mg/dL)	116 -80-
Vitamin D (ng/mL)	11 -17-
Leucocytes (n°/μL)	8000 -4000-
Lymphocytes (n°/μL)	1200 -400-

SD: standard deviation; IQR: interquartile range; NYHA: New York Heart Association; mMRC: Medical Research Council. BMI: body mass index.

3.1. Oxidative Stress Markers

Median catalase and GR activity were 53 nmol/min/mL (IQR = 20–83), and 9.8 U/mL (IQR = 6.6–13.2), respectively. Total antioxidant activity against ROS was 2.4 mM Trolox equivalents (IQR = 1.8–3). Finally, median SOD activity was 4.6 U/mL (IQR = 2.8–6.6).

Differences of oxidative stress markers in patients with sarcopenia, frailty, or those with both conditions with respect to those without sarcopenia, robust, or those without both conditions are detailed in Table 2.

Table 2. Differences of oxidative stress markers, telomere length, and apoptosis markers in patients with multimorbidity according to their sarcopenia and frailty assessment.

Molecular Parameter	Sarcopenia and Frailty Assessment		p
Sarcopenia	Not Sarcopenic	Sarcopenic	
Oxidative stress marker			
CAT	52 (12.6–82) *	58 (29.4–87.8)	0.16
GR	9.8 (6.8–13.4)	9.9 (5.5–13)	0.45
TAC-ROS	2.42 (1.8–3)	2.29 (1.75–2.8)	0.12
SOD	4.4 (2.7–6.5)	5.8 (3.7–6.9)	0.02
Absolute telomere length	4.96 (0.7–19)	1.65 (0.6–3.9)	0.001
Apoptosis (WBC DNA fragmentation)	No evidence	No evidence	-
Frailty	Robust	Frail	
Oxidative stress marker			
CAT	55.6 (21.7–80)	51.4 (19–83.5)	0.6
GR	9.1 (5.3–9)	10.2 (6.9–13.5)	0.12
TAC-ROS	3.5 (1.6–9)	3.3 (1.9–3)	0.044
SOD	3.8 (2.3–6.2)	5.1 (3.2–7)	0.002
Absolute telomere length	5.7 (1.7–19)	1.5 (0.6–3.4)	<0.0001
Apoptosis (WBC DNA fragmentation)	No evidence	No evidence	-
Sarcopenia and Frailty	Not Sarcopenic and Robust	Sarcopenic and Frail	
Oxidative stress marker			
CAT	46.4 (46.5–77.5)	51.5 (26.2–79)	0.2
GR	9.7 (6.7–13.2)	10.1 (5.9–14)	0.5
TAC-ROS	2.4 (1.8–3.1)	2.2 (1.8–2.8)	0.08
SOD	4.4 (2.8–6.4)	5.7 (4.1–6.4)	0.0012
Absolute telomere length	6.5 (0.7–20)	1.5 (0.6–3.8)	<0.0001
Apoptosis (WBC DNA fragmentation)	No evidence	No evidence	-

CAT: catalase (nmol/min/mL); GR: Glutathione reductase (U/mL); TAC-ROS: total antioxidant activity against reactive oxygen species (mM Trolox equivalents); SOD: superoxide dismutase (U/mL); absolute telomere length (kbases/telomere); * Interquartile range; WBC: white blood cells; DNA: deoxyribonucleic acid.

3.2. Absolute Telomere Length Analysis

Mean aTL was 2 kbases per telomere (IQR = 0.1–55). Differences of aTL in patients with sarcopenia, frailty, or those with both conditions with respect to those without sarcopenia, robust, or those without both conditions are also detailed in Table 2.

3.3. Apoptosis

Apoptosis by means of DNA fragmentation analysis was not present in any of the patients included in the study.

3.4. Functional Parameters, Death Risk by PROFUND Index and Survival according to Different Molecular Parameters

A worse functional status by means of lower Barthel's index score was associated to shorter telomere length (Beta = 1.25 (1.07–1.34)); $p = 0.001$, but not with any of the oxidative stress markers.

A higher death risk by means of PROFUND index was associated to shorter telomere length (Beta = 0.5 (0.14–0.65); $p = 0.001$) and to a higher GR activity (Beta = 1.7 (1.2–2); $p = 0.04$). On the other hand, a lower number of survival days was associated to shorter telomere length (Beta = 1.2 (1.01–1.32); $p = 0.003$) and to a higher GR activity (Beta = 0.3 (0.1–0.24)); $p = 0.02$).

4. Discussion

In the present study, we have detected enhanced oxidative stress and significant telomere shortening in PP with sarcopenia, frailty, or both syndromes combined. On the contrary, no evidence of apoptosis was detected.

Sarcopenia was prevalent in our cohort of polypathological patients and was associated to a significant higher SOD activity; other oxidative stress markers activity was also elevated, and the TAC-ROS decreased, but differences in these last were not significant. In the same way, we observed a significant telomere length shortening in these patients compared to other PP without sarcopenia. These results are highly concordant with the pathogenesis of sarcopenia in the elderly as already demonstrated by other authors [24–27]. Many authors have compared these markers among elderly and young people [28]; in the present study we have also detected important differences among elderly patients with chronic conditions with or without sarcopenia. These findings could have two major clinical applications: first, to use them as biological markers of sarcopenia in the elderly compared to persons of the same age; and second, to guide future treatments towards these targets in order to avoid or delay the development of sarcopenia. With respect to oxidative stress, SOD was the marker with the largest differences among PP with or without sarcopenia. As a matter of fact, SOD has been already strongly linked to muscular weakness, muscular wasting, and sarcopenia in clinical and experimental scenarios [29–31]; in this sense, among others, probably SOD could be the optimal oxidative stress marker in the evaluation of sarcopenia.

Frailty was also highly prevalent in the studied PP cohort and was associated to a significant increase in SOD activity and a decreased plasma TAC-ROS. It was also associated to a significant telomere length shortening compared to other PP without frailty. The deep relation between sarcopenia and frailty is already known; they share molecular and physiological pathways, symptoms, signs, and clinical phenotypes [32,33], so the presence of these molecular alterations in both of them is biologically coherent. In this case, we also observed a decreased antioxidant fitness of the plasma in frail PP. As main differences, frailty is more age related, whereas sarcopenia is also related to disease, starvation, and disuse [34]; additionally, despite criteria defining the two conditions overlap, frailty requires weight loss, whereas sarcopenia requires muscle loss [34,35].

In PP with sarcopenia and/or frailty we have observed the coexistence of telomere shortening and enhanced oxidative stress. There is accumulating evidence of the role of oxidative stress in DNA damage and telomere shortening with aging and chronic diseases [36]. These changes have been observed in humans, as well as in mouse models and cell cultures [36]. There are probably mixed mechanisms in this narrow relation of oxidative stress and telomere length. In aging and in many chronic conditions, processes associated to chronic inflammation play a nuclear role. Chronic inflammation is characterized by higher oxidative stress in affected tissues and circulating plasma. This may lead to direct cell DNA damage, including telomere regions. Additionally, inflammatory states are associated to enhanced necrosis and cellular regeneration cycles, and this increased cell turnover directly affects telomere length [37–42]. Many authors already point out that targeting oxidative stress could be of notable benefit in telomere length maintenance, especially in populations with chronic conditions like patients in the present study [39–42].

We did not detect any DNA fragmentation in our patients' leucocytes, so no apoptosis evidence could be detected in PP's blood samples by this technique. Apoptosis pathways have been classically associated to sarcopenia and frailty and nowadays are considered one of the main causes of these two syndromes [43,44]. As a matter of fact, there is multiple evidence of apoptosis presence in muscle tissue of experimental animal models, as well as in humans with sarcopenia [45–49]. Nevertheless, no information is available about the presence of apoptosis evidence in blood leukocytes of patients with sarcopenia and/or frailty. Some authors have described indirect apoptosis pathways data in blood leucocytes in elderly and in patients with dementia (like less resistance to experimental apoptosis inducers; senescence of CD8+ T-cells; and increased expression of HLA-DR, CD95, and Bcl-2 in CD3+ lymphocytes) [50]. Recently, increased ROS production and DNA fragmentation has been observed in blood monocytes of atherosclerotic mice, uprising again the interrelations of oxidative stress and apoptosis signaling [51]. Apoptosis will for sure be present in muscle tissues of patients with sarcopenia and frailty, like enhanced oxidative stress and telomere shortening. Nevertheless, according to our data, an easy detection of its presence in blood samples from these patients is probably not useful in the clinical setting, and demonstrating it in tissue specimens is not clinically justified.

A poorer functional status, higher mortality risk, and less survival days in the 12-month follow-up were associated to shorter telomere length; besides, mortality risk and survival days were also associated to enhanced GR activity. These data are in concordance with previous studies in which telomere shortening has been associated to poorer survival in cancer, diabetes, cardiovascular diseases, and even to higher all-cause mortality [52–56]; additionally, oxidative stress has also been related to poor health outcomes in many clinical scenarios, and to all-cause mortality [57–60]. Our data confirm this deleterious relationships with sarcopenia and frailty in patients with multimorbidity, as well as the association to poorer functional status. Some authors have already claimed the clinical usefulness of biomarkers' panels including aTL, if we want to accurately assess and predict outcomes in vulnerable aged populations [61]. We suggest including also oxidative stress markers in these panels, mainly GR, TAC-ROS, and SOD.

This study has some limitations that should be noted. The results could be limited by the number of patients, but on the other hand, the cohort was recruited in various centers, was homogeneous, and probably represents adequately hospital-based populations with moderate–severe multimorbidity. Additionally, the studied biomarkers are also associated to some of the chronic conditions of the included patients and could raise the question of their real correlation to sarcopenia and frailty; this issue always underlies the frailty and sarcopenia phenotypes, since they have multiple concurrent causes, with a prominent role of debilitating chronic diseases; in our opinion, they behave as parts of the same clinical-molecular syndrome; as a matter of fact, the term "inflamm-aging" is already established, and probably in the future, it will be necessary to add chronic conditions and call it "inflamm-chronic-aging".

In conclusion, oxidative stress and telomere shortening, but not apoptosis markers, were enhanced in blood samples of polypathological patients with sarcopenia and/or frailty with respect to those patients without these two geriatric syndromes. Telomere shortening was associated to functional decline, and both, oxidative stress markers and telomere shortening, were associated to higher mortality risks and decreased survival. Both of these biomarkers could be useful in the clinical evaluation of vulnerable patients prone to sarcopenia and frailty and of potential interest as therapeutic targets.

Author Contributions: Conceptualization, M.B.-W. and M.O.-B.; Formal analysis, M.B.-W.; Investigation, M.B.-W., R.G.-D., Á.G.-M., S.V.-S., J.D.-M., F.S. and M.S.-M.; Methodology, M.B.-W., R.G.-D. and J.D.-M.; Supervision, M.O.-B.; Visualization, M.O.-B.; Writing–original draft, M.B.-W.; Writing–review & editing, Á.G.-M. and M.O.-B. All authors have contributed substantially to the work. All authors have read and agreed to the published version of the manuscript.

Funding: This research received no external funding.

Acknowledgments: Special thanks to all researchers from the proteo project listed below. Máximo Bernabeu-Wittel (1), Álvaro González-Molina (1), Rocío Fernández-Ojeda (2), Jesús Díez-Manglano (3), Fernando Salgado-Ordóñez (4), María Soto-Martín (5), Marta Muniesa (6), Manuel Ollero-Baturone (1), Juan Gómez-Salgado (7), Sofía Vidal-Serrano (2), Adriana Rivera-Sequeiros (2), Antonio Fernández-Moyano (2), Lourdes Moreno-Gaviño (1), Dolores Nieto-Martín (1), Nieves Ramírez-Duque (1), Esther del Corral-Beamonte (3), Pablo Martínez-Rodés (3), María Sevil-Puras (3), Rosa Bernal-López (4), Ricardo Gómez-Huelgas (4), Bosco Barón-Franco (5). Hospitals: (1) Hospital Universitario Virgen del Rocío, Sevilla, Spain; (2) Hospital San Juan de Dios del Aljarafe, Sevilla, Spain; (3) Hospital Royo Villanova, Zaragoza, Spain; (4) Hospital Regional, Málaga, Spain; (5) Hospital Juan Ramón Jiménez, Huelva, Spain; (6) Hospital San Juan de Dios de Pamplona, Pamplona, Spain; (7) School of Nursery, University of Huelva, Spain.

Conflicts of Interest: The authors declare no conflict of interest.

References

1. Colombo, F.; García-Goñi, M.; Schwierz, C. Addressing multimorbidity to improve healthcare and economic sustainability. *J. Comorb.* **2016**, *6*, 21–27. [CrossRef] [PubMed]
2. Yarnall, A.J.; Sayer, A.A.; Clegg, A.; Rockwood, K.; Parker, S.; Hindle, J.V. New horizons in multimorbidity in older adults. *Age Ageing* **2017**, *46*, 882–888. [CrossRef] [PubMed]
3. Puth, M.T.; Weckbecker, K.; Schmid, M.; Münster, E. Prevalence of multimorbidity in Germany: Impact of age and educational level in a cross-sectional study on 19,294 adults. *BMC Public Health* **2017**, *17*, 826. [CrossRef] [PubMed]
4. Fabbri, E.; Zoli, M.; Gonzalez-Freire, M.; Salive, M.E.; Studenski, S.A.; Ferrucci, L. Aging and multimorbidity: New tasks, priorities, and frontiers for integrated gerontological and clinical research. *J. Am. Med. Dir. Assoc.* **2015**, *16*, 640–647. [CrossRef]
5. Von Haehling, S.; Morley, J.E.; Anker, S.D. An overview of sarcopenia: Facts and numbers on prevalence and clinical impact. *J. Cachex Sarcopenia Muscle* **2010**, *1*, 129–133. [CrossRef]
6. Ligthart-Melis, G.C.; Luiking, Y.C.; Kakourou, A.; Cederholm, T.; Maier, A.B.; de van der Schueren, M.A.E. Frailty, Sarcopenia, and Malnutrition Frequently (Co-)occur in Hospitalized Older Adults: A Systematic Review and Meta-analysis. *J. Am. Med. Dir. Assoc.* **2020**. online ahead of print. [CrossRef]
7. Bernabeu-Wittel, M.; González-Molina, Á.; Fernández-Ojeda, R.; Díez-Manglano, J.; Salgado, F.; Soto-Martín, M.; Muniesa, M.; Ollero-Baturone, M.; Gómez-Salgado, J. Impact of sarcopenia and frailty in a multicenter cohort of polypathological patients. *J. Clin. Med.* **2019**, *8*, 535. [CrossRef]
8. Davies, B.; García, F.; Ara, I.; Artalejo, F.R.; Rodriguez-Mañas, L.; Walter, S. Relationship between sarcopenia and frailty in the toledo study of healthy aging: A population based cross-sectional study. *J. Am. Med. Dir. Assoc.* **2018**, *19*, 282–286. [CrossRef]
9. Shafiee, G.; Keshtkar, A.; Soltani, A.; Ahadi, Z.; Larijani, B.; Heshmat, R. Prevalence of sarcopenia in the world: A systematic review and meta-analysis of general population studies. *J. Diabetes Metab. Disord.* **2017**, *16*, 21. [CrossRef]
10. Marty, E.; Liu, Y.; Samuel, A.; Or, O.; Lane, J. A review of sarcopenia: Enhancing awareness of an increasingly prevalent disease. *Bone* **2017**, *105*, 276–286. [CrossRef]
11. Tournadre, A.; Vial, G.; Capel, F.; Soubrier, M.; Boirie, Y. Sarcopenia. *Jt. Bone Spine* **2019**, *86*, 309–314. [CrossRef]
12. Xue, Q.L. The frailty syndrome: Definition and natural history. *Clin. Geriatr. Med.* **2011**, *27*, 1–15. [CrossRef] [PubMed]
13. Wou, F.; Conroy, S. The frailty syndrome. *Medicine* **2013**, *41*, 13–15. [CrossRef]
14. Wang, J.; Maxwell, C.A.; Yu, F. Biological processes and biomarkers related to frailty in older adults: A state-of-the-science literature review. *Biol. Res. Nurs.* **2019**, *21*, 80–106. [CrossRef] [PubMed]
15. Cruz-Jentoft, A.J.; Baeyens, J.P.; Bauer, J.M.; Boirie, Y.; Cederholm, T.; Landi, F.; Martin, F.C.; Michel, J.-P.; Rolland, Y.; Schneider, S.M.; et al. Sarcopenia: European consensus on definition and diagnosis. Report of the European Working Group on Sarcopenia in Older People. *Age Ageing* **2010**, *39*, 412–423. [CrossRef]
16. Fried, L.P.; Tangen, C.M.; Walston, J.; Newman, A.B.; Hirsch, C.; Gottdiener, J.; Seeman, T.; Tracy, R.; Kop, W.J.; Burke, G.; et al. Frailty in older adults: Evidence for a phenotype. *J. Gerontol. Ser. A Boil. Sci. Med. Sci.* **2001**, *56*, M146–M157. [CrossRef]
17. Johansson, L.H.; Borgh, L.A.H. A spectrophotometric method for determination of catalase activity in small tissue samples. *Anal. Biochem.* **1988**, *174*, 331–336. [CrossRef]
18. Wheeler, C.R.; Salzman, J.A.; Elsayed, N.M.; Omaye, S.T.; Korte, D.W. Automated assays for superoxide dismutase, catalase, glutathione peroxidase, and glutathione reductase activity. *Anal. Biochem.* **1990**, *184*, 193–199. [CrossRef]
19. Carlberg, I.; Mannervik, B. Glutathione reductase. *Met. Enzymol.* **1985**, *113*, 484–490.
20. Miller, N.; Rice-Evans, C. Factors influencing the antioxidant activity deteimrned by the ABTS[+] radical cation assay. *Free Radic. Res.* **1997**, *26*, 195–199. [CrossRef]
21. Koracevic, D.; Harris, G.; Rayner, A.; Blair, J.; Watt, B.; Koracevic, G.; Djordjevic, V.; Andrejevic, S.; Cosic, V. Method for the measurement of antioxidant activity in human fluids. *J. Clin. Pathol.* **2001**, *54*, 356–361. [CrossRef] [PubMed]

22. O'Callaghan, N.J.; Fenech, M. A quantitative PCR method for measuring absolute telomere length. *Biol. Proc. Online* **2011**, *13*, 3–13. [CrossRef] [PubMed]
23. Allen, P.D.; Newland, A.C. Electrophoretic DNA analysis for the detection of apoptosis. *Mol. Biotechnol.* **1998**, *9*, 247–251. [CrossRef] [PubMed]
24. Liguori, I.; Russo, G.; Curcio, F.; Bulli, G.; Aran, L.; Della-Morte, D.; Gargiulo, G.; Testa, G.; Francesco, C.; Domenico, B.; et al. Oxidative stress, aging, and diseases. *Clin. Interv. Aging* **2018**, *13*, 757–772. [CrossRef] [PubMed]
25. Marzetti, E.; Calvani, R.; Cesari, M.; Buford, T.W.; Lorenzi, M.; Behnke, B.J.; Leeuwenburgh, C. Mitochondrial dysfunction and sarcopenia of aging: From signaling pathways to clinical trials. *Int. J. Biochem. Cell Biol.* **2013**, *45*, 2288–2301. [CrossRef]
26. Kameda, M.; Teruya, T.; Yanagida, M.; Kondoh, H. Frailty markers comprise blood metabolites involved in antioxidation, cognition, and mobility. *Proc. Natl. Acad. Sci. USA* **2020**, *117*, 9483–9489. [CrossRef]
27. Marzetti, E.; Lorenzi, M.; Antocicco, M.; Bonassi, S.; Celi, M.; Mastropaolo, S.; Settanni, S.; Valdiglesias, V.; Landi, F.; Bernabei, R.; et al. Shorter telomeres in peripheral blood mononuclear cells from older persons with sarcopenia: Results from an exploratory study. *Front. Aging Neurosci.* **2014**, *6*, 233. [CrossRef]
28. Fasching, C.L. Telomere length measurement as a clinical biomarker of aging and disease. *Crit. Rev. Clin. Lab. Sci.* **2018**, *55*, 443–465. [CrossRef]
29. Muller, F.L.; Song, W.; Liu, Y.; Chaudhuri, A.; Pieke-Dahl, S.; Strong, R.; Huang, T.T.; Epstein, C.J.; Roberts, L.J., 2nd; Csete, M.; et al. Absence of CuZn superoxide dismutase leads to elevated oxidative stress and acceleration of age-dependent skeletal muscle atrophy. *Free Radic. Biol. Med.* **2006**, *40*, 1993–2004. [CrossRef]
30. Barreiro, E.; Coronell, C.; Laviña, B.; Ramírez-Sarmiento, A.; Orozco-Levi, M.; Gea, J. PENAM Project. Aging, sex differences, and oxidative stress in human respiratory and limb muscles. *Free Radic. Biol. Med.* **2006**, *41*, 797–809. [CrossRef]
31. Belenguer-Varea, Á.; Tarazona-Santabalbina, F.J.; Avellana-Zaragoza, J.A.; Martínez-Reig, M.; Mas-Bargues, C.; Inglés, M. Oxidative stress and exceptional human longevity: Systematic review. *Free Radic. Biol. Med.* **2019**. [CrossRef] [PubMed]
32. Reijnierse, E.M.; Trappenburg, M.C.; Blauw, G.J.; Verlaan, S.; de van der Schueren, M.A.; Meskers, C.G.; Maier, A.B. Common ground? The concordance of sarcopenia and frailty definitions. *J. Am. Med. Dir. Assoc.* **2015**, *17*, 371. [CrossRef] [PubMed]
33. Carmeli, E. Frailty and primary sarcopenia: A review. *Adv. Exp. Med. Biol.* **2017**, *1020*, 53–68. [PubMed]
34. Cederholm, T. Overlaps between frailty and sarcopenia definitions. *Nestle Nutr. Inst. Workshop Ser.* **2015**, *83*, 65–69. [PubMed]
35. Cruz-Jentoft, A.J.; Kiesswetter, E.; Drey, M.; Sieber, C.C. Nutrition, frailty, and sarcopenia. *Aging Clin. Exp. Res.* **2017**, *29*, 43–48. [CrossRef]
36. Barnes, R.P.; Fouquerel, R.P.; Opresko, P.L. The impact of oxidative DNA damage and stress on telomere homeostasis. *Mech. Ageing Dev.* **2019**, *177*, 37–45. [CrossRef]
37. Richter, T.; von Zglinicki, T. A continuous correlation between oxidative stress and telomere shortening in fibroblasts. *Exp. Gerontol.* **2007**, *42*, 1039–1042. [CrossRef]
38. Reichert, S.; Stier, A. Does oxidative stress shorten telomeres in vivo? A review. *Biol. Lett.* **2017**, *13*, 20170463. [CrossRef]
39. Markkanen, E. Not breathing is not an option: How to deal with oxidative DNA damage. *DNA Repair* **2017**, *59*, 82–105. [CrossRef]
40. Martens, D.S.; Nawrot, T.S. Air pollution stress and the aging phenotype: The telomere connection. *Curr. Environ. Health Rep.* **2016**, *3*, 258–269. [CrossRef]
41. Von Zglinicki, T. Oxidative stress shortens telomeres. *Trends Biochem. Sci.* **2002**, *27*, 339–344. [CrossRef]
42. Sfeir, A.; Kosiyatrakul, S.T.; Hockemeyer, D.; MacRae, S.L.; Karlseder, J.; Schildkraut, C.L.; de Lange, T. Mammalian telomeres resemble fragile sites and require TRF1 for efficient replication. *Cell* **2009**, *138*, 90–103. [CrossRef] [PubMed]

43. Marzetti, E.; Calvani, R.; Bernabei, R.; Leeuwenburgh, C. Apoptosis in skeletal myocytes: A potential target for interventions against sarcopenia and physical frailty—A mini-review. *Gerontology* **2012**, *58*, 99–106. [CrossRef] [PubMed]
44. Marzetti, E.; Leeuwenburgh, C. Skeletal muscle apoptosis, sarcopenia and frailty at old age. *Exp. Gerontol.* **2006**, *41*, 1234–1238. [CrossRef]
45. Du, J.; Wang, X.; Miereles, C.; Bailey, J.L.; Debigare, R.; Zheng, B.; Price, S.R.; Mitch, W.E. Activation of caspase-3 is an initial step triggering accelerated muscle proteolysis in catabolic conditions. *J. Clin. Investig.* **2004**, *113*, 115–123. [CrossRef]
46. Argiles, J.M.; Lopez-Soriano, F.J.; Busquets, S. Apoptosis signalling is essential and precedes protein degradation in wasting skeletal muscle during catabolic conditions. *Int. J. Biochem. Cell Biol.* **2008**, *40*, 1674–1678. [CrossRef]
47. Schindowski, K.; Leutner, S.; Müller, W.E.; Eckert, A. Age-related changes of apoptotic cell death in human lymphocytes. *Neurobiol. Aging* **2000**, *21*, 661–670. [CrossRef]
48. Effros, R.B. Replicative senescence of CD8 T cells: Effect on human ageing. *Exp. Gerontol.* **2004**, *39*, 517–524. [CrossRef]
49. Hodkinson, C.F.; O'Connor, J.M.; Alexander, H.D.; Bradbury, I.; Bonham, M.P.; Hannigan, B.M.; Gilmore, W.S.; Strain, J.J.; Wallace, J.M. Whole blood analysis of phagocytosis, apoptosis, cytokine production, and leukocyte subsets in healthy older men and women: The ZENITH study. *J. Gerontol. A Biol. Sci. Med. Sci.* **2006**, *61*, 907–917. [CrossRef]
50. Leuner, K.; Schulz, K.; Schütt, T.; Pantel, J.; Prvulovic, D.; Rhein, V.; Savaskan, E.; Czech, C.; Eckert, A.; Müller, W.E. Peripheral mitochondrial dysfunction in Alzheimer's disease: Focus on lymphocytes. *Mol. Neurobiol.* **2012**, *46*, 194–204. [CrossRef]
51. Jacinto, T.A.; Meireles, G.S.; Dias, A.T.; Aires, R.; Porto, M.L.; Gava, A.L.; Gava, A.L.; Meyrelles, S.S. Increased ROS production and DNA damage in monocytes are biomarkers of aging and atherosclerosis. *Biol. Res.* **2018**, *51*, 33. [CrossRef] [PubMed]
52. Pusceddu, I.; Kleber, M.; Delgado, G.; Herrmann, W.; März, W.; Herrmann, M. Telomere length and mortality in the Ludwigshafen Risk and Cardiovascular Health study. *PLoS ONE* **2018**, *13*, e0198373. [CrossRef] [PubMed]
53. Bonfigli, A.R.; Spazzafumo, L.; Prattichizzo, F.; Bonafè, M.; Mensà, E.; Micolucci, L.; Giuliani, A.; Fabbietti, P.; Testa, R.; Boemi, M.; et al. Leukocyte telomere length and mortality risk in patients with type 2 diabetes. *Oncotarget* **2016**, *7*, 50835–50844. [CrossRef] [PubMed]
54. Bendix, L.; Thinggaard, M.; Fenger, M.; Kolvraa, S.; Avlund, K.; Linneberg, A.; Osler, M. Longitudinal changes in leukocyte telomere length and mortality in humans. *J. Gerontol. A Biol. Sci. Med. Sci.* **2014**, *69*, 231–239. [CrossRef] [PubMed]
55. Weischer, M.; Nordestgaard, B.G.; Cawthon, R.M.; Freiberg, J.J.; Tybjærg-Hansen, A.; Bojesen, S.E. Short telomere length, cancer survival, and cancer risk in 47102 individuals. *J. Natl. Cancer Instig.* **2013**, *105*, 459–468. [CrossRef]
56. Wang, Q.; Zhan, Y.; Pedersen, N.L.; Fang, F.; Hägg, S. Telomere length and all-cause mortality: A meta-analysis. *Ageing Res. Rev.* **2018**, *48*, 11–20. [CrossRef]
57. Schöttker, B.; Saum, K.U.; Jansen, E.H.; Boffetta, P.; Trichopoulou, A.; Holleczek, B.; Dieffenbach, A.K.; Brenner, H. Oxidative stress markers and all-cause mortality at older age: A population-based cohort study. *J. Gerontol. A Biol. Sci. Med. Sci.* **2015**, *70*, 518–524. [CrossRef]
58. Xuan, Y.; Gào, X.; Anusruti, A.; Holleczek, B.; Jansen, E.H.J.M.; Muhlack, D.C.; Brenner, H.; Schöttker, B. Association of serum markers of oxidative stress with incident major cardiovascular events, cancer incidence, and all-cause mortality in type 2 diabetes patients: Pooled results from two cohort studies. *Diabetes Care* **2019**, *42*, 1436–1445. [CrossRef]
59. Gao, X.; Gào, X.; Zhang, Y.; Holleczek, B.; Schöttker, B.; Brenner, H. Oxidative stress and epigenetic mortality risk score: Associations with all-cause mortality among elderly people. *Eur. J. Epidemiol.* **2019**, *34*, 451–462. [CrossRef]

60. Xuan, Y.; Bobak, M.; Anusruti, A.; Jansen, E.H.J.M.; Pająk, A.; Tamosiunas, A.; Saum, K.-U.; Holleczek, B.; Gao, X.; Brenner, H.; et al. Association of serum markers of oxidative stress with myocardial infarction and stroke: Pooled results from four large European cohort studies. *Eur. J. Epidemiol.* **2019**, *34*, 471–481. [CrossRef]
61. Lorenzi, M.; Bonassi, S.; Lorenzi, T.; Giovannini, S.; Bernabei, R.; Onder, G. A review of telomere length in sarcopenia and frailty. *Biogerontology* **2018**, *19*, 209–221. [CrossRef] [PubMed]

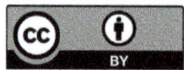

© 2020 by the authors. Licensee MDPI, Basel, Switzerland. This article is an open access article distributed under the terms and conditions of the Creative Commons Attribution (CC BY) license (http://creativecommons.org/licenses/by/4.0/).

Measures Derived from Panoramic Ultrasonography and Animal-Based Protein Intake Are Related to Muscular Performance in Middle-Aged Adults

Nathaniel R. Johnson [1], Christopher J. Kotarsky [2], Kyle J. Hackney [1], Kara A. Trautman [3], Nathan D. Dicks [4], Wonwoo Byun [5], Jill F. Keith [6], Shannon L. David [1] and Sherri N. Stastny [1,*]

1. Department of Health, Nutrition, and Exercise Sciences, North Dakota State University, Fargo, ND 58105, USA; nathaniel.johnson.4@ndsu.edu (N.R.J.); Kyle.hackney@ndsu.edu (K.J.H.); shannon.david@ndsu.edu (S.L.D.)
2. Department of Health and Human Physiological Sciences, Skidmore College; ckotarsk@skidmore.edu
3. Department of Health and Exercise Science, Gustavus Adolphus College, St. Peter, MN 56082, USA; karat@gustavus.edu
4. Department of Nutrition, Dietetics and Exercise Science, Concordia College, Moorhead, MN 56562, USA; ndicks@cord.edu
5. Department of Health and Kinesiology, University of Utah, Salt Lake City, UT 84112, USA; won.byun@utah.edu
6. Department of Family and Consumer Sciences, University of Wyoming, Laramie, WY 82071, USA; jkeith5@uwyo.edu
* Correspondence: sherri.stastny@ndsu.edu; Tel.: +1-701-231-7479

Abstract: Ultrasonography advantageously measures skeletal muscle size and quality, but some muscles may be too large to capture with standardized brightness mode (B-mode) imaging. Panoramic ultrasonography can capture more complete images and may more accurately measure muscle size. We investigated measurements made using panoramic compared to B-mode ultrasonography images of the rectus femoris with muscular performance. Concurrently, protein intake plays an important role in preventing sarcopenia; therefore, we also sought to investigate the association between animal-based protein intake (ABPI) and muscular performance. Ninety-one middle-aged adults were recruited. Muscle cross-sectional area (CSA) and thickness were obtained using B-mode and panoramic ultrasound and analyzed with Image J software. Muscular performance was assessed using isokinetic dynamometry, a 30-s chair test, and handgrip strength. Three-day food diaries estimated dietary intakes. Linear regression models determined relationships between measures from ultrasonography and muscular performance. Mixed linear models were used to evaluate the association between ABPI and muscular performance. Muscle CSA from panoramic ultrasonography and ABPI were positively associated with lower-body strength (β ± S.E.; CSA, 42.622 ± 20.024, $p = 0.005$; ABPI, 65.874 ± 19.855, $p = 0.001$), lower-body endurance (β ± S.E.; CSA, 595 ± 200.221, $p = 0.001$; ABPI, 549.944 ± 232.478, $p = 0.020$), and handgrip strength (β ± S.E.; CSA, 6.966 ± 3.328, $p = 0.004$; ABPI, 0.349 ± 0.171, $p = 0.045$). Panoramic ultrasound shows promise as a method for assessing sarcopenia. ABPI is related to better muscular performance.

Keywords: panoramic ultrasound; echogenicity; specific force; isokinetic dynamometry; protein intake; muscle quality; strength; endurance

1. Introduction

Earlier and more frequent assessments of muscle strength, mass, size, and quality and physical performance could help prevent sarcopenia by indicating a need for treatment or other intervention. According to the European Working Group on Sarcopenia in Older People 2, low muscle strength is the first criteria of sarcopenia, and low muscle mass or quality is the second; both must be assessed to determine sarcopenia [1]. Low physical performance in addition to low muscle strength and quantity is considered severe sarcopenia [1]. Measures of muscle strength, such as handgrip strength and physical performance (e.g., 30-s chair stand), however, can be performed with minimal equipment and are used across various settings [1]. Although several methods can be used to accurately assess muscle quantity and quality such as computed tomography (CT), magnetic resonance imaging (MRI), and dual x-ray absorptiometry, these techniques require expensive equipment and are not portable, limiting their utility. Ultrasonography is a portable and relatively low-cost method of assessing muscle size [2], making it a potentially useful tool for evaluating sarcopenia for clinical or research purposes [3,4]. Beyond this, ultrasonography records a measure of muscle quality in the form of echogenicity or echo intensity [5–7], making ultrasound a potentially more powerful tool than bioelectrical impedance for assessing sarcopenia or signs of pre-sarcopenia in middle age.

Others have used ultrasonography to successfully diagnose sarcopenia [7–9]. However, two of these studies were performed with either frail elderly patients or older adults diagnosed with chronic kidney disease [8,9]. Not only are the causes of sarcopenia thought to start earlier in life [1], making middle-aged adults a population of interest, but also, older adults often have smaller muscles that can be captured using a traditional ultrasound image at 50% of leg length. Although Ismail and colleagues [7] were able to discriminate between those with sarcopenia and those without in a younger cohort, they did this by using longitudinal and not transverse images of the rectus femoris. The crux of the issue is that in populations that have greater muscle mass at the midpoint of the thigh, such as younger populations, the entire transverse rectus femoris may be too large to capture in one image [10]. Assuming the goal is to image the entire transverse rectus femoris, then there are two workarounds: one is to use a feature, like the panoramic feature, to record the entire rectus femoris at the midpoint of the thigh, and the other is to move the imaging site distally down the leg where the rectus femoris has smaller transverse sections. Other researchers have validated panoramic ultrasound of the quadriceps with MRI [11], but to our knowledge, the relationship between ultrasonographic measures of the transverse rectus femoris captured using the panoramic feature and muscular performance, in particular that of the knee extensors, has not been investigated. Because muscle strength is more closely related to sarcopenia than muscle mass [1,12], the association warranted investigation.

Beyond this, specific force, the amount of force produced per unit of muscle, like echogenicity [6], is considered a measure of muscle quality [12]. Although echogenicity of the rectus femoris is related to muscle quality assessed using CT [8], and to a lesser extent knee extensor strength [13], the echogenicity of the rectus femoris has not been directly related to the specific force of the muscle. However, Ismail and colleagues [7] reported a significant relationship between echogenicity of rectus femoris and handgrip strength relative to bodyweight, a crude measure of specific force. If echogenicity and specific force reflect the muscle quality of the rectus femoris, then they should be closely related. We also sought to determine this relationship.

Outside of assessing the condition, nutrition is another important consideration for preventing and treating sarcopenia. Although there are many nutritional factors that can impact sarcopenia [14], dietary protein is perhaps of greatest interest because of its ability to stimulate muscle protein synthesis [15]. Recently though, the role of protein intake in performance has come into question, with one group finding no relationship between protein intake and measures of muscular performance, such as handgrip strength, knee extensor strength, and 30-s chair stand test performance [16]. Foods from animal and plant sources, of course, differ in their digestibility and amino acid content [17], and therefore in their ability to stimulate muscle protein synthesis [18]. Due to the differential impact that animal-based protein has on muscle protein synthesis, we secondarily sought to determine the relationship between animal-based protein intake (ABPI) and lower-body strength and endurance, handgrip strength, and 30-s chair stand performance, measures of muscular performance.

2. Materials and Methods

This was a cross-sectional study conducted in the North Dakota State University Healthy Aging Lab from October 2016 to December 2018. A total of 50 women and 41 men from the local community were recruited using e-mail, flyers, and word-of-mouth to visit the research lab for two sessions. During the first session, anthropometric, ultrasonographic, and performance variables were measured, and accelerometers and three-day food diaries were provided. Within seven to 14 days, participants returned their accelerometers and their completed food diaries to the lab. Participants were between 40 and 67 years of age, not currently using any nicotine product, free of any untreated or nonresponsive diseases or conditions including neuromuscular disease or conditions that might undermine muscle health, such as diabetes, ambulatory without any assistance, and had to include both animal-based and plant-based foods in their diets. Participants were screened using the 2011 Physical Activity Readiness Questionnaire [19], a more detailed health history questionnaire, and an orthostatic hypotension test. Participants were also instructed to refrain from exercise and strenuous physical activity at least 48 h prior to the first session. The study was approved by the North Dakota State University Institutional Review Board (#HE26929 & 26153) and complied with the Helsinki Declaration of 1983. Written informed consent was obtained from all participants in this study.

2.1. Participant Heath Screening and Anthropometric Measures

To screen participants for orthostatic hypotension, related to regulatory and safety concerns, resting blood pressure and standing blood pressure were measured manually with a stethoscope and Diagnostix 703 sphygmomanometer (American Diagnostic Corporation, Hauppauge, NY, USA). Those whose blood pressure dropped by more than 10 mm Hg, either systolic or diastolic, from resting to standing during the orthostatic hypotension test were excluded ($n = 0$). Following the orthostatic hypotension test, anthropometric variables were measured. Age (years) was self-reported. Height (cm) was measured using a stadiometer (Seca 213, Chino, CA, USA) and body mass (kg) was recorded using a digital balance (Denver Instrument DA-150, Arvada, CO, USA).

2.2. Ultrasonography

Images of the right rectus femoris muscle were captured using a Philips ultrasound system (model HD11 XE; Bothell, WA, USA) with a L12-5 50 mm linear array probe by three trained research assistants. Images were taken while participants were standing at marked sites 50% and 75% of the measured distance from the superior iliac spine of the hip to the lateral condyle of the knee. Participants were instructed to use their left leg as a base of support, while relaxing their right, resulting in a slight bend in the right knee. Previous works have shown high test–retest reliability of ultrasound measures of muscle thickness of healthy adults taken in the standing position [20,21]. A more recent study found the intraclass correlation coefficient (ICC) for standing measures of the anterior thigh muscles was 0.89, while the ICC for the same measures taken while participants were recumbent was 0.90 [22]. Following generous application of ultrasonic gel, the probe was placed on the skin perpendicular to the leg, and light, consistent pressure was applied to avoid excessive depression of the dermal surface until a full, clear image was obtained. The probe was removed from participants' skin between each image acquisition, and markings were used to ensure the same area was measured. Because our participants were younger and likely have greater muscle size, the panoramic feature was used at the 50% site to record the entire transverse rectus femoris [10]. For panoramic ultrasonography, the lateral side of the right rectus femoris was identified, and the probe was moved medially until the entire transverse rectus femoris was recorded. B-mode image captures were taken at the 75% site where transverse sections of the rectus femoris are smaller. Three images were captured at each site using a frequency of 37 Hz with a standardized depth of 7 cm and gain of 100%.

After each image was captured, a 1 cm line was added to each image to act as a known distance during analysis. Images were transferred to personal computers, calibrated, and analyzed. ImageJ software (National, Institutes of Health, Bethesda, MD, USA, version 1.42) was used to analyze echogenicity, cross-sectional area (CSA), and muscle thickness [23]. Echogenicity was defined as the mean pixel intensity of the rectus femoris measured in arbitrary units (A.U.) ranging between 0 (i.e., black) and 255 (i.e., white). Anatomical muscle CSA was determined by tracing the inside of the epimysium of the rectus femoris using the polygon tool. Rectus femoris thickness was assessed with a single measurement using the straight-line tool; using ImageJ, a line was made through the largest, middle portion of the muscle perpendicular to the skin. Intraclass correlation coefficients (ICC) were used to examine the reliability of these analyses. All three research assistants completed reliability training prior to being allowed to be an operator for the testing in the study. The test–retest reliability of three images obtained by the research assistants using ICCs and 95% confidence intervals were as follows: panoramic muscle thickness = 0.98 (0.90, 0.95), B-mode muscle thickness = 0.98 (0.97, 0.99), panoramic muscle area = 0.95 (0.93, 0.96), B-mode muscle area = 0.97 (0.97, 0.98), panoramic muscle echogenicity = 0.98 (0.97, 0.98), and B-mode echogenicity = 0.81 (0.75, 0.87). For consistency, these measurements were all analyzed by the same member of the research team. The mean of each participant's values across the three images at each site (i.e., 50% and 75%) was used in our analyses. Figure 1 displays an example of muscle thickness and CSA captured and analyzed at each site.

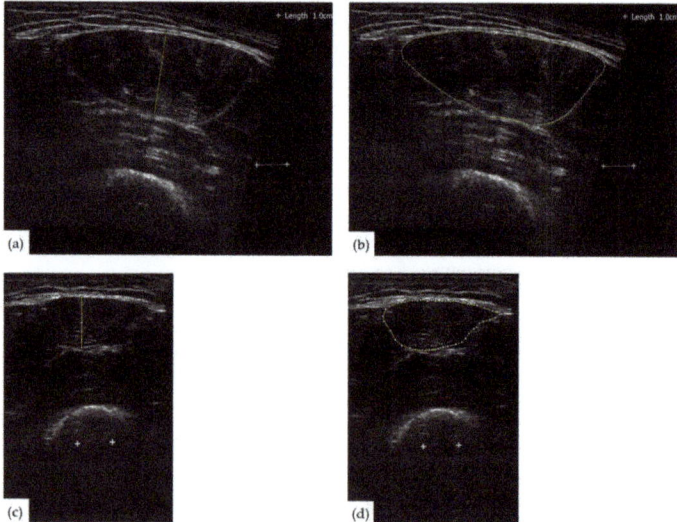

Figure 1. Examples of rectus femoris muscle thickness and CSA captured via ultrasonography for one participant. (**a**) Rectus femoris muscle thickness at 50% of leg length captured using the panoramic feature. (**b**) Same as A but showing muscle CSA. (**c**) Rectus femoris muscle thickness at 75% of leg length captured using a standardized B-mode image. (**d**) Same as C but showing muscle CSA.

2.3. Performance Measures

Participants performed a self-paced, low to moderate intensity warm-up for five minutes using a cycle ergometer. Muscle strength and endurance of the lower body were tested using isokinetic dynamometry on a Biodex Pro IV System (Biodex Medical Systems, Shirley, NY, USA). Lower body muscular strength was assessed using peak torque performed during a three-repetition test at 60° per second for knee extension–flexion and a three-repetition test at 30° per second for plantar-dorsiflexion. Lower body muscular endurance was evaluated using the total amount of work performed during a 21-repetition test at 180° per second for knee extension–flexion and 60° per second for plantar-dorsiflexion [24]. Muscular strength and then endurance were first assessed in upper leg (i.e., knee extension–flexion) and then in the lower leg (i.e., plantar-dorsiflexion).

A warm-up set was completed before each lower-body strength test (i.e., knee extension–flexion and plantar-dorsiflexion); participants were instructed to perform three repetitions at ≤75% of their perceived maximal effort. Thirty seconds of rest was given between all extension-flexion tests. One minute of rest was provided between plantar-dorsiflexion tests. To optimize performance, participants were encouraged to employ "all-out effort" by research staff during all muscle function tests. To better capture muscular performance of the entire right leg, peak torques from the isokinetic strength test and total work from the isokinetic endurance test were added together to create summed peak torque and summed total work (i.e., knee extension + knee flexion + plantarflexion + dorsiflexion).

Maximal handgrip strength (kg) was assessed using an analog Jamar Handheld Dynamometer (Bolingbrook, IL, USA). Participants were instructed to grasp the dynamometer in their dominant hand and to keep their elbow at their side with a 90° bend between the upper arm and forearm, while standing. Participants were told to squeeze the dynamometer as hard as possible for two to three seconds. Each participant performed three maximal attempts; the highest grip strength was used.

Participants then performed a 30-s chair stand test on a chair with a 43 cm floor-to-seat height. All trials were performed with participants' arms crossed and feet at a comfortable distance apart (i.e., about hip to shoulder width). With a straight back, participants were instructed to fully sit down and stand-up for each repetition, and practice repetitions were performed to ensure adequate performance during the test. The total number of repetitions completed in 30-s period was recorded, and the 30-s period began when participants started to rise.

2.4. Physical Activity Assessment

Following performance testing, participants were given accelerometers and three-day food diaries. Physical activity was recorded using Actigraph (ActiGraph Corp, Pensacola, FL, USA) GT9X accelerometers. Participants were instructed to wear accelerometers on their right hip during all waking hours, excluding activities where the device may get wet (e.g., bathing or swimming), for a period of one week and to keep a sleep log to record the time that the accelerometer was removed at night and put back on in the morning. The raw acceleration data were collected at 80 Hz and processed in R software (http://cran.r-project.org, accessed on 6 September 2016) using the GGIR package (version 1.10-10) [25]. Non-wear time was defined as intervals of at least 90 min of zero counts with allowance of a two-minute interval of non-zero counts within a 30-min window [26]; thus, only valid time during waking hours of each day was included for statistical analyses. Although accelerometry captures many aspects of physical activity (e.g., sedentary time, light physical activity, etc.), we decided to use moderate-to-vigorous physical activity (MVPA) in our analyses because of its relationship with performance variables [27,28].

2.5. Nutrition Analysis

After performance testing, participants were also given three-day food diaries, received training on how to record dietary intakes by a member of the research team, and were required to watch a prerecorded training video. Dietary intakes from three-day food diaries, including nutritional supplements, were entered into Food Processor Nutrition Analysis Software (ESHA Research, Salem, OR, USA), which uses FoodData Central (USDA National Nutrient Database) by trained research assistants. Data entry was then line-by-line verified by a registered dietitian. Animal- and plant-based protein intakes were estimated using a line-by-line examination of dietary intake by a registered dietitian. Food items that contained less than 1 g of total protein were excluded from these calculations. Foods containing both animal- and plant-based protein were split according to their ingredients to distinguish protein sources. Animal-based protein sources included meat, fish and seafood, dairy, eggs, poultry, and wild game.

2.6. Statistical Analyses

Alpha was set at 0.05, and all statistics were performed in SPSS version 27 (IBM, Armonk, NY, USA). All data are available as a supplemental file.

2.6.1. Primary Analyses: Measures from Ultrasonography and Their Relationships with Muscular Performance and the Association between Rectus Femoris Echogenicity and Specific Force

Three male participants could not be included in analyses of ultrasonography because our ultrasound machine suffered a catastrophic failure near the very end of the data collection window, precluding ultrasonography for these male participants. Thus, all analyses related to ultrasonography have 88 as opposed to 91 participants.

We used multiple-linear regression models to determine the relationships between variables derived from ultrasonography (i.e., rectus femoris muscle thickness, echogenicity, and CSA) using the two different methodologies (i.e., panoramic versus B-mode images) and sites (i.e., 50% and 75% of right leg length) with measures of muscular performance. Each of these variables from ultrasonography were assessed in separate multiple-linear regression models. Although we consider summed peak torque and summed total work to be more representative of lower-body performance, we specifically included knee extensor peak torque and total work in these analyses, because ultrasonography was used to measure the rectus femoris, one of the knee extensors. Separate multiple-linear regression models were also used to evaluate the relationship between echogenicity and specific force of the rectus femoris, two measures of muscle quality. All aforementioned regression models were adjusted for gender (i.e., 0 = women, 1 = men), age, and body mass in kilograms divided by the square of height in meters (BMI), because these variables are routinely collected in both clinical and research settings.

2.6.2. Secondary Analyses: Animal-Based Protein Intake and Muscular Performance

All participants completed a three-day food diary, completed all performance measures (i.e., isokinetic dynamometry, handgrip strength, and 30-s chair stand test), and wore an accelerometer. For our analyses investigating nutritional variables, we first used simple linear regression models to verify that our estimates of animal-based and plant-based protein intakes together agreed with total protein intake. Animal-based and plant-based protein intakes, determined by line-by-line analysis of three-day food diaries by a registered dietitian and expressed either as relative intakes or percentages of energy intakes, were entered as predictor variables, and total protein, without partitioning into animal- or plant-based protein intakes, was the outcome variable.

Analyses of nutritional data are complicated by the shared variance of many variables. Energy intake and macronutrient intakes, which we examined in this work, are directly related, that is, a person's macronutrient intake, withstanding alcohol, determines their energy intake (i.e., protein + carbohydrates + fat = energy). Therefore, when analyzing dietary variables, relative energy (kcals/kg/day) and the relative intakes of all the macronutrients (g/kg/day) cannot be entered simultaneously. We used Pearson Product–Moment Coefficients to examine the collinearity of both relative macronutrient intakes and macronutrient intakes as percentages of energy intake with one another and with relative energy intake. Although there are other methodologies, we chose to include relative energy intake (kcal/kg/day) in our analyses and to express the intake of the macronutrients as percentages of energy intake. This method allowed us to control for both relative energy intake and macronutrient intakes in our statistical models.

Mixed linear models were used to evaluate the impact of ABPI on muscular performance. The 41 men and 50 women were first blocked according to self-reported gender (0 = women, 1 = men). Then, each gender was split at their median of energy intake from animal-based protein. More specifically, gender and ABPI (below median = 0, above median = 1) were entered as fixed factors. Age, BMI, MVPA, relative energy intake, and percent energy from protein, fat, and carbohydrates were entered as continuous covariates.

Models were evaluated for equality of error of variance using Levene's Test of Equality of Variance and for heteroscedasticity using White's Test of Heteroscedasticity; mixed models that were significantly unequal in their variances or heteroscedastic were transformed using the square root function. Out of an abundance of caution, we chose to use the HC3 method to calculate the standard errors of our variables, as it is more robust to unequal variances, heteroscedasticity, and multicollinearity than the ordinary least squares method [29]. We did not hypothesize that there would be interaction between gender and ABPI, so only main effects were examined in these mixed models. For those models in which ABPI is significant, we evaluated effect size using partial eat squared. We also sought to verify that ABPI and not total protein intake is important to performance. We verified our results by performing the same aforementioned methods, but we split each gender at median of total protein intake as a percentage of energy intake and included ABPI as a percentage of energy intake as a continuous covariate.

Estimates of physical activity from accelerometry are considered valid when the devices are worn for 10 h per day for at least four days [28], and three participants failed to meet these criteria despite our instruction to wear the devices during all waking hours for one week. Nonetheless, all other participants achieved at least four or more days including one weekend day with an average of 10 or more hours of time wearing the device. These three participants who failed to wear accelerometers as directed represent a small portion of our sample (3.3%), and physical activity was included in our mixed models as a covariate; physical activity is not the focus of this work, but we feel it is essential to control for in our mixed models evaluating ABPI. For these reasons and due to small sample size, particularly when split into groups, we decided to include these three participants, using their limited physical activity data in our analyses.

2.6.3. Descriptive Statistics

For our descriptive statistics, we described the four groups from the secondary analyses in our all of our tables, even though we chose not to investigate the association between ABPI and measures from ultrasonography, because the three men who were precluded from ultrasonography were, coincidentally, above the median for animal-based protein intake as a percentage of energy. Within these tables, we chose to use the Brown–Forsythe method for comparisons, because we did not assume equal variances. We compared those above the median of ABPI as a percentage of energy to those below the median within each gender, so we did not adjust for multiple comparisons.

3. Results

Table 1 describes participants self-reported age, measured height, weight, and calculated BMI. There were no statistically significant differences between those below or above the median of ABPI as a percentage of total energy within each gender.

Table 1. Self-reported age and anthropometrics for 41 men and 50 women.

	Women			Men		
	Total (n = 50)	Below Median ABPI (n = 25)	Above Median ABPI (n =25)	Total (n = 41)	Below Median ABPI (n = 21)	Above Median ABPI (n =20)
Age (years)	54.00	55.00	54.00	51.00	55.00	50.00
Height (cm)	165.20	164.00	165.50	181.00	176.70	181.05
Weight (kg)	68.30	67.33	69.12	87.7	85.20	92.36
BMI	25.11	24.43	25.54	26.57	26.57	26.32

All values are medians. Comparisons within gender and between those below and above the median for animal-based protein intake (ABPI) as a percentage of energy intake were made using the Brown–Forsythe method.

Table 2 describes right rectus femoris muscle thickness, echogenicity, and CSA measured using the panoramic ultrasonography at 50% and B-mode images at 75% of the distance of the right leg. Within each gender, there were no statistically significant differences in these measures between those above the median of ABPI and those below.

Table 2. Rectus femoris muscle thickness, echogenicity, and cross-sectional area assessed via ultrasonography captured using the panoramic feature at 50% and with regular B-mode images at 75% of the right leg in 88 middle-aged men and women.

	Women			Men		
	Total (n = 50)	Below Median ABPI (n = 25)	Above Median ABPI (n =25)	Total (n = 38)	Below Median ABPI (n = 21)	Above Median ABPI (n =17)
Muscle Thickness at 50% (cm)	2.109	2.038	2.178	2.339	2.275	2.345
Muscle Thickness at 75% (cm)	0.707	0.710	0.706	0.994	0.918	1.070
Echogenicity at 50% (A.U.)	96.70	97.86	96.64	35.90	34.85	41.73
Echogenicity at 75% (A.U.)	91.99	93.34	90.63	81.99	74.56	84.54
Muscle CSA at 50% (cm^2)	7.384	6.569	7.861	10.593	10.470	10.963
Muscle CSA at 75% (cm^2)	0.957	0.790	1.055	1.934	1.660	2.088

All values are medians. CSA = Muscle Cross-Sectional Area. A.U. = Arbitrary Units. Comparisons within gender and between those below and above the median for animal-based protein intake (ABPI) as a percentage of energy intake were made using the Brown–Forsythe method.

Table 3 presents the results of the seperate multiple-linear regression models investigating the relationship between different measures derived from ultrasonography and muscular performance. Measures of rectus femoris size assessed using panoramic ultrasonography were less related to knee extensor performance but more strongly related to overall muscular performance. More specifically, both muscle thickness (p = 0.302) and CSA (p = 0.056) assessed using the panoramic feature of the right leg were unrelated to knee extensor peak torque, whereas the same measures assessed using a B-mode image at of the right leg were related to knee extensor peak torque. Similarly, muscle thickness assessed using the panoramic feature was unrelated to knee extensor total work (p = 0.197). Although muscle CSA captured with the panoramic feature was related to knee extensor total work (p = 0.049), it was less closely related than muscle CSA (p = 0.013) or thickness (p = 0.036) assessed with a B-mode image at 75% of leg length. Conversely, measures of muscle thickness (p = 0.001) and CSA (p = 0.004) derived from panoramic ultrasound were significantly related to handgrip strength performance, whereas the same measures collected using B-mode were not. Muscle CSA from panoramic ultrasound was also most closely related to summed peaked torque (p = 0.005), a relationship that was only close to significance (p = 0.051) with a B-mode image. Both methodologies (i.e., panoramic and B-mode) produced measures of muscle thickness and CSA that were associated with summed total work.

Echogenicity of rectus femoris was unrelated to both knee extensor and summed peak torque but was significantly associated with knee extensor total work when captured using either panoramic (p = 0.001) or B-mode images (p = 0.004). Echogenicity of the rectus femoris from both panoramic (p = 0.008) and B-mode (p = 0.007) images was also associated with handgrip strength. Interestingly, although echogenicity was related to knee extensor total work, it was not related to summed total work when using either methodology. No ultrasonographic measure was associated with 30-s chair stand performance.

Table 4 describes our evaluation of echogenicity with specific force, two measures of muscle quality. Echogenicity was not related to specific force in any regression model nor was any model significant. We found measures from the 50% site, taken using the panoramic feature, created better fitting models. In fact, echogenicity assessed at 50% trended toward significance (p = 0.077).

Table 3. The associations between different ultrasonographic measures of the right rectus femoris using the panoramic feature (50% of leg upper length) and a B-mode image (75% of upper leg length) in a sample of 88 middle-aged men and women when controlling for age, gender, and BMI.

Variable Entered	Dependent Variable											
	Knee Extensor Peak Torque (Nm)		Summed Peak Torque (Nm)		Knee Extensor Total Work (J)		Summed Total Work (J)		30-s Chair Stand Test (Repetitions)		Handgrip Strength (kg)	
	R	B ± S.E.	R	B ± S.E.	R	B ± S.E.	R	B ± S.E.	R	B ± S.E.	R	B ± S.E.
Muscle Thickness at 50% (cm)	0.816 $p < 0.001$	11.098 ± 10.286 $p = 0.302$	0.861 $p < 0.001$	42.622 ± 20.024 $p = 0.036$	0.707 $p < 0.001$	174.654 ± 134.410 $p = 0.197$	0.850 $p < 0.001$	595.980 ± 200.221 $p = 0.004$	0.353 $p = 0.025$	1.348 ± 1.415 $p = 0.334$	0.900 $p < 0.001$	6.966 ± 3.328 $p = 0.001$
Muscle Thickness at 75% (cm)	0.826 $p < 0.001$	23.166 ± 9.955 $p = 0.022$	0.862 $p < 0.001$	42.533 ± 19.076 $p = 0.025$	0.719 $p < 0.001$	269.252 ± 126.430 $p = 0.036$	0.849 $p < 0.001$	555.550 ± 191.981 $p = 0.005$	0.347 $p = 0.029$	0.963 ± 1.357 $p = 0.480$	0.885 $p < 0.001$	0.307 ± 2.131 $p = 0.886$
Echogenicity at 50% (A.U.)	0.822 $p < 0.001$	−0.271 ± 0.141 $p = 0.059$	0.854 $p < 0.001$	−0.237 ± 0.275 $p = 0.389$	0.854 $p < 0.001$	−5.809 ± 1.710 $p = 0.001$	0.836 $p < 0.001$	−3.622 ± 2.804 $p = 0.200$	0.349 $p = 0.027$	−0.016 ± 0.019 $p = 0.412$	0.895 $p < 0.001$	−0.078 ± 0.029 $p = 0.008$
Echogenicity at 75% (A.U.)	0.817 $p < 0.001$	−0.142 ± 0.129 $p = 0.274$	0.853 $p < 0.001$	−0.058 ± 0.248 $p = 0.815$	0.853 $p < 0.001$	−4.763 ± 1.550 $p = 0.003$	0.834 $p < 0.001$	−4.763 ± 1.550 $p = 0.370$	0.376 $p = 0.012$	−0.027 ± 0.017 $p = 0.113$	0.895 $p < 0.001$	−0.071 ± 0.026 $p = 0.007$
Muscle CSA at 50% (cm^2)	0.823 $p < 0.001$	3.406 ± 1.754 $p = 0.056$	0.867 $p < 0.001$	9.915 ± 3.271 $p = 0.005$	0.717 $p < 0.001$	44.281 ± 22.142 $p = 0.049$	0.860 $p < 0.001$	126.648 ± 32.205 $p < 0.001$	0.349 $p = 0.028$	0.193 ± 0.237 $p = 0.418$	0.897 $p < 0.001$	1.050 ± 0.354 $p = 0.004$
Muscle CSA at 75% (cm^2)	0.828 $p < 0.001$	8.120 ± 3.245 $p = 0.014$	0.860 $p < 0.001$	12.464 ± 6.294 $p = 0.051$	0.726 $p < 0.001$	104.435 ± 40.951 $p = 0.013$	0.844 $p < 0.001$	153.621 ± 63.783 $p = 0.018$	0.341 $p = 0.034$	0.165 ± 0.445 $p = 0.713$	0.885 $p < 0.001$	−0.154 ± 0.698 $p = 0.826$

S.E. = standard error. Age: years. Gender: Women = 0, Men = 1; CSA = Muscle Cross-Sectional Area; BMI: kg/m^2. Summed peak torque was calculated by adding the peak torques recorded during the isokinetic strength test, 60° per second for knee extension-flexion and 30° per second for plantar-dorsiflexion. Summed isokinetic endurance was calculated by adding total work performed during a 21-repetition test at 180° per second for the knee extension-flexion and 60° per second for plantar-dorsiflexion. The height of the chair for the 30-s chair stand test was 43 cm.

Table 4. Association of echogenicity assessed via ultrasonography captured using the panoramic feature and B-mode images of the right leg with various assessments of knee extensor specific force in 88 middle-aged men and women.

Variable Entered	Specific Force Variable	R	$F_{4,83}$	Age (Beta ± S.E.)	Gender (Beta ± S.E.)	BMI (Beta ± S.E.)	Entered Variable (Beta ± S.E.)
Echogenicity at 50% (A.U.)	Peak KE Torque by Muscle Thickness at 50% (Nm/cm)	0.299	2.030 $p = 0.098$	−0.799 ± 3.154 $p = 0.801$	−106.185 ± 54.253 $p = 0.054$	10.527±4.306 $p = 0.017$	−1.381 ± 0.770 $p = 0.077$
	Peak KE Torque by Muscle CSA at 50% (Nm/cm^2)	0.311	2.226 $p = 0.073$	−0.625 ± 2.187 $p = 0.776$	−5.110 ± 37.627 $p = 0.892$	6.163±2.986 $p = 0.042$	−0.831 ± 0.534 $p = 0.123$
Echogenicity at 75% (A.U.)	Peak KE Torque by Muscle Thickness at 75% (Nm/cm)	0.239	1.253 $p = 0.295$	−0.074 ± 3.181 $p = 0.982$	−45.255 ± 41.943 $p = 0.284$	9.403±4.341 $p = 0.033$	−0.370 ± 0.702 $p = 0.600$
	Peak KE Torque by Muscle CSA at 75% (Nm/cm^2)	0.267	1.594 $p = 0.184$	−0.161 ± 2.199 $p = 0.535$	32.388 ± 28.991 $p = 0.267$	5.416±3.001 $p = 0.075$	−0.131 ± 0.485 $p = 0.788$

A.U. = Arbitrary Units. S.E. = Standard Error. Age: years. Gender: Women = 0; Men = 1. BMI: kg/m^2.

Table 5 describes the nutritional variables assessed from three-day food diaries for study participants. There were significant differences in macronutrient intake between those above the median for ABPI as a percentage of energy intake and those below within each gender; relative carbohydrate intake, carbohydrate intake as percentage of energy, protein intake as percentage of energy, relative ABPI, ABPI as a percentage of energy, and relative plant-based protein intake were all significantly different in both men and women. Those above the median consumed less carbohydrates, more protein, and more animal based protein than those below. In women, there were also significant differences in relative fat and calcium intake with those above the median consuming less fat and more calcium. In men, on the other hand, there was a significant difference in relative energy intake with those below the median of ABPI consuming more energy.

Table 6 lists physical activity variables recorded using accelerometry. Excluding wear days, which were greater in men below the median compared to men above the median, there were no significant differences between those above the median of animal-based protein as percentage of energy intake and those below.

Regression models examining estimates of animal-based and plant-based protein intakes with total protein intake showed good agreement between our estimates and total protein. Estimates of relative animal-based and relative plant-based protein intakes explained 98.4% of the variance in relative protein intake (F2,88 = 2788.702, $p < 0.001$), and estimates of animal- and plant-based protein intakes as percentages of energy explained 94.0% of the variance in protein as a percentage of energy (F2,88 = 683.550, $p < 0.001$).

Table 7 shows Pearson Product–Moment Correlations between relative macronutrient intakes, macronutrient intakes as percentages of energy intake, and relative energy intake. Relative macronutrient intakes showed stronger relationships with relative energy intake than macronutrient intakes expressed as a percentage of energy intake. Withstanding the association between percent of energy from fats and carbohydrates, macronutrient intakes expressed as percentages of energy were less strongly correlated amongst one another than relative macronutrient intakes. These results suggest macronutrient intakes should be expressed as percentages of energy intake in statistical models including relative energy intake to limit collinearity.

Table 5. Dietary intakes accessed from three-day food diaries in 41 middle-aged men and 50 middle-aged women.

	Women			Men		
	Total (n = 50)	Below Median ABPI (n = 25)	Above Median ABPI (n = 25)	Total (n = 41)	Below Median ABPI (n = 21)	Above Median ABPI (n = 20)
Relative Energy (kcal/kg/day)	24.46	30.51	22.51	28.41	31.08 *	26.73
Relative Fat (g/kg/day)	1.04	1.14 *	0.90	1.15	1.20	0.99
Fat Percent Energy (%)	35.66	37.03	34.88	34.85	34.02	35.63
Relative Carbohydrate (g/kg/day)	2.85	3.22 **	2.30	3.56	4.12 **	2.81
Carbohydrate Percent Energy (%)	46.20	48.56 *	44.36	46.86	48.82 ***	41.16
Relative Protein (g/kg/day)	1.19	1.15 *	1.25	1.28	1.28	1.24
Protein Percent Energy (%)	17.99	14.40 **	21.27	17.35	14.54 ***	18.65
Relative Animal Protein (g/kg/day)	0.77	0.61 ***	1.00	0.87	0.82 *	0.96
Animal Protein Percent Energy (%)	11.99	8.59 ***	16.08	11.74	10.39 ***	15.16
Relative Plant Protein (g/kg/day)	0.31	0.37 *	0.27	0.34	0.39 **	0.29
Plant Protein Percent Energy (%)	4.92	5.23	4.81	4.56	4.77	4.26
Vitamin D (IU/day)	155.28	105.58	236.41	149.70	206.52	135.49
Calcium (mg/day)	849.06	743.91 **	951.94	1166.69	1103.57	1212.28
Mg (mg/day)	202.96	196.17	210.15	315.96	254.04	332.94
Mn (mg/day)	1.67	1.50	1.98	2.03	2.31	1.89
Vitamin K (mcg/day)	72.01	88.31	59.97	70.72	52.02	77.98
Fe (mg/day)	12.49	12.51	12.03	16.10	18.43	14.80
Vitamin C (mg/day)	107.42	84.78	115.31	79.03	86.42	54.11
Vitamin E (mg/day)	7.716	7.00	13.06	7.71	5.37	8.10
P (mg/day)	772.54	809.96	765.45	1314.39	1265.21	1349.81
K (mg/day)	1693.39	1692.27	1754.97	2577.01	2577.01	2576.71

All values are medians. Comparisons between those below and above the median for animal-based protein intake (ABPI) as a percentage of energy intake within gender were made using the Brown–Forsythe method. * $p < 0.05$; ** $p < 0.01$; *** $p < 0.001$.

Table 6. Physical activity variables assessed using accelerometry in 41 middle-aged men and 50 middle-aged women.

	Women			Men		
	Total (n = 50)	Below Median ABPI (n = 25)	Above Median ABPI (n = 25)	Total (n = 41)	Below Median ABPI (n = 21)	Above Median ABPI (n = 20)
Wear Days (days)	7.00	6.00	7.007	7.00	7.00 *	6.00
Wear Time (min/day)	867.04	869.50	864.57	895.33	895.71	891.87
Sedentary Time (min/day)	559.58	556.00	563.001	613.14	606.00	620.91
Light Physical Activity (min/day)	265.13	285.83	260.33	242.38	269.43	210.11
Moderate Physical Activity (min/day)	27.46	30.67	22.00	27.86	31.83	25.85
Vigorous Physical Activity (min/day)	0.15	0.14	0.29	0.33	2.00	0.00
Moderate to Vigorous Physical Activity (min/day)	31.05	31.20	27.14	33.25	33.83	27.00

All values are medians. Comparisons between those below and above the median for animal-based protein intake (ABPI) as a percentage of energy intake within gender were made using the Brown–Forsythe method. * $p < 0.05$.

Table 7. Pearson Product–Moment Correlations of macronutrient intakes, including animal-based protein, and relative energy intake in 41 middle-aged men and 50 middle-aged women.

Variable	Variable								
	Relative Energy Intake	Relative Fat (g/kg/day)	Fat Percent Energy (%)	Relative Carbohydrate (g/kg/day)	Carbohydrate Percent Energy (%)	Relative Protein (g/kg/day)	Protein Percent Energy (%)	Relative Animal Protein (g/kg/day)
Relative Fat (g/kg/day)	0.819 $p < 0.001$	-	-	-	-	-	-	-
Fat Percent Energy (%)	−0.120 $p = 0.258$	0.435 $p < 0.001$	-	-	-	-	-	-
Relative Carbohydrate (g/kg/day)	0.911 $p < 0.001$	0.534 $p < 0.001$	-0.440 $p < 0.001$	-	-	-	-	-
Carbohydrate Percent Energy (%)	0.315 $p = 0.002$	−0.188 $p = 0.074$	−0.845 $p < 0.001$	0.648 $p < 0.001$	-	-	-	-
Relative Protein (g/kg/day)	0.755 $p < 0.001$	0.617 $p < 0.001$	−0.144 $p = 0.174$	0.570 $p < 0.001$	−0.019 $p = 0.858$	-	-	-
Protein Percent Energy (%)	−0.353 $p = 0.001$	−0.351 $p = 0.001$	−0.114 $p = 0.281$	−0.438 $p < 0.001$	−0.438 $p < 0.001$	0.297 $p = 0.004$	-	-
Relative Animal Protein (g/kg/day)	0.548 $p < 0.001$	0.452 $p < 0.001$	−0.122 $p = 0.248$	0.357 $p = 0.001$	−0.138 $p = 0.191$	0.922 $p < 0.001$	0.473 $p < 0.001$	-
Animal Protein Percent Energy (%)	−0.350 $p < 0.001$	−0.332 $p = 0.001$	−0.082 $p = 0.439$	−0.440 $p < 0.001$	−0.431 $p < 0.001$	0.277 $p = 0.008$	0.916 $p < 0.001$	0.550 $p < 0.001$

Table 8 and Figure 2 present the results of our investigation of the relationship between ABPI with performance measures. To create homoscedastic models with equal variances, data from the handgrip strength test (kg) and the 30-s chair stand test (repetitions) were transformed using the square root function. Using these transformed variables, all of these mixed models had equal variances according to Levene's Test and were homoscedastic according to White's test (i.e., $p > 0.05$).

Table 8. Animal-based protein intake and muscular performance in middle-aged men and women.

Performance Variable	R	$F_{9,81}$	Age (Beta ± S.E.)	Gender (Beta ± S.E.)	BMI (Beta ± S.E.)	MVPA (Beta ± S.E.)	Relative Energy (Beta ± S.E.)	Fat Percent Energy (Beta ± S.E.)	Carbohydrate Percent Energy (Beta ± S.E.)	Protein Percent Energy (Beta ± S.E.)	Animal-Based Protein Intake Median Split (Beta ± S.E.)
Summed Isokinetic Peak Torque (Nm)	0.887	33.111 $p < 0.001$	−3.767 ± 1.138 $p = 0.001$	190.543 ± 13.850 $p < 0.001$	1.694 ± 1.874 $p = 0.369$	0.287 ± 0.395 $p = 0.469$	−0.829 ± 0.862 $p = 0.339$	−3.754 ± 8.467 $p = 0.659$	−3.889 ± 8.351 $p = 0.643$	−5.769 ± 8.007 $p = 0.473$	65.874 ± 19.855 $p = 0.001$
Summed Isokinetic Work (J)	0.870	28.032 $p < 0.001$	−46.224 ± 11.546 $p < 0.001$	1671.298 ± 126.695 $p < 0.001$	29.436 ± 19.814 $p = 0.141$	2.842 ± 4.617 $p = 0.540$	16.825 ± 9.500 $p = 0.080$	−100.977 ± 76.033 $p = 0.188$	−95.794 ± 76.033 $p = 0.204$	−92.620 ± 71.011 $p = 0.196$	549.944 ± 232.478 $p = 0.020$
Transformed 30-Second Chair Stand (repetitions #)	0.437	2.128 $p = 0.036$	0.004 ± 0.010 $p = 0.700$	0.316 ± 0.128 $p = 0.016$	−0.024 ± 0.013 $p = 0.081$	0.000 ± 0.003 $p = 0.940$	0.008 ± 0.009 $p = 0.859$	−0.092 ± 0.077 $p = 0.237$	−0.103 ± 0.076 $p = 0.182$	−0.095 ± 0.076 $p = 0.214$	0.086 ± 0.156 $p = 0.584$
Transformed Handgrip Strength (kg)	0.913	45.026 $p < 0.001$	−0.029 ± 0.008 $p = 0.001$	1.898 ± 0.105 $p < 0.001$	0.001 ± 0.018 $p = 0.956$	0.003 ± 0.003 $p = 0.295$	−0.008 ± 0.008 $p = 0.323$	−0.083 ± 0.042 $p = 0.052$	−0.091 ± 0.041 $p = 0.027$	−0.111 ± 0.040 $p = 0.007$	0.349 ± 0.171 $p = 0.045$

S.E. = standard error. Age: years. Gender: Women = 0, Men = 1. BMI: kg/m^2. Relative energy intake: kcal/kg/day. Animal-based protein intake was split at the median of percent energy from animal-based protein within both men and women; below median = 0, above median = 1. Nutritional variables were assessed using three-day food diaries. Summed isokinetic peak torque was calculated by adding the peak torques recorded during the isokinetic strength test, 60° per second for knee extension–flexion and 30° per second for plantar-dorsiflexion. Summed isokinetic endurance was calculated by adding total work performed during a 21-repetition test at 180° per second for the knee extension–flexion and 60° per second for plantar-dorsiflexion. Total repetitions performed during the 30-s chair stand test and handgrip strength were transformed using the square root function. The height of the chair for the 30-s chair stand test was 43 cm.

Our mixed models explained 78.6% of the variance of summed peak torque performed during the isokinetic strength test, 75.7% of the variance of summed work performed during the isokinetic endurance test, and 83.3% of the variance in handgrip strength transformed using the square root function, indicating good model fit for these performance variables. However, our mixed model investigating the results of the 30-s chair stand test only explained 19.1% of the variance in this measure, indicating relatively poor model fit. Nonetheless, all models were significant.

Animal-based protein intake was significant to mixed models evaluating lower-body muscular strength, lower-body muscular endurance, and handgrip strength. Those consuming above the median of animal-based protein as percentage of energy intake performed better on these tests of muscular strength and endurance than those below the median. The effect sizes assessed using partial eta squared of the ABPI median split were 0.120, 0.065, and 0.049 for summed lower-body peak torque, summed lower-body total work, and handgrip strength, respectively. Animal-based protein intake was not related to performance in the 30-s chair stand test.

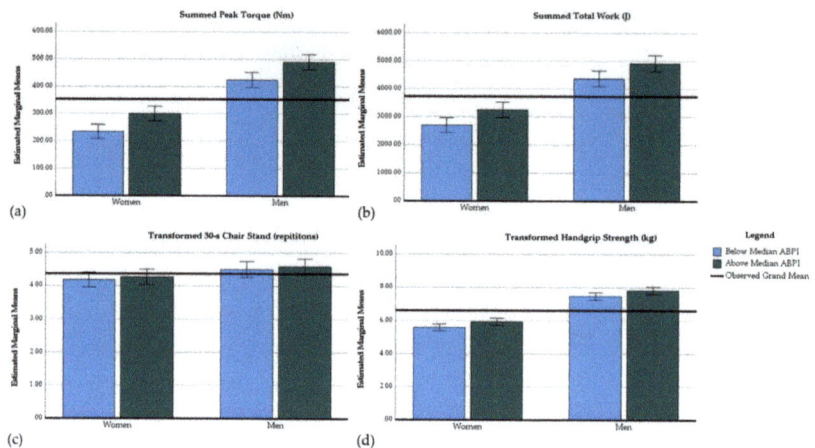

Figure 2. Animal-based protein intake and muscular performance. Animal-based protein intake was split at the median of percent energy from animal-based protein within both men and women; below median = 0, above median = 1. Covariates included age, gender, BMI, MVPA, relative energy intake, and percentages of energy intake from fat, carbohydrate, and protein. All bars are means, and error bars represent 95% confidence intervals. (**a**) Summed isokinetic peak torque by gender and animal-based protein intake. Summed isokinetic peak torque was calculated by adding the peak torques recorded during the isokinetic strength test, 60° per second for knee extension–flexion and 30° per second for plantar-dorsiflexion. (**b**) Summed isokinetic endurance by gender and animal-based protein intake. Summed isokinetic endurance was calculated by adding total work performed during a 21-repetition test at 180° per second for the knee extension–flexion and 60° per second for plantar-dorsiflexion. (**c**) Square root transformed 30-s chair stand test repetitions by gender and animal-based protein intake. The height of the chair for the 30-s chair stand test was 43 cm. (**d**) Square root transformed handgrip strength by gender and animal-based protein intake.

Because ABPI was significant to lower-body muscular strength, lower-body muscular endurance, and handgrip strength, we wanted to verify that these findings were due to ABPI and not to greater total protein intake. Although we did control for total protein intake as percentage of energy in our mixed models where participants were split at the median of ABPI, Table 9 shows our analyses where participants were split at the median of total protein intake as percentage of energy intake and ABPI as a percent of energy intake was entered as a continuous covariate. With the exception of square root transformed 30-s chair stand repetitions, all of these mixed models had equal variances according to Levene's Test and were homoscedastic according to White's test (i.e., $p > 0.05$). Square root transformed 30-s chair stand performance was homoscedastic but showed unequal variances between groups ($p = 0.024$) according to Levene's test. Because our earlier analysis of square root transformed 30-s chair stand performance (i.e., Table 8) showed equal variances between groups, was homoscedastic, and produced nonsignificant results regarding protein intake and ABPI, we did not transform 30-s chair stand performance using a different methodology (e.g., Log). In other words, square root transformed 30-s chair stand performance was included in Table 9 despite showing unequal variances between groups, although the HC3 method is considered to be more robust to violations of unequal variance [28]. Total protein intake split at the median of energy intake was not significant to any performance variable, whereas APBI split at the median was significant to lower-body muscular strength, lower-body muscular endurance, and handgrip strength, indicating that APBI is more closely related to muscular performance than total protein intake.

Table 9. Total protein intake and muscular performance in middle-aged men and women.

Performance Variable	R	$F_{9,81}$	Age (Beta ± S.E.)	Gender (Beta ± S.E.)	BMI (Beta ± S.E.)	MVPA (Beta ± S.E.)	Relative Energy (Beta ± S.E.)	Fat Percent Energy (Beta ± S.E.)	Carbohydrate Percent Energy (Beta ± S.E.)	ABPI Energy (Beta ± S.E.)	Total Protein Intake Median Split (Beta ± S.E.)
Summed Isokinetic Peak Torque (Nm)	0.871	28.366 $p < 0.001$	−4.013 ± 1.171 $p = 0.001$	189.571 ± 14.575 $p < 0.001$	2.003 ± 2.029 $p = 0.326$	0.194 ± 0.427 $p = 0.651$	−0.792 ± 0.962 $p = 0.413$	−0.049 ± 4.836 $p = 0.992$	−0.681 ± 4.576 $p = 0.882$	1.754 ± 3.637 $p = 0.631$	19.397 ± 23.176 $p = 0.405$
Summed Isokinetic Work (J)	0.856	24.638 $p < 0.001$	−47.751 ± 12.387 $p < 0.001$	1654.781 ± 134.463 $p < 0.001$	32.111 ± 22.256 $p = 0.153$	2.090 ± 5.296 $p = 0.694$	16.687 ± 10.609 $p = 0.120$	−24.735 ± 61.303 $p = 0.688$	−24.971 ± 58.990 $p = 0.673$	29.836 ± 43.397 $p = 0.494$	−2.405 ± 258.849 $p = 0.993$
Transformed 30-Second Chair Stand (repetitions #)	0.409	1.806 $p = 0.080$	0.004 ± 0.011 $p = 0.728$	0.313 ± 0.130 $p = 0.018$	−0.024 ± 0.013 $p = 0.084$	0.000 ± 0.003 $p = 0.958$	0.007 ± 0.009 $p = 0.466$	−0.011 ± 0.043 $p = 0.803$	−0.024 ± 0.040 $p = 0.549$	0.003 ± 0.043 $p = 0.939$	−0.112 ± 0.172 $p = 0.519$
Transformed Handgrip Strength (kg)	0.904	40.523 $p < 0.001$	−0.030 ± 0.009 $p = 0.001$	1.901 ± 0.121 $p < 0.001$	0.004 ± 0.0019 $p = 0.834$	0.002 ± 0.003 $p = 0.680$	−0.008 ± 0.008 $p = 0.360$	−0.018 ± 0.043 $p = 0.683$	−0.031 ± 0.042 $p = 0.459$	0.000 ± 0.032 $p = 0.997$	0.187 ± 0.197 $p = 0.953$

S.E. = standard error. ABPI = animal-based protein intake. Age: years. Gender: Women = 0, Men = 1. BMI: kg/m². Relative energy intake: kcal/kg/day. Total protein intake was split at the median of percent energy from protein within both men and women; below median = 0, above median = 1. Nutritional variables were assessed using three-day food diaries. Summed isokinetic peak torque was calculated by adding the peak torques recorded during the isokinetic strength test, 60° per second for knee extension–flexion and 30° per second for plantar-dorsiflexion. Summed isokinetic endurance was calculated by adding total work performed during a 21-repetition test at 180° per second for the knee extension–flexion and 60° per second for plantar-dorsiflexion. Total repetitions performed during the 30-s chair stand test and handgrip strength were transformed using the square root function. The height of the chair for the 30-s chair stand test was 43 cm.

4. Discussion

We found that measures of muscle size from standardized B-mode ultrasound images better captured the performance of the knee extensors, whereas measures of muscle size assessed from panoramic images were more closely related to overall muscular performance, producing significant associations between muscle size with summed peak torque and handgrip strength. However, our methodology differed from that of others who have utilized panoramic ultrasound. We took panoramic images of the rectus femoris at one location (i.e., 50% of leg length) as opposed to using a template to image the entire length of the quadriceps, although one research group advocated for an investigation of a single site at the mid-quadriceps [11].

Nonetheless, the lack of a significant relationship between muscle thickness and CSA measured using the panoramic feature and knee extensor strength is surprising, considering these measures of muscle size were more closely related both to lower-body strength (i.e., summed peak torque) and upper-body strength. Low muscle strength is the first criterion of sarcopenia according to the European Working Group on Sarcopenia in Older People 2 and should be, albeit not necessarily linearly, related to muscle mass [1]. In other words, changes in muscle mass or size are not as meaningful as changes in muscle strength. Measures of muscle size or mass that are unrelated to muscle strength then may have limited utility in assessing or screening for sarcopenia. Despite the fact measures from panoramic ultrasonography lacked face validity in the form of a significant relationship with knee extensor peak torque, our findings suggest that the panoramic feature is a suitable method for assessing sarcopenia in those with greater muscle at the midpoint of thigh, as it is related to both lower-body and upper-body strength.

We also report that in our sample echogenicity was unrelated to both knee extensor, strength, overall lower-body strength, and rectus femoris specific force, another measure of muscle quality. Although Strasser and colleagues [13] reported a significant correlation between echogenicity and knee extensor strength, the relationship was only found in younger and not older adults. In contrast, Akima and colleagues [30] found a significant relationship between echogenicity and sit-to-stand performance in older Japanese men and women. However, in a subsequent work, the same research group reported no relationship between echogenicity and knee extensor strength [6]. We also did not find a significant relationship between echogenicity and knee extensor strength, and we were the first, at least to our knowledge, to directly compare the echogenicity of the rectus femoris to the muscle's specific force. None of the relationships were significant. However, we did find an association between echogenicity with handgrip strength and knee extensor muscular endurance. Echogenicity has been related to both intramuscular fat [31] and fibrous tissue [32] content of muscle. In a large study of older Italian men and women, De Stefano and colleagues [33] reported a negative association between intramuscular fat and physical performance but found that those who were overweight or "Class I" obese had greater knee extensor strength than those with a normal BMI, suggesting that intramuscular fat plays a greater role in physical performance than in maximal strength. Our findings regarding echogenicity support that view. Echogenicity, then, is not closely related to specific force as it is with other muscular qualities such as endurance, because specific force is dependent on maximal muscle strength.

Our secondary findings regarding dietary intake indicate a positive relationship between ABPI and muscle strength when controlling for gender, age, BMI, relative energy intake, and macronutrient composition. More specifically, those above the median of ABPI as percentage of energy intake showed greater lower-body strength and endurance and greater handgrip strength than those below. Although greater protein intake is thought to be protective from developing sarcopenia [34–36], a recent cross-sectional study of older Danish adults utilizing methods similar to ours (e.g., three-day food diary and physical activity assessment) reported that protein intake was not related to knee extensor strength, handgrip strength, and 30-s chair stand test performance [16]. In contrast to their methodology where participants were divided into groups based on relative protein intake, we split ours according to ABPI as a percentage of energy intake. Although recommendations for protein intake are made on a g/kg basis [36], an advantage of expressing intakes as percentages of energy intake is that one can control for relative energy intakes and for macronutrient composition in the same statistical model. There is a high degree of collinearity between relative intakes of macronutrients and relative energy intake. In fact, one of the main findings from Højfeldt and colleagues' study of older Danish adults was that relative protein intakes and relative energy intakes are related [16]. Collinearity can bias estimates of betas in multivariate analyses [37]. Although there is still a degree of collinearity between macronutrient intakes as percentages of energy and relative energy intakes, we addressed this issue by using the HC3 method of calculating standard errors, which is more robust to collinearity and heteroscedasticity [29]. Outside of expressing intakes as percentages of energy, our methodology also differed because we evaluated ABPI. Plant-based proteins generally contain amino acids that are oxidized to be used as energy to a greater extent than higher quality animal-based proteins [18]. Thus, total protein intake is likely less strongly related to muscle mass and strength than protein intake from higher quality sources, and our findings particularly support this notion. When split at its median, total protein intake as a percentage of energy intake was not related to lower-body strength, lower-body endurance, and handgrip strength, whereas ABPI split at the median was positively associated with all these measures.

There are some limitations to our investigations. We cannot determine from our primary results if the panoramic feature inaccurately quantified muscle size, because our study lacked a measure of criterion validity in the form rectus femoris muscle thickness and cross-sectional area assessed using MRI or CT. Another caveat to our findings regarding ultrasonography is the skill of our sonographers. Although our sonographers were trained and showed good reliability, ICCs were greater than 0.95 for all measures other than B-mode echo intensity, which was equal to 0.81; they were and are not professional sonographers. Panoramic ultrasound is a more difficult method to perform, as the probe must be moved while keeping light, consistent pressure during imaging. Our results regarding panoramic ultrasonography and knee extensor performance may indicate, then, that the method should only be performed by those with highest levels of skill. Nonetheless, measures from panoramic ultrasonography were related to summed peak torque and handgrip strength, indicating these measures were related to overall performance. Another potential limitation was the assessment of anatomical as opposed to physiological CSA, as physiological CSA of pennate muscles, such as the rectus femoris, is thought to be more closely related to strength [10].

Regarding the limitations of our secondary analysis, this was a cross-sectional study incapable of establishing causality, the self-reported nature of our food-diary recording limits its accuracy, and we included three participants' physical activity data despite the fact these participants did not have enough valid wear days. Our secondary investigation did have some strengths. We objectively measured and controlled for physical activity. We verified our partitioning of protein intake into animal- and plant-based sources using regression models. We included relative energy and macronutrient intakes in our mixed models to control for differences in participants' diets outside of ABPI. Lastly, we confirmed the importance of ABPI to muscular performance by performing another set on analyses where participants were spilt at the median of percent energy from total protein.

5. Conclusions

We report that measures of muscle thickness and CSA derived from panoramic ultrasonography are more closely related to overall strength than the same measures derived from B-mode ultrasound images. Thus, panoramic images may be a suitable method to measure muscle size and estimate overall muscle mass when the entire transverse area of a muscle cannot be measured with a standardized B-mode image. However, measures of muscle size from B-mode images were more closely related to the performance of knee extensors alone, suggesting that B-mode images may be better measures of individual muscles or muscle groups. Echogenicity of the rectus femoris was unrelated to its specific force and to overall lower-body strength. Instead, echogenicity was related to handgrip strength and knee extensor endurance. Finally, we found a positive relationship between ABPI and lower-body strength, lower-body endurance, and handgrip strength when controlling for physical activity and diet.

Supplementary Materials: The following are available online at https://www.mdpi.com/2077-0383/10/5/988/s1: Supplementary Data File.

Author Contributions: Conceptualization: W.B., S.L.D., K.J.H., J.F.K., and S.N.S.; methodology: W.B., K.J.H., and S.N.S.; validation: W.B., K.J.H., and S.N.S.; formal analysis: W.B., C.J.K., and S.N.S.; investigation: N.D.D., N.R.J., C.J.K., and K.A.T.; resources: W.B., S.L.D., K.J.H., J.F.K., and S.N.S.; data curation: N.R.J.; writing—original draft preparation: N.R.J.; writing—review and editing: W.B., N.D.D., S.L.D., K.J.H., J.F.K., C.J.K., S.N.S., and K.A.T.; visualization: C.J.K. and N.R.J.; supervision: W.B., S.L.D., K.J.H., J.F.K., and S.N.S; project administration: K.J.H. and S.N.S.; funding acquisition: W.B., S.L.D., K.J.H., J.K., and S.N.S. All authors have read and agreed to the published version of the manuscript.

Funding: This project was funded by the Beef Checkoff through the National Cattlemen's Beef Association and the Minnesota Beef Council FAR26929.

Institutional Review Board Statement: The study was approved by the North Dakota State University Institutional Review Board (#HE26929 & 26153) and complied with the Helsinki Declaration of 1983.

Informed Consent Statement: Written informed consent was obtained from all participants in this study.

Data Availability Statement: Data is available as a Supplemental Data File.

Acknowledgments: We are grateful for the undergraduate and graduate students who helped complete the project.

Conflicts of Interest: This project was funded by the National Cattlemen's Beef Association. The sponsor had no role in the design, execution, interpretation, or writing of the study.

References

1. Cruz-Jentoft, A.J.; Bahat, G.; Bauer, J.; Boirie, Y.; Bruyère, O.; Cederholm, T.; Cooper, C.; Landi, F.; Rolland, Y.; Sayer, A.A.; et al. Sarcopenia: Revised European consensus on definition and diagnosis. *Age Ageing* **2019**, *48*, 16–31. [CrossRef] [PubMed]
2. Stokes, T.; Tripp, T.R.; Murphy, K.; Morton, R.W.; Oikawa, S.Y.; Lam Choi, H.; McGrath, J.; McGlory, C.; MacDonald, M.J.; Phillips, S.M. Methodological considerations for and validation of the ultrasonographic determination of human skeletal muscle hypertrophy and atrophy. *Physiol. Rep.* **2021**, *9*, 1–12. [CrossRef]
3. Ponti, F.; de Cinque, A.; Fazio, N.; Napoli, A.; Guglielmi, G.; Bazzocchi, A. Ultrasound imaging, a stethoscope for body composition assessment. *Quant. Imaging Med. Surg.* **2020**, *10*, 1699–1722. [CrossRef] [PubMed]
4. Stringer, H.J.; Wilson, D. The Role of Ultrasound as a Diagnostic Tool for Sarcopenia. *J. Frailty Aging* **2018**, *7*, 258–261. [CrossRef] [PubMed]
5. Fukumoto, Y.; Ikezoe, T.; Yamada, Y.; Tsukagoshi, R.; Nakamura, M.; Mori, N.; Kimura, M.; Ichihashi, N. Skeletal muscle quality assessed from echo intensity is associated with muscle strength of middle-aged and elderly persons. *Eur. J. Appl. Physiol.* **2012**, *112*, 1519–1525. [CrossRef] [PubMed]
6. Yoshiko, A.; Kaji, T.; Sugiyama, H.; Koike, T.; Oshida, Y.; Akima, H. Muscle quality characteristics of muscles in the thigh, upper arm and lower back in elderly men and women. *Eur. J. Appl. Physiol.* **2018**, *118*, 1385–1395. [CrossRef] [PubMed]
7. Ismail, C.; Zabal, J.; Hernandez, H.J.; Woletz, P.; Manning, H.; Teixeira, C.; DiPietro, L.; Blackman, M.R.; Harris-Love, M.O. Diagnostic ultrasound estimates of muscle mass and muscle quality discriminate between women with and without sarcopenia. *Front. Physiol.* **2015**, *6*, 1–10. [CrossRef] [PubMed]
8. Salim, S.Y.; Al-Khathiri, O.; Tandon, P.; Baracos, V.E.; Churchill, T.A.; Warkentin, L.M.; Khadaroo, R.G. Thigh ultrasound used to identify frail elderly patients with sarcopenia undergoing surgery: A pilot study. *J. Surg. Res.* **2020**, *256*, 422–432. [CrossRef]
9. Wilkinson, T.J.; Gore, E.F.; Vadaszy, N.; Nixon, D.G.D.; Watson, E.L.; Smith, A.C. Utility of ultrasound as a valid and accurate diagnostic tool for sarcopenia. *J. Ultrasound Med.* **2020**, 1–11. [CrossRef] [PubMed]
10. Perkisas, S.; Baudry, S.; Bauer, J.; Beckwée, D.; De Cock, A.M.; Hobbelen, H.; Jager-Wittenaar, H.; Kasiukiewicz, A.; Landi, F.; Marco, E.; et al. Application of ultrasound for muscle assessment in sarcopenia: Towards standardized measurements. *Eur. Geriatr. Med.* **2018**, *9*, 739–757. [CrossRef]
11. Scott, J.M.; Martin, D.S.; Ploutz-Snyder, R.; Matz, T.; Caine, T.; Downs, M.; Hackney, K.; Buxton, R.; Ryder, J.W.; Ploutz-Snyder, L. Panoramic ultrasound: A novel and valid tool for monitoring change in muscle mass. *J. Cachexia. Sarcopenia Muscle* **2017**, *8*, 475–481. [CrossRef]
12. Barbat-Artigas, S.; Rolland, Y.; Vellas, B.; Aubertin-Leheudre, M. Muscle quantity is not synonymous with muscle quality. *J. Am. Med. Dir. Assoc.* **2013**, *14*, 852.e1–852.e7. [CrossRef] [PubMed]
13. Strasser, E.M.; Draskovits, T.; Praschak, M.; Quittan, M.; Graf, A. Association between ultrasound measurements of muscle thickness, pennation angle, echogenicity and skeletal muscle strength in the elderly. *Age (Omaha)* **2013**, *35*, 2377–2388. [CrossRef]
14. Abiri, B.; Vafa, M. Nutrition and sarcopenia: A review of the evidence of nutritional influences. *Crit. Rev. Food Sci. Nutr.* **2019**, *59*, 1456–1466. [CrossRef] [PubMed]
15. Deer, R.R.; Volpi, E. Protein intake and muscle function in older adults. *Curr. Opin. Clin. Nutr. Metab. Care* **2015**, *18*, 248–253. [CrossRef]
16. Højfeldt, G.; Nishimura, Y.; Mertz, K.; Schacht, S.R.; Lindberg, J.; Jensen, M.; Hjulmand, M.; Lind, M.V.; Jensen, T.; Jespersen, A.P.; et al. Daily protein and energy intake are not associated with muscle mass and physical function in healthy older individuals—a cross-sectional study. *Nutrients* **2020**, *12*, 1–16. [CrossRef] [PubMed]
17. Gilbert, J.-A.; Bendsen, N.T.; Tremblay, A.; Astrup, A. Effect of proteins from different sources on body composition. *Nutr. Metab. Cardiovasc. Dis.* **2011**, *21* (Suppl. 2), B16–B31. [CrossRef]
18. Berrazaga, I.; Micard, V.; Gueugneau, M.; Walrand, S. The role of the anabolic properties of plant-versus animal-based protein sources in supporting muscle mass maintenance: A critical review. *Nutrients* **2019**, *11*, 1825. [CrossRef] [PubMed]
19. Godin, G. International launch of the PAR-Q+ and ePARmed-X+ The Physical Activity Readiness Questionnaire for Everyone (PAR-Q+) and Electronic Physical Activity Readiness Medical Examination (ePARmed-X+). *Health Fit. J. Canada* **2011**, *4*, 18–22.
20. Abe, T.; Kondo, M.; Kawakami, Y.; Fukunaga, T. Prediction equations for body composition of Japanese adults by B-mode ultrasound. *Am. J. Hum. Biol.* **1994**, *6*, 161–170. [CrossRef] [PubMed]
21. Reimers, C.D.; Harder, T.; Saxe, H. Age-related muscle atrophy does not affect all muscles and can partly be compensated by physical activity: An ultrasound study. *J. Neurol. Sci.* **1998**, *159*, 60–66. [CrossRef]
22. Thoirs, K.; English, C. Ultrasound measures of muscle thickness: Intra-examiner reliability and influence of body position. *Clin. Physiol. Funct. Imaging* **2009**, *29*, 440–446. [CrossRef]
23. Schneider, C.A.; Rasband, W.S.; Eliceiri, K.W. NIH Image to ImageJ: 25 years of image analysis. *Nat. Methods* **2012**, *9*, 671–675. [CrossRef] [PubMed]

24. English, K.L.; Lee, S.M.C.; Loehr, J.A.; Ploutz–Snyder, R.J.; Ploutz–Snyder, L.L. Isokinetic strength changes following long-duration spaceflight on the ISS. *Aerosp. Med. Hum. Perform.* **2015**, *86*, 68–77. [CrossRef]
25. Migueles, J.H.; Rowlands, A.V.; Huber, F.; Sabia, S.; van Hees, V.T. GGIR: A research community–driven open source R package for generating physical activity and sleep outcomes from multi-day raw accelerometer data. *J. Meas. Phys. Behav.* **2019**, *2*, 188–196. [CrossRef]
26. Choi, L.; Liu, Z.; Matthews, C.E.; Buchowski, M.S. Validation of accelerometer wear and nonwear time classification algorithm. *Med. Sci. Sports Exerc.* **2011**, *43*, 357–364. [CrossRef]
27. Chalé-Rush, A.; Guralnik, J.M.; Walkup, M.P.; Miller, M.E.; Rejeski, W.J.; Katula, J.A.; King, A.C.; Glynn, N.W.; Manini, T.M.; Blair, S.N.; et al. Relationship between physical functioning and physical activity in the lifestyle interventions and independence for elders pilot. *J. Am. Geriatr. Soc.* **2010**, *58*, 1918–1924. [CrossRef] [PubMed]
28. Spartano, N.L.; Lyass, A.; Larson, M.G.; Tran, T.; Andersson, C.; Blease, S.J.; Esliger, D.W.; Vasan, R.S.; Murabito, J.M. Objective physical activity and physical performance in middle-aged and older adults. *Exp. Gerontol.* **2019**, *119*, 203–211. [CrossRef]
29. Aslam, M. Using heteroscedasticity-consistent standard errors for the linear regression model with correlated regressors. *Commun. Stat. Simul. Comput.* **2014**, *43*, 2353–2373. [CrossRef]
30. Akima, H.; Yoshiko, A.; Tomita, A.; Ando, R.; Saito, A.; Ogawa, M.; Kondo, S.; Tanaka, N.I. Relationship between quadriceps echo intensity and functional and morphological characteristics in older men and women. *Arch. Gerontol. Geriatr.* **2017**, *70*, 105–111. [CrossRef] [PubMed]
31. Young, H.J.; Jenkins, N.T.; Zhao, Q.; Mccully, K.K. Measurement of intramuscular fat by muscle echo intensity. *Muscle Nerve* **2015**, *52*, 963–971. [CrossRef] [PubMed]
32. Pillen, S.; Tak, R.O.; Zwarts, M.J.; Lammens, M.M.Y.; Verrijp, K.N.; Arts, I.M.P.; van der Laak, J.A.; Hoogerbrugge, P.M.; van Engelen, B.G.M.; Verrips, A. Skeletal muscle ultrasound: Correlation between fibrous tissue and echo intensity. *Ultrasound Med. Biol.* **2009**, *35*, 443–446. [CrossRef] [PubMed]
33. De Stefano, F.; Zambon, S.; Giacometti, L.; Sergi, G.; Corti, M.C.; Manzato, E.; Busetto, L. Obesity, muscular strength, muscle composition and physical performance in an elderly population. *J. Nutr. Health Aging* **2015**, *19*, 785–791. [CrossRef]
34. Hurt, R.T.; McClave, S.A.; Martindale, R.G.; Ochoa Gautier, J.B.; Coss-Bu, J.A.; Dickerson, R.N.; Heyland, D.K.; Hoffer, L.J.; Moore, F.A.; Morris, C.R.; et al. Summary points and consensus recommendations from the International Protein Summit. *Nutr. Clin. Pract.* **2017**, *32*, 142S–151S. [CrossRef] [PubMed]
35. Paddon-Jones, D.; Short, K.R.; Campbell, W.W.; Volpi, E.; Wolfe, R.R. Role of dietary protein in the sarcopenia of aging. *Am. J. Clin. Nutr.* **2008**, *87*, 1562–1566. [CrossRef] [PubMed]
36. Bauer, J.; Biolo, G.; Cederholm, T.; Cesari, M.; Cruz-Jentoft, A.J.; Morley, J.E.; Phillips, S.; Sieber, C.; Stehle, P.; Teta, D.; et al. Evidence-based recommendations for optimal dietary protein intake in older people: A position paper from the PROT-AGE Study Group. *J. Am. Med. Dir. Assoc.* **2013**, *14*, 542–559. [CrossRef] [PubMed]
37. Wonsuk, Y.; Robert, M.; Sejong, B.; Karan, S.; He, Q.; James, W.L.J. A study of effects of multicollinearity in the multivariable analysis. *Int. J. Appl. Sci. Technol.* **2013**, *6*, 9–19.

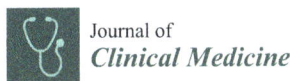 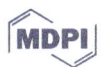

Article

Correlations between the Quality of Life Domains and Clinical Variables in Sarcopenic Osteoporotic Postmenopausal Women

Mariana Cevei [1], Roxana Ramona Onofrei [2,*], Felicia Cioara [1] and Dorina Stoicanescu [3]

[1] Psychoneuro Sciences and Rehabilitation Department, Faculty of Medicine & Pharmacy, University of Oradea, 410087 Oradea, Romania; cevei_mariana@yahoo.com (M.C.); felicia_cioara@yahoo.com (F.C.)
[2] Department of Rehabilitation, Physical Medicine and Rheumatology, "Victor Babeş" University of Medicine and Pharmacy Timişoara, 300041 Timişoara, Romania
[3] Microscopic Morphology Department, "Victor Babeş" University of Medicine and Pharmacy Timişoara, 300041 Timişoara, Romania; dstoicanescu@yahoo.com
* Correspondence: onofrei.roxana@umft.ro

Received: 30 December 2019; Accepted: 4 February 2020; Published: 6 February 2020

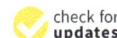

Abstract: (1) Background: both sarcopenia and osteoporosis are major health problems in postmenopausal women. The aim of the study was to evaluate the quality of life (QoL) and the associated factors for sarcopenia in osteoporotic postmenopausal women, diagnosed according to EWGSOP2 criteria. (2) Methods: the study sample comprised 122 osteoporotic postmenopausal women with low hand grip strength and was divided into two groups: group 1 (probable sarcopenia) and group 2 (sarcopenia). QoL was assessed using the validated Romanian version of SarQol questionnaire. (3) Results: the D1, D4, D5, D7 and total SarQoL scores were significantly lower in women from group 2 compared to group 1. In group 2, women older than 70 years had significant lower values for D1, D3, D4, D6 and total SarQoL scores. Age, history of falls and the presence of confirmed and severe sarcopenia were predictors for overall QoL. (4) Conclusions: the frequency of sarcopenia was relatively high in our sample, with body mass index and history of falls as predictors for sarcopenia. Older osteoporotic postmenopausal women, with previous falls and an established sarcopenia diagnosis (low muscle strength and low muscle mass), were more likely to have a decreased quality of life.

Keywords: sarcopenia; quality of life; osteoporosis; postmenopausal women

1. Introduction

Sarcopenia is characterized by decreased muscle strength, loss of muscle mass and poor physical performance [1]. The condition is associated with aging. Aging is a complex process, involving many variables that interact with each other and include, besides genetic factors, lifestyle and chronic diseases. Even if sarcopenia is more common among older individuals, it can also occur earlier in life. It typically begins in the fourth decade of life, but the decline is accelerated after the sixth decade [2,3].

The decrease in muscle strength and muscle mass contributes to the loss of the ability to live independently and thus becomes an important public health problem. Sarcopenia is associated with physical disability, poor physical performance, functional decline, falls, and hospitalization [4]. Multimorbidity is frequent in older individuals and some diseases, such as heart failure or chronic obstructive pulmonary disease, accelerate the loss of muscle strength and mass, creating a vicious cycle [5]. All these have a major impact on the patient's quality of life [6]. Sarcopenia also increases the risk of falls. There is a high risk for hip fractures, as loss of muscle mass is frequently associated with loss of bone [5]. The high risk of falls in sarcopenic patients was found to be regardless of age, gender and other confounding factors [7]. In turn, falls are associated with functional deterioration, physical disability, impairment in activities of daily living, increased morbidity and mortality [8]. In a meta-analysis that included 17 studies, a significant association between sarcopenia and fractures was found, independent of study design, study population, gender, sarcopenia definition, geographical area or study quality [9].

Considering the specificities of older individuals, a sarcopenia-specific quality of life questionnaire (SarQoL) has been developed [10,11] and validated [12]. The Romanian version of the SarQoL® was validated in 2017 [13]. Previous studies have reported the associated factors and the effects on the quality of life in adults with sarcopenia, using different diagnostic criteria. Only a few studies used the revised criteria of the European Working Group on Sarcopenia in Older People (EWGSOP2) [14–16]. The purpose of the present study was to evaluate the quality of life and the associated factors for sarcopenia in Romanian osteoporotic postmenopausal women, using the EWGSOP2 diagnostic criteria.

2. Materials and Methods

2.1. Study Design and Participants

Participants for this observational study were recruited from the postmenopausal women admitted to Medical Rehabilitation Clinical Hospital Băile Felix, România. To be selected, participants had to be previously diagnosed with primary osteoporosis (T-score ≤ −2.5, evaluated by DXA) and to have low hand grip strength. Low hand grip strength was defined according to the EWGSOP2 recommended cut-off of < 16 kg for women and was used to quantify the loss of muscle strength [1]. Criteria for exclusion were: (1) severe mobility disorders of the weight-bearing joints and cases with neurological conditions that affect balance and gait; (2) inability to walk for at least 10 min without a walking aid; (3) history of hip or knee arthroplasty; (4) inflammatory musculoskeletal conditions; (5) malignancies; (6) infectious diseases, (7) diabetic neuropathy; (8) cognitive impairments.

All participants provided written informed consent. The study complied with the Declaration of Helsinki and was approved by the Local Ethics Commission for Scientific Research of Medical Rehabilitation Clinical Hospital Băile Felix, România (4016/30.04.2018).

2.2. Assessments

Socio-demographic and clinical data (age, weight, height, body mass index, marital status, occupational status, years of menopause, history of and tendency towards falls, history of osteoporotic fractures, clinical conditions) were collected by interview and from medical documents. From the medical documents, the appendicular lean muscle mass determined by dual-energy X-ray absorptiometry was recorded for each participant in the study. Based on these results, and according to the recommended EWGSOP2 cut-off points for skeletal muscle mass index (appendicular lean mass/height^2), the participants were categorized as having low muscle mass (<5.5 kg/m^2) and normal muscle mass [1].

2.2.1. Physical Performance

Physical performance was examined by the Timed Up&Go test, with the G-Walk system (BTS Bioengineering, Milan, Italy). It uses a validated wireless inertial sensor, made up of four inertial platforms, each composed of a tri-axial accelerometer, a tri-axial gyroscope and a magnetometer [17]. The G-sensor was attached to the participants fifth lumbar vertebra. The subjects were asked to stand up from a chair, to walk along a 3 m pathway at a self-selected speed, turn around and walk back to the chair and sit down. The recorded data were transmitted to the PC through a Bluetooth connection and processed by the BTS G-studio software (BTS Bioengineering, Milan, Italy). Women who scored ≥ 20 s were considered to have low physical performance.

Cases with low muscle strength were classified as having probable sarcopenia. We considered all participants that met the two EWGSOP2 diagnostic criteria-low muscle strength and low muscle mass—to have confirmed sarcopenia. Women with confirmed sarcopenia and low physical performance were categorized as having severe sarcopenia, according to the EWGSOP2 revised criteria [1]. We divided the study sample in two groups: group 1 comprised participants with probable sarcopenia ($n = 58$) and group 2, those with an established sarcopenia diagnosis, which included participants with confirmed and severe sarcopenia, according to EWGSOP2 ($n = 64$).

2.2.2. Quality of Life

The quality of life was assessed using the validated Romanian version of SarQol questionnaire (Sarcopenia Quality of Life). This is a multidimensional questionnaire, evaluating seven domains of health-related quality of life—physical and mental health (D1), locomotion (D2), body composition (D3), functionality (D4), activities of daily living (D5), leisure activities (D6) and fears (D7) [10]. The 22 questions are rated on a 4-point Likert scale. Each domain is scored from 0 to 100 and an overall score is calculated. A higher score reflects a higher quality of life [12]. The SarQol questionnaire has good internal consistency and construct validity, good discriminative power and good responsiveness [12–14,18].

2.3. Statistical Analysis

The statistical analysis was performed using the Medcalc Statistical Software version 19.1 (MedCalc Software bv, Ostend, Belgium). All data were tested for normality with the Shapiro–Wilk's test. Descriptive statistics were calculated for all socio-demographics' characteristics (frequencies, means and standard deviation), SarQoL scores and TUG (median and interquartile range (IQR)). Between-groups differences were assessed using the independent t-test and Mann–Whitney test, respectively. Categorical data were compared using Chi-squared test. Logistic regression analysis was used to identify the factors associated with sarcopenia. Odds ratios (OR), 95% confidence intervals (CI) and p values were reported. Spearman rank correlation coefficient was used to assess the relationship between socio-demographic and clinical factors and the SarQoL scores. Variables that demonstrated significance were then entered into a stepwise multiple linear regression analysis to assess the predictors of quality of life, with SarQoL domains and total scores as a dependent variable. The significance level was set at $p < 0.05$ for all tests.

3. Results

The study sample comprised 122 women (mean age 67.02 ± 8.3 years) (ranging between 48 and 83 years) that met the inclusion criteria and agreed to participate in the study. More than half of the participants (52.46%) were diagnosed with confirmed and severe sarcopenia.

Table 1 summarizes the characteristics of the participants. There were no significant differences between the two groups in participants' characteristics, except for weight, BMI and fall history. There was a higher percent of overweight and obese women in group 1 compared to group 2 ($p < 0.0001$). The proportion of overweight or obese women in our sample was 69.67%. A total of 93.10% of participants with probable sarcopenia and 48.43% of those with sarcopenia were overweight or obese. Women with sarcopenia had a higher frequency of history of falls than those with probable sarcopenia ($p = 0.03$).

Table 1. Socio-Demographic and Clinical Characteristics.

	All (n = 122)	Group 1 (n = 58)	Group 2 (n = 64)	p
Age, years	67.02 ± 8.03	66.48 ± 7.76	67.5 ± 8.79	NS
<60 years	26 (21.31)	10 (17.24)	16 (25)	
60–69 years	49 (40.16)	29 (50)	20 (31.25)	NS
>70 years	47 (38.53)	19 (32.76)	28 (43.75)	
Weight, kg	67.82 ± 11.02	72.34 ± 9.56	63.72 ± 10.69	<0.0001
Height, cm	157.93 ± 6.19	158 ± 6.18	157.9 ± 6.25	NS
BMI, kg/m^2	27.22 ± 4.28	29.07 ± 3.71	25.55 ± 4.1	<0.0001
Underweight (<18.5 kg/m^2)	3 (2.46)	1 (1.72)	2 (3.13)	
Normal (18.5–24.9 kg/m^2)	34 (27.87)	3 (5.17)	31 (48.44)	<0.0001
Overweight (25–29.9 kg/m^2)	55 (45.08)	33 (56.9)	22 (34.37)	
Obese (>30 kg/m^2)	30 (24.59)	21 (36.21)	9 (14.06)	
Years of menopause	19.66 ± 9.1	19.21 ± 8.25	20.08 ± 9.85	NS
Tendency to fall	55 (45.08)	24 (41.38)	31 (48.44)	NS
Fall history	28 (22.95)	8 (13.79)	20 (31.25)	0.02
Osteoporotic fractures history	30 (24.59)	18 (31.03)	12 (18.75)	NS
Number of comorbitites	5.85 ± 2.07	6 ± 1.97	5.72 ± 2.17	NS
Education				NS
Primary education (<8 classes)	52 (42.63)	23 (39.66)	29 (45.31)	
High school	50 (40.98)	27 (46.55)	23 (35.94)	
University	20 (16.39)	8 (13.79)	12 (18.75)	
Marital status				NS
Married	73 (59.84)	39 (67.24)	34 (53.13)	
Single	49 (40.16)	19 (32.76)	30 (46.88)	
Occupational status				NS
Working	46 (37.7)	23 (39.66)	23 (35.94)	
Retired	76 (62.3)	35 (60.34)	41 (64.06)	
Physical performance				
TUG (s)	19.6 (15.17–25.5)	19.45 (14.75–25.13)	19.65 (15.65–26.74)	NS
TUG>20s	61 (50)	28 (48.27)	33 (51.56)	NS

Data are presented as mean ± SD, number (percentage) or median [IQR]

The associations between the socio-demographic and clinical factors and the presence of sarcopenia were analysed by logistic regression. The factors significantly associated with sarcopenia were BMI (OR 0.79, 95%CI 0.71–0.88, $p < 0.0001$) and the history of falls (OR 2.84, 95%CI 1.13–7.09, $p = 0.003$). After adjusting for covariates (age, marital status, number of comorbidities and years since menopause), multiple logistic regression showed that BMI (OR 0.77, 95%CI 0.69–0.87, $p < 0.0001$) and the history of falls (OR 3.95, 95%CI 1.38–11.29, $p = 0.01$) together can predict the sarcopenic status. A lower BMI associated with at least one fall in the past would predispose osteoporotic postmenopausal women to sarcopenia.

Table 2 presents the total scores, as well as each domain scores of the SarQoL questionnaire. The D1, D4, D5, D7 and total SarQoL scores were significantly lower in women from group 2 compared to group 1.

In the whole study sample, significant lower scores were observed for D1, D4, D5, D7 and total SarQoL scores in the > 70 years group compared to the other two age groups, and for D2 and D3 in the > 70 years compared to the < 60 years group. In the probable sarcopenia group, no significant differences in all the SarQoL scores were observed between age groups. In group 2, women older than 70 years had significantly lower values for D1, D3, D4, D6 and total SarQoL scores than those from the other two age groups. For the D5 and D7 domains, women from group 2, older than 70 years, had significantly lower scores than those younger than 60 years ($p < 0.05$). When comparing the SarQoL scores between the two groups based on age, significantly lower scores were recorded only in the >70 years old group for D3, D4, D5 and total scores.

Table 2. Results of the SarQol Questionnaire in the Three Age Groups.

SarQoL Domains	All (n = 122)	Group 1 (n = 58)	Group 2 (n = 64)	p [a]
D1	52.20 (45.50–65.50)	56.65 (48.90–72.20)	54.10 (49.45–62.20)	0.01
<60 years	58.30 (51.38–75.50)	66.65 (54.68–79.13)	53.85 (48.9–69.73)	NS
60–69	57.80 (48.90–67.20)	58.90 (52.20–71.1)	55.50 (42.25–65.60)	NS
>70 years	47.80 (37.80–55.50) [b,c]	52.20 (45.50–58.9)	47.80 (35.25–51.93) [b,c]	NS
D2	55.60 (47.20–66.70)	56.95 (50–70.10)	55.60 (42.38–63.90)	NS
<60 years	59.70 (55.60–70.10)	68.05 (54.85–73.60)	58.30 (55.60–66)	NS
60–69	55.60 (50–68.05)	55.60 (50–72.20)	53.50 (47.20–63.90)	NS
>70 years	50 (38.90–61.10) [c]	55.60 (50–63.90)	47.20 (31.28–61.10)	NS
D3	54.20 (45.80–66.70)	58.3 (48.95–66.07)	54.20 (41.70–65.65)	NS
<60 years	60.40 (53.15–70.80)	64.6 (50–68.78)	58.30 (54.20–70.80)	NS
60–69	58.30 (45.8–70.80)	58.30 (45.80–68.75)	58.30 (46.85–73.95)	NS
>70 years	50 (37.50–62.50) [c]	50 (50–66.7)	45.80 (37.50–57.28) [b,c]	<0.05
D4	63.50 (53.32–75)	67.3 (57.7–78.6)	59.60 (50–70.80)	0.01
<60 years	69.60 (66.35–78.65)	73.10 (67.3–80.38)	68.75 (62.75–77.85)	NS
60–69	63.50 (56.45–78.7)	63.50 (57.70–78.80)	63 (52.78–75.98)	NS
>70 years	55.80 (48.10–69.20) [b,c]	65.40 (55.80–71.20)	50 (45.18–55.80) [b,c]	<0.05
D5	48.25 (37.30–60.17)	53.30 (43.30–66.25)	43.30 (33.30–55.60)	0.001
<60 years	56.70 (44.58–66.65)	59.15 (56.28–80.53)	51.65 (43–63.65)	NS
60–69	48.30 (41.70–63.80)	51.70 (42.50–66.30)	48.30 (34.20–61.45)	NS
>70 years	40 (33.30–50) [b,c]	46.70 (38.30–60.70)	35.85 (30.83–45.45) [c]	<0.05
D6	33.30 (16.60–33.3)	33.30 (16.60–52.85)	33.3 (16.6–33.3)	NS
<60 years	33.30 (16.60–37.45)	33.30 (12.45–41.60)	33.30 (33.30–45.75)	NS
60–69	33.30 (33.30–55.80)	33.30 (16.60–66.50)	33.30 (33.30–33.30)	NS
>70 years	33.30 (0–33.30) [b]	33.30 (16.60–33.30)	24.95 (0–33.30) [b,c]	NS
D7	87.50 (75–87.50)	87.5 (84.38–100)	87.50 (75–87.50)	0.006
<60 years	87.50 (87.50–100)	87.5 (87.50–100)	87.50 (77.08–96.88)	NS
60–69	87.5 (75–100)	87.5 (81.25–100)	87.50 (75–87.50)	NS
>70 years	75 (62.50–87.50) [b,c]	87.5 (75–87.50)	75 (62.50–87.50) [c]	NS
Total	55.45 (46.57–65.10)	57.90 (51.23–67.23)	53.33 (44.23–59.20)	0.003
<60 years	60.75 (54.30–68.05)	65.30 (59.33–76.2)	59 (54.30–66.98)	NS
60–69	56.30 (49.85–66.45)	59.90 (51.45–67.85)	56.30 (46.15–64.60)	NS
>70 years	48.10 (39.60–57.80) [b,c]	56.10 (48.10–59.90)	45.25 (38.75–52.75) [b,c]	<0.05

Data are presented as median and (IQR); p [a] relates to group 1–group 2 comparison (p < 0.05); [b] relates to the > 70 years and 60–69 years comparison (p < 0.05); [c] relates to the >70 years and <60 years (p < 0.05).

Physical performance did not differ significantly between the two groups. Low physical performance assessed with TUG (TUG > 20 s) was observed in 28 women from group 1 (48.27%) and in 34 women from group 2 (53.12%). According to the EWGSOP2 criteria, 53.12% women from group 2 were classified as having severe sarcopenia when using TUG performance. No age differences were observed between those with confirmed sarcopenia and those with severe sarcopenia.

In the whole study sample and in the probable sarcopenia group, significant greater TUG scores were observed in women older than 70 years compared to those younger than 60 years (21.8(17.9–30.6) vs. 16.3(13.3–21.38) s, p = 0.001 for the whole sample; 25.10(19.06–33.3) vs. 13.90(9.54–17.18) s, p < 0.001 for the probable sarcopenia group).

Significant negative correlations were found between SarQoL domains and total scores and some of the socio-anthropometric data for the whole study sample (Table 3). The history of falls and the number of comorbidities were negatively correlated with all SarQoL scores, except the D6 domains.

Table 3. Correlations between Sarqol Domaines and Clinical Variables.

	SarQoL D1	SarQoL D2	SarQoL D3	SarQoL D4	SarQoL D5	SarQoL D6	SarQoL D7	SarQoL Total
Age	−0.339 *	−0.238	−0.141	−0.318 *	−0.339 *	−0.062	−0.392 *	−0.392 *
BMI	−0.374 *	−0.171	−0.196	−0.302 *	−0.207	−0.184	−0.214	−0.297 *
Years of menopause	−0.379 *	−0.205	−0.153	−0.264 *	−0.303 *	0.017	−0.323 *	−0.314 *
No of comorbidities	−0.455 *	−0.312 *	−0.425 *	−0.396 *	−0.305 *	−0.204	−0.307 *	−0.381 *
Tendency to fall	−0.110	−0.113	−0.092	−0.077	−0.006	−0.059	−0.197	−0.086
Falls history	−0.406 *	−0.315 *	−0.344 *	−0.330 *	−0.263 *	−0.148	−0.361 *	−0.372 *
Osteoporotic fractures history	−0.061	0.08	−0.008	−0.059	−0.057	−0.150	0.005	−0.03
TUG	−0.206	−0.19	−0.137	−0.217	−0.236	0.053	−0.307 *	−0.244

Data represents the Spearman correlation coefficient; * $p < 0.05$

The stepwise multiple linear regression analysis with SarQoL total score as a dependent variable revealed a negative association with age, history of falls and being sarcopenic (adjusted $R^2 = 0.238$; $F_{3,118} = 13.59$, $p < 0.0001$). Being older, sarcopenic with at least one fall in the past would negatively affect the quality of life of osteoporotic postmenopausal women. Table 4 shows the results of the regression analysis for all the SarQoL scores. In all regression models, history of falls was negatively correlated with all quality of life questionnaire domains, indicating that osteoporotic postmenopausal women with low muscle strength and falls in the past will have a poorer quality of life.

Table 4. Multiple Linear Regression Analysis with the Total and the Seven Domain Scores of SarQoL as Dependent Variables.

Independent Variable	B	SE	Beta	T	p	R^2	Adjusted R^2	Model Significance
SarQoL Total Score								
1. Age	−0.443	0.149	−0.268	−3.023	0.003	0.256	0.238	$F_{3,118} = 13.59$ $p < 0.0001$
2. Fall history	−10.318	2.946	−0.306	−3.502	0.0001			
3. Sarcopenia (confirmed and severe)	−5.140	2.365	−0.196	0.031	0.03			
SarQoL D1								
1. Age	−0.425	0.17	−0.222	−2.483	0.01	0.248	0.228	$F_{3,118} = 12.97$ $p < 0.0001$
2. Number of comorbidities	−1.454	0.66	−0.198	−2.202	0.02			
3. Fall history	−11.562	3.262	−0.310	−3.544	0.0006			
SarQoL D2								
1. Fall history	−15.035	3.608	−0.355	−4.167	0.0001	0.126	0.119	$F_{1,120} = 17.3$ $p = 0.0001$
SarQoL D3								
1. Number of comorbidities	−1.628	0.653	−0.222	−2.491	0.01	0.135	0.116	$F_{2,119} = 9$ $p = 0.0002$
2. Fall history	−9.679	3.208	−2.66	−3.017	0.003			
SarQoL D4								
1. Age	−0.474	0.145	−0.286	−3.259	0.001	0.261	0.249	$F_{2,119} = 21.07$ $p < 0.0001$
2. Fall history	−12.440	2.865	−0.369	−4.341	<0.0001			
SarQoL D5								
1. Age	−0.540	0.190	−0.252	−2.838	0.006	0.189	0.168	$F_{3,118} = 9.186$ $p < 0.0001$
2. Fall history	−7.976	3.820	−0.188	−2.088	0.01			
3. Sarcopenia (confirmed and severe)	−7.522	3.066	−0.220	−2.453	0.01			
SarQoL D6								
1. Fall history	−12.402	4.671	−0.235	−2.655	0.009	0.055	0.047	$F_{1,120} = 7.04$ $p = 0.009$
SarQoL D7								
1. Years of menopause	−0.458	0.137	−0.293	−3.344	0.001	0.187	0.174	$F_{2,119} = 13.75$ $p < 0.0001$
2. Fall history	−8.802	2.954	−0.263	−2.980	0.003			

4. Discussion

The main aim of this study was to assess the relationship between sarcopenia and the quality of life in osteoporotic postmenopausal women. Both sarcopenia and osteoporosis are major health problems in postmenopausal women, negatively affecting the quality of life [19–21], the incidence of falls, and mortality [22–25]. To the best of our knowledge, there are no studies investigating the quality of life in Romanian postmenopausal osteoporotic women diagnosed with sarcopenia according to the updated EWGSOP diagnostic criteria.

There are several definitions, diagnostic criteria and cut-offs used for the diagnosis of sarcopenia [1,26–31]. In our study, we used the revised EWGSOP2 criteria. The percentage of confirmed and severe sarcopenia in osteoporotic postmenopausal women aged between 48 and 83 years at the time of assessment was 52.46%. Similar results were also found in other studies, showing the association of sarcopenia and osteoporosis [32–37]. Walsh et al., reported a similar prevalence of sarcopenia of 50% in osteoporotic postmenopausal women, using the loss of muscle mass for the sarcopenia diagnosis [38]. Hamad et al. found that sarcopenia was present in 74.6% of postmenopausal women with osteoporosis, supporting the results of Yoshimura that osteoporosis increases the risk of sarcopenia [39,40]. Studies indicate that the prevalence of sarcopenia increases with age [41,42]. In our study, the percentage of osteoporotic postmenopausal women diagnosed with sarcopenia increased with age, with 43.75% of women being older than 70 years. The true prevalence of sarcopenia cannot be correctly estimated, since various definitions, cut-offs or populations were used across studies.

History of falls and BMI were significantly associated with the presence of sarcopenia in osteoporotic postmenopausal women. Our results showed that osteoporotic postmenopausal women with at least one fall in the past had a significantly higher risk of developing sarcopenia. Similar results were presented by Clynes et al., who reported an association of falls in the last year and sarcopenia, diagnosed using the IWGS (International Working Group of Sarcopenia) definition, but not the EWGSOP one [43]. In their meta-analysis, Yeung et al. also reported a positive association between sarcopenia and falls [9]. Sepulveda-Loyola et al. found a strong association between osteosarcopenia (defined as the concomitant presence of osteoporosis/osteopenia with sarcopenia [44]) and falls and fractures history in community-dwelling older adults [45]. Other prospective studies have reported the association between sarcopenia and the incidence and risk of falls [7,46–48].

We found that BMI was lower in sarcopenic women than in those with probable sarcopenia from group 1. There was a higher percent of overweight and obese women with probable sarcopenia compared to those with an established sarcopenia diagnosis. In the sarcopenic group, we identified 14.06% cases of sarcopenic obesity. In recent years, the prevalence of obesity combined with sarcopenia had increased, resulting in a high-risk geriatric syndrome. Affected individuals are at risk of synergistic complications from both sarcopenia and obesity [49].

The logistic regression results in our study showed that osteoporotic postmenopausal women with a higher body mass index had a significantly reduced risk of developing sarcopenia. Similar results were found in previous studies [50–52], although in these studies the comparisons were made with non-sarcopenic subjects. Other studies also reported the protective effect of high body mass against sarcopenia in Asian population [53–55]. Moreno-Aguilar et al. found that a higher BMI represents a protective factor against the presence of osteosarcopenia [56]. Despite these findings, in a recent meta-analysis Shen et al. suggested, as well as Gonzales et al. in 2017, that BMI should not be used for making clinically important decisions at the individual patient level, since it could not differentiate between body weight components (body fat and lean mass) [57,58].

The SarQoL questionnaire is a specific health-related quality of life questionnaire for sarcopenia and muscle impairments [59]. Previous studies have demonstrated the ability of SarQoL to discriminate sarcopenic individuals with regard to their quality of life, as long as for the diagnosis of sarcopenia both muscle mass and muscle strength criteria were used [12,13,59–61]. The present study showed that osteoporotic postmenopausal women with probable and established sarcopenia had a reduced quality of life, as assessed with the SarQoL questionnaire. Our results were slightly lower than those obtained in previous studies by the sarcopenic participants [12,14,59–62]. We have to mention that, in previous studies, the EWGSOP criteria were used for establishing the diagnosis of sarcopenia, with a few exceptions where the revised EWGSOP2 criteria were used [14,62,63]. We found that the domains of physical and mental health (D1), functionality (D4), activities of daily living (D5), fears

(D7) and total SarQoL scores were significantly lower in women with sarcopenia than those with probable sarcopenia. For locomotion (D2), body composition (D3) and leisure activities (D6) domains we have not found significant differences between sarcopenic groups. Similar results were found for the D6 domain in the study of Gasparik et al., with no significant differences between sarcopenic and non-sarcopenic participants when using the Romanian version of the SarQoL, as well as in the study of Konstantynowicz et al., who used the Polish version of the SarQoL [13,60]. The reason could be due to the fact that Romanian and Polish older people are not involved in many leisure activities [60].

In our study, osteoporotic postmenopausal women with sarcopenia who were older than 70 years had significantly lower values for physical and mental health (D1), body composition (D3), functionality (D4), leisure (D6) and total SarQoL scores than the younger ones. In the probable sarcopenia cases, the SarQoL scores were not influenced by age.

The negative impact of sarcopenia on quality of life has been largely investigated, although different criteria and questionnaires were used. The physical function domain of the quality of life has been proved to be impaired in sarcopenic patients, as assessed by the SF-36 questionnaire [52,64–67].

The multiple regression analysis in the present study showed a significant impact of age, history of falls and the presence of sarcopenia on the overall quality of life of postmenopausal osteoporotic women, as assessed with the SarQoL questionnaire. Older osteoporotic postmenopausal women with previous falls were more likely to have lower scores on physical and mental health (D1), functionality (D4) and activities of daily living (D5) domains. In association with the history of falls, the number of comorbidities was found to be a predictor only in the physical and mental health domain (D1) and body composition domain scores, respectively. Years since menopause, along with the history of falls, negatively influenced the fear domain (D7) score.

Several limitations of this study should be addressed. The study sample comprised only osteoporotic postmenopausal women with low grip strength, and no control group (premenopausal, non-sarcopenic) was included. Another issue that has to be mentioned is that the number of comorbidities was quite high and could influence the quality of life. The sample could have also been biased compared to the normal population, since the subjects were recruited from a rehabilitation clinic.

5. Conclusions

In summary, in our sample of osteoporotic postmenopausal women, the frequency of sarcopenia, as defined with the EWGSOP2 criteria, was relatively high. The body mass index and the history of falls could predict, together, sarcopenia in osteoporotic postmenopausal women. Our results showed that osteoporotic postmenopausal women with at least one fall in the past and a lower body mass index had a significantly higher risk of developing sarcopenia. History of falls and the number of comorbidities were negatively correlated with all quality of life questionnaire domains, indicating that postmenopausal women with low muscle strength and falls in the past will have a poorer quality of life. Older osteoporotic postmenopausal women, with previous falls and a confirmed sarcopenia diagnosis (low muscle strength and low muscle mass) were more likely to have a decreased quality of life. Future studies are required to identify women at risk, in order to reduce the prevalence of sarcopenia and its negative effects.

Author Contributions: Conceptualization, M.C., D.S. and R.R.O.; methodology, M.C., D.S., F.C. and R.R.O.; formal analysis, M.C., D.S., F.C. and R.R.O.; investigation, M.C. and F.C.; data curation, D.S. and R.R.O.; writing—original draft preparation, M.C., D.S., F.C. and R.R.O.; writing—review and editing, M.C., D.S. and R.R.O.; visualization, M.C., D.S., F.C. and R.R.O.; supervision, M.C. All authors have read and agreed to the published version of the manuscript.

Conflicts of Interest: The authors declare no conflict of interest.

References

1. Cruz-Jentoft, A.J.; Bahat, G.; Bauer, J.; Boirie, Y.; Bruyère, O.; Cederholm, T.; Cooper, C.; Landi, F.; Rolland, Y.; Sayer, A.A.; et al. Sarcopenia: Revised European consensus on definition and diagnosis. *Age Ageing* **2019**, *48*, 16–31. [CrossRef] [PubMed]
2. Han, A.; Bokshan, S.; Marcaccio, S.; DePasse, J.; Daniels, A. Diagnostic Criteria and Clinical Outcomes in Sarcopenia Research: A Literature Review. *J. Clin. Med.* **2018**, *7*, 70. [CrossRef] [PubMed]
3. Roubenoff, R.; Hughes, V.A. Sarcopenia: Current concepts. *J. Gerontol. Ser. A Biol. Sci. Med. Sci.* **2000**, *55*, M716–M724. [CrossRef] [PubMed]
4. Beaudart, C.; Rizzoli, R.; Bruyère, O.; Reginster, J.Y.; Biver, E. Sarcopenia: Burden and challenges for public health. *Arch. Public Health* **2014**, *72*, 45. [CrossRef]
5. Morley, J.E.; Anker, S.D.; von Haehling, S. Prevalence, incidence, and clinical impact of sarcopenia: Facts, numbers, and epidemiology—Update 2014. *J. Cachexia. Sarcopenia Muscle* **2014**, *5*, 253–259. [CrossRef]
6. Rizzoli, R.; Reginster, J.Y.; Arnal, J.F.; Bautmans, I.; Beaudart, C.; Bischoff-Ferrari, H.; Biver, E.; Boonen, S.; Brandi, M.L.; Chines, A.; et al. Quality of life in sarcopenia and frailty. *Calcif. Tissue Int.* **2013**, *93*, 101–120. [CrossRef]
7. Landi, F.; Liperoti, R.; Russo, A.; Giovannini, S.; Tosato, M.; Capoluongo, E.; Bernabei, R.; Onder, G. Sarcopenia as a risk factor for falls in elderly individuals: Results from the ilSIRENTE study. *Clin. Nutr.* **2012**, *31*, 652–658. [CrossRef]
8. Terroso, M.; Rosa, N.; Torres Marques, A.; Simoes, R. Physical consequences of falls in the elderly: A literature review from 1995 to 2010. *Eur. Rev. Aging Phys. Act.* **2014**, *11*, 51–59. [CrossRef]
9. Yeung, S.S.Y.; Reijnierse, E.M.; Pham, V.K.; Trappenburg, M.C.; Lim, W.K.; Meskers, C.G.M.; Maier, A.B. Sarcopenia and its association with falls and fractures in older adults: A systematic review and meta-analysis. *J. Cachexia. Sarcopenia Muscle* **2019**, *10*, 485–500. [CrossRef]
10. Beaudart, C.; Biver, E.; Reginster, J.Y.; Rizzoli, R.; Rolland, Y.; Bautmans, I.; Petermans, J.; Gillain, S.; Buckinx, F.; Van Beveren, J.; et al. Development of a self-administrated quality of life questionnaire for sarcopenia in elderly subjects: The SarQoL. *Age Ageing* **2015**, *44*, 960–966. [CrossRef]
11. Beaudart, C.; Reginster, J.Y.; Geerinck, A.; Locquet, M.; Bruyère, O. Current review of the SarQoL®: A health-related quality of life questionnaire specific to sarcopenia. *Expert Rev. Pharm. Outcomes Res.* **2017**, *17*, 335–341. [CrossRef] [PubMed]
12. Beaudart, C.; Biver, E.; Reginster, J.Y.; Rizzoli, R.; Rolland, Y.; Bautmans, I.; Petermans, J.; Gillain, S.; Buckinx, F.; Dardenne, N.; et al. Validation of the SarQoL®, a specific health-related quality of life questionnaire for Sarcopenia. *J. Cachexia. Sarcopenia Muscle* **2017**, *8*, 238–244. [CrossRef] [PubMed]
13. Ildiko, G.A.; Gabriela, M.; Charlotte, B.; Olivier, B.; Raluca-Monica, P.; Jean-Yves, R.; Maria, P.I. Psychometric performance of the Romanian version of the SarQoL®, a health-related quality of life questionnaire for sarcopenia. *Arch. Osteoporos.* **2017**, *12*. [CrossRef] [PubMed]
14. Alekna, V.; Kilaite, J.; Tamulaitiene, M.; Geerinck, A.; Mastaviciute, A.; Bruyère, O.; Reginster, J.Y.; Beaudart, C. Validation of the Lithuanian version of sarcopenia-specific quality of life questionnaire (SarQoL®). *Eur. Geriatr. Med.* **2019**. [CrossRef]
15. Franzon, K.; Zethelius, B.; Cederholm, T.; Kilander, L. The impact of muscle function, muscle mass and sarcopenia on independent ageing in very old Swedish men. *BMC Geriatr.* **2019**, *19*, 153. [CrossRef]
16. Su, Y.; Hirayama, K.; Han, T.; Izutsu, M.; Yuki, M. Sarcopenia Prevalence and Risk Factors among Japanese Community Dwelling Older Adults Living in a Snow-Covered City According to EWGSOP2. *J. Clin. Med.* **2019**, *8*, 291. [CrossRef]
17. Available online: https://www.btsbioengineering.com/products/g-walk-inertial-motion-system. (accessed on 7 October 2019).
18. Geerinck, A.; Bruyère, O.; Locquet, M.; Reginster, J.Y.; Beaudart, C. Evaluation of the Responsiveness of the SarQoL® Questionnaire, a Patient-Reported Outcome Measure Specific to Sarcopenia. *Adv. Ther.* **2018**, *35*, 1842–1858. [CrossRef]
19. Stoicanescu, D.L.; Cevei, M.L.; Guler, N. Physical function limitation in osteoporotic cases. *Osteoporos. Int.* **2018**, *29*, 416–417.
20. Cevei, M.; Stoicanescu, D.; Suciu, R.; Cioara, F. Immobilization osteoporosis and sarcopenia in patients with vertebromedullary trauma. *Osteoporos. Int.* **2019**, *30*, 444.

21. Go, S.W.; Cha, Y.H.; Lee, J.A.; Park, H.S. Association between sarcopenia, bone density, and health-related quality of life in korean men. *Korean J. Fam. Med.* **2013**, *34*, 281–288. [CrossRef]
22. Beaudart, C.; Zaaria, M.; Pasleau, F.; Reginster, J.Y.; Bruyère, O. Health outcomes of sarcopenia: A systematic review and meta-analysis. *PLoS ONE* **2017**, *12*, e0169548. [CrossRef] [PubMed]
23. Lang, T.; Streeper, T.; Cawthon, P.; Baldwin, K.; Taaffe, D.R.; Harris, T.B. Sarcopenia: Etiology, clinical consequences, intervention, and assessment. *Osteoporos. Int.* **2010**, *21*, 543–559. [CrossRef] [PubMed]
24. Sim, M.; Prince, R.L.; Scott, D.; Daly, R.M.; Duque, G.; Inderjeeth, C.A.; Zhu, K.; Woodman, R.J.; Hodgson, J.M.; Lewis, J.R. Sarcopenia Definitions and Their Associations With Mortality in Older Australian Women. *J. Am. Med. Dir. Assoc.* **2019**, *20*, 76–82. [CrossRef] [PubMed]
25. Greco, E.A.; Pietschmann, P.; Migliaccio, S. Osteoporosis and sarcopenia increase frailty syndrome in the elderly. *Front. Endocrinol. (Lausanne)* **2019**, *10*, 255. [CrossRef]
26. Cruz-Jentoft, A.J.; Baeyens, J.P.; Bauer, J.M.; Boirie, Y.; Cederholm, T.; Landi, F.; Martin, F.C.; Michel, J.-P.; Rolland, Y.; Schneider, S.M.; et al. Sarcopenia: European consensus on definition and diagnosis: Report of the European Working Group on Sarcopenia in Older People. *Age Ageing* **2010**, *39*, 412–423. [CrossRef]
27. Fielding, R.A.; Vellas, B.; Evans, W.J.; Bhasin, S.; Morley, J.E.; Newman, A.B.; Abellan van Kan, G.; Andrieu, S.; Bauer, J.; Breuille, D.; et al. Sarcopenia: An Undiagnosed Condition in Older Adults. Current Consensus Definition: Prevalence, Etiology, and Consequences. International Working Group on Sarcopenia. *J. Am. Med. Dir. Assoc.* **2011**, *12*, 249–256. [CrossRef]
28. Morley, J.E.; Abbatecola, A.M.; Argiles, J.M.; Baracos, V.; Bauer, J.; Bhasin, S.; Cederholm, T.; Stewart Coats, A.J.; Cummings, S.R.; Evans, W.J.; et al. Sarcopenia With Limited Mobility: An International Consensus. *J. Am. Med. Dir. Assoc.* **2011**, *12*, 403–409. [CrossRef]
29. Delmonico, M.J.; Harris, T.B.; Lee, J.S.; Visser, M.; Nevitt, M.; Kritchevsky, S.B.; Tylavsky, F.A.; Newman, A.B. Alternative definitions of sarcopenia, lower extremity performance, and functional impairment with aging in older men and women. *J. Am. Geriatr. Soc.* **2007**, *55*, 769–774. [CrossRef]
30. Muscaritoli, M.; Anker, S.D.; Argilés, J.; Aversa, Z.; Bauer, J.M.; Biolo, G.; Boirie, Y.; Bosaeus, I.; Cederholm, T.; Costelli, P.; et al. Consensus definition of sarcopenia, cachexia and pre-cachexia: Joint document elaborated by Special Interest Groups (SIG) cachexia-anorexia in chronic wasting diseases and nutrition in geriatrics. *Clin. Nutr.* **2010**, *29*, 154–159. [CrossRef]
31. Studenski, S.A.; Peters, K.W.; Alley, D.E.; Cawthon, P.M.; McLean, R.R.; Harris, T.B.; Ferrucci, L.; Guralnik, J.M.; Fragala, M.S.; Kenny, A.M.; et al. The FNIH Sarcopenia Project: Rationale, Study Description, Conference Recommendations, and Final Estimates. *J. Gerontol. Ser. A* **2014**, *69*, 547–558. [CrossRef]
32. Sjöblom, S.; Suuronen, J.; Rikkonen, T.; Honkanen, R.; Kröger, H.; Sirola, J. Relationship between postmenopausal osteoporosis and the components of clinical sarcopenia. *Maturitas* **2013**, *75*, 175–180. [CrossRef] [PubMed]
33. Miyakoshi, N.; Hongo, M.; Mizutani, Y.; Shimada, Y. Prevalence of sarcopenia in Japanese women with osteopenia and osteoporosis. *J. Bone Miner. Metab.* **2013**, *31*, 556–561. [CrossRef] [PubMed]
34. He, H.; Liu, Y.; Tian, Q.; Papasian, C.J.; Hu, T.; Deng, H.-W. Relationship of sarcopenia and body composition with osteoporosis. *Osteoporos. Int.* **2016**, *27*, 473–482. [CrossRef] [PubMed]
35. Nielsen, B.R.; Abdulla, J.; Andersen, H.E.; Schwarz, P.; Suetta, C. Sarcopenia and osteoporosis in older people: A systematic review and meta-analysis. *Eur. Geriatr. Med.* **2018**, *9*, 419–434. [CrossRef]
36. Tarantino, U.; Baldi, J.; Celi, M.; Rao, C.; Liuni, F.M.; Iundusi, R.; Gasbarra, E. Osteoporosis and sarcopenia: The connections. *Aging Clin. Exp. Res.* **2013**, *25*, 93–95. [CrossRef]
37. Reiss, J.; Iglseder, B.; Alzner, R.; Mayr-Pirker, B.; Pirich, C.; Kässmann, H.; Kreutzer, M.; Dovjak, P.; Reiter, R. Sarcopenia and osteoporosis are interrelated in geriatric inpatients. *Z. Gerontol. Geriatr.* **2019**, *52*, 688–693. [CrossRef]
38. Walsh, M.C.; Hunter, G.R.; Livingstone, M.B. Sarcopenia in premenopausal and postmenopausal women with osteopenia, osteoporosis and normal bone mineral density. *Osteoporos. Int.* **2006**, *17*, 61–67. [CrossRef]
39. Hamad, B.; Basaran, S.; Coskun Benlidayi, I. Osteosarcopenia among postmenopausal women and handgrip strength as a practical method for predicting the risk. *Aging Clin. Exp. Res.* **2019**. [CrossRef]
40. Yoshimura, N.; Muraki, S.; Oka, H.; Iidaka, T.; Kodama, R.; Kawaguchi, H.; Nakamura, K.; Tanaka, S.; Akune, T. Is osteoporosis a predictor for future sarcopenia or vice versa? Four-year observations between the second and third ROAD study surveys. *Osteoporos. Int.* **2017**, *28*, 189–199. [CrossRef]

41. Volpato, S.; Bianchi, L.; Cherubini, A.; Landi, F.; Maggio, M.; Savino, E.; Bandinelli, S.; Ceda, G.P.; Guralnik, J.M.; Zuliani, G.; et al. Prevalence and Clinical Correlates of Sarcopenia in Community-Dwelling Older People: Application of the EWGSOP Definition and Diagnostic Algorithm. *J. Gerontol. Ser. A* **2013**, *69*, 438–446. [CrossRef]
42. Cruz-Jentoft, A.J.; Landi, F.; Schneider, S.M.; Zúñiga, C.; Arai, H.; Boirie, Y.; Chen, L.-K.; Fielding, R.A.; Martin, F.C.; Michel, J.-P.; et al. Prevalence of and interventions for sarcopenia in ageing adults: A systematic review. Report of the International Sarcopenia Initiative (EWGSOP and IWGS). *Age Ageing* **2014**, *43*, 748–759. [CrossRef] [PubMed]
43. Clynes, M.A.; Edwards, M.H.; Buehring, B.; Dennison, E.M.; Binkley, N.; Cooper, C. Definitions of Sarcopenia: Associations with Previous Falls and Fracture in a Population Sample. *Calcif. Tissue Int.* **2015**, *97*, 445–452. [CrossRef] [PubMed]
44. Huo, Y.R.; Suriyaarachchi, P.; Gomez, F.; Curcio, C.L.; Boersma, D.; Muir, S.W.; Montero-Odasso, M.; Gunawardene, P.; Demontiero, O.; Duque, G. Phenotype of Osteosarcopenia in Older Individuals With a History of Falling. *J. Am. Med. Dir. Assoc.* **2015**, *16*, 290–295. [CrossRef] [PubMed]
45. Sepúlveda-Loyola, W.; Phu, S.; Bani Hassan, E.; Brennan-Olsen, S.L.; Zanker, J.; Vogrin, S.; Conzade, R.; Kirk, B.; Al Saedi, A.; Probst, V.; et al. The Joint Occurrence of Osteoporosis and Sarcopenia (Osteosarcopenia): Definitions and Characteristics. *J. Am. Med. Dir. Assoc.* **2019**. [CrossRef] [PubMed]
46. Bischoff-Ferrari, H.A.; Orav, J.E.; Kanis, J.A.; Rizzoli, R.; Schlögl, M.; Staehelin, H.B.; Willett, W.C.; Dawson-Hughes, B. Comparative performance of current definitions of sarcopenia against the prospective incidence of falls among community-dwelling seniors age 65 and older. *Osteoporos. Int.* **2015**, *26*, 2793–2802. [CrossRef] [PubMed]
47. Mori, H.; Tokuda, Y. Differences and overlap between sarcopenia and physical frailty in older community-dwelling Japanese. *Asia Pac. J. Clin. Nutr.* **2019**, *28*, 157–165.
48. Gadelha, A.B.; Neri, S.G.R.; Oliveira RJ, d.e.; Bottaro, M.; David AC, d.e.; Vainshelboim, B.; Lima, R.M. Severity of sarcopenia is associated with postural balance and risk of falls in community-dwelling older women. *Exp. Aging Res.* **2018**, *44*, 258–269. [CrossRef]
49. Batsis, J.A.; Villareal, D.T. Sarcopenic obesity in older adults: Aetiology, epidemiology and treatment strategies. *Nat. Rev. Endocrinol.* **2018**, *14*, 513–537. [CrossRef]
50. Akune, T.; Muraki, S.; Oka, H.; Tanaka, S.; Kawaguchi, H.; Nakamura, K.; Yoshimura, N. Exercise habits during middle age are associated with lower prevalence of sarcopenia: The ROAD study. *Osteoporos. Int.* **2014**, *25*, 1081–1088. [CrossRef]
51. Fukuoka, Y.; Narita, T.; Fujita, H.; Morii, T.; Sato, T.; Sassa, M.H.; Yamada, Y. Importance of physical evaluation using skeletal muscle mass index and body fat percentage to prevent sarcopenia in elderly Japanese diabetes patients. *J. Diabetes Investig.* **2019**, *10*, 322–330. [CrossRef]
52. Beaudart, C.; Reginster, J.Y.; Petermans, J.; Gillain, S.; Quabron, A.; Locquet, M.; Slomian, J.; Buckinx, F.; Bruyère, O. Quality of life and physical components linked to sarcopenia: The SarcoPhAge study. *Exp. Gerontol.* **2015**, *69*, 103–110. [CrossRef] [PubMed]
53. Yu, R.; Wong, M.; Leung, J.; Lee, J.; Auyeung, T.W.; Woo, J. Incidence, reversibility, risk factors and the protective effect of high body mass index against sarcopenia in community-dwelling older Chinese adults. *Geriatr. Gerontol. Int.* **2014**, *14*, 15–28. [CrossRef] [PubMed]
54. Han, P.; Zhao, J.; Guo, Q.; Wang, J.; Zhang, W.; Shen, S.; Wang, X.; Dong, R.; Ma, Y.; Kang, L.; et al. Incidence, risk factors, and the protective effect of high body mass index against sarcopenia in suburb-dwelling elderly Chinese populations. *J. Nutr. Health Aging* **2016**, *20*, 1056–1060. [CrossRef] [PubMed]
55. Kim, H.; Suzuki, T.; Kim, M.; Kojima, N.; Yoshida, Y.; Hirano, H.; Saito, K.; Iwasa, H.; Shimada, H.; Hosoi, E.; et al. Incidence and predictors of sarcopenia onset in community-dwelling elderly japanese women: 4-Year follow-up study. *J. Am. Med. Dir. Assoc.* **2015**, *16*, e1–e85. [CrossRef]
56. Moreno-Aguilar, M.; Molina, M.M.; Hernandez, M.F.H. Inverse Association Between Body Mass Index and Osteosarcopenia in Community Dwelling Elderly. *Surg. Obes. Relat. Dis.* **2017**, *13*, 190. [CrossRef]
57. Shen, Y.; Chen, J.; Chen, X.; Hou, L.S.; Lin, X.; Yang, M. Prevalence and Associated Factors of Sarcopenia in Nursing Home Residents: A Systematic Review and Meta-analysis. *J. Am. Med. Dir. Assoc.* **2019**, *20*, 5–13. [CrossRef]
58. Gonzalez, M.C.; Correia, M.I.T.D.; Heymsfield, S.B. A requiem for BMI in the clinical setting. *Curr. Opin. Clin. Nutr. Metab. Care* **2017**, *20*, 314–321. [CrossRef]

59. Beaudart, C.; Locquet, M.; Reginster, J.Y.; Delandsheere, L.; Petermans, J.; Bruyère, O. Quality of life in sarcopenia measured with the SarQoL®: Impact of the use of different diagnosis definitions. *Aging Clin. Exp. Res.* **2018**, *30*, 307–313. [CrossRef]
60. Konstantynowicz, J.; Abramowicz, P.; Glinkowski, W.; Taranta, E.; Marcinowicz, L.; Dymitrowicz, M.; Reginster, J.-Y.; Bruyere, O.; Beaudart, C. Polish Validation of the SarQoL®, a Quality of Life Questionnaire Specific to Sarcopenia. *J. Clin. Med.* **2018**, *7*, 323. [CrossRef]
61. Geerinck, A.; Scheppers, J.; Beaudart, C.; Bruyère, O.; Vandenbussche, W.; Bautmans, R.; Delye, S.; Bautmans, I. Translation and validation of the dutch sarqol®, a quality of life questionnaire specific to sarcopenia. *J. Musculoskelet. Neuronal Interact.* **2018**, *18*, 463–472.
62. Geerinck, A.; Alekna, V.; Beaudart, C.; Bautmans, I.; Cooper, C.; De Souza Orlandi, F.; Konstantynowicz, J.; Montero-Errasquín, B.; Topinková, E.; Tsekoura, M.; et al. Standard error of measurement and smallest detectable change of the Sarcopenia Quality of Life (SarQoL) questionnaire: An analysis of subjects from 9 validation studies. *PLoS ONE* **2019**, *14*. [CrossRef] [PubMed]
63. Fábrega-Cuadros, R.; Martínez-Amat, A.; Cruz-Díaz, D.; Aibar-Almazán, A.; Hita-Contreras, F. Psychometric Properties of the Spanish Version of the Sarcopenia and Quality of Life, a Quality of Life Questionnaire Specific for Sarcopenia. *Calcif. Tissue Int.* **2019**. [CrossRef] [PubMed]
64. Patel, H.P.; Syddall, H.E.; Jameson, K.; Robinson, S.; Denison, H.; Roberts, H.C.; Edwards, M.; Dennison, E.; Cooper, C.; Aihie Sayer, A. Prevalence of sarcopenia in community-dwelling older people in the UK using the European Working Group on Sarcopenia in Older People (EWGSOP) definition: Findings from the Hertfordshire Cohort Study (HCS). *Age Ageing* **2013**, *42*, 378–384. [CrossRef] [PubMed]
65. Manrique-Espinoza, B.; Salinas-Rodríguez, A.; Rosas-Carrasco, O.; Gutiérrez-Robledo, L.M.; Avila-Funes, J.A. Sarcopenia Is Associated With Physical and Mental Components of Health-Related Quality of Life in Older Adults. *J. Am. Med. Dir. Assoc.* **2017**, *18*, e1–e636. [CrossRef]
66. Kull, M.; Kallikorm, R.; Lember, M. Impact of a New Sarco-Osteopenia Definition on Health-related Quality of Life in a Population-Based Cohort in Northern Europe. *J. Clin. Densitom.* **2012**, *15*, 32–38. [CrossRef]
67. Trombetti, A.; Reid, K.F.; Hars, M.; Herrmann, F.R.; Pasha, E.; Phillips, E.M.; Fielding, R.A. Age-associated declines in muscle mass, strength, power, and physical performance: Impact on fear of falling and quality of life. *Osteoporos. Int.* **2016**, *27*, 463–471. [CrossRef]

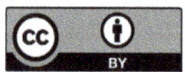

© 2020 by the authors. Licensee MDPI, Basel, Switzerland. This article is an open access article distributed under the terms and conditions of the Creative Commons Attribution (CC BY) license (http://creativecommons.org/licenses/by/4.0/).

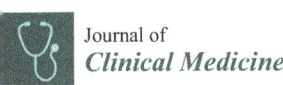

Article

Using the Updated EWGSOP2 Definition in Diagnosing Sarcopenia in Spanish Older Adults: Clinical Approach

Anna Arnal-Gómez [1,2], Maria A. Cebrià i Iranzo [1,3,4,*], Jose M. Tomas [5,6], Maria A. Tortosa-Chuliá [7,8], Mercè Balasch-Bernat [1,4], Trinidad Sentandreu-Mañó [1,6], Silvia Forcano [3] and Natalia Cezón-Serrano [1,4]

- [1] Department of Physiotherapy, University of Valencia, 46010 Valencia, Spain; anna.arnal@uv.es (A.A.-G.); merce.balasch@uv.es (M.B.-B.); trinidad.sentandreu@uv.es (T.S.-M.); natalia.cezon@uv.es (N.C.-S.)
- [2] Research Unit in Clinical Biomechanics (UBIC), University of Valencia, 46010 Valencia, Spain
- [3] Hospital Universitari i Politècnic La Fe, 46026 Valencia, Spain; sforcanosanjuan@gmail.com
- [4] Physiotherapy in Motion, MultiSpeciality Research Group (PTinMOTION), University of Valencia, 46010 Valencia, Spain
- [5] Department of Methodology for the Behavioral Sciences, University of Valencia, 46010 Valencia, Spain; Jose.M.Tomas@uv.es
- [6] Advanced Research Methods Applied to Quality of Life Promotion (ARMAQoL), University of Valencia, 46010 Valencia, Spain
- [7] Department of Applied Economics, University of Valencia, 46022 Valencia, Spain; angeles.tortosa@uv.es
- [8] Psychological Development, Health and Society (PSDEHESO), University of Valencia, 46022 Valencia, Spain
- * Correspondence: angeles.cebria@uv.es; Tel.: +34-963-983-853 (ext. 51233)

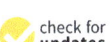

Citation: Arnal-Gómez, A.; Cebrià i Iranzo, M.A.; Tomas, J.M.; Tortosa-Chuliá, M.A.; Balasch-Bernat, M.; Sentandreu-Mañó, T.; Forcano, S.; Cezón-Serrano, N. Using the Updated EWGSOP2 Definition in Diagnosing Sarcopenia in Spanish Older Adults: Clinical Approach. *J. Clin. Med.* **2021**, *10*, 1018. https://doi.org/10.3390/jcm10051018

Academic Editor: Gianluca Testa

Received: 30 December 2020
Accepted: 18 February 2021
Published: 2 March 2021

Publisher's Note: MDPI stays neutral with regard to jurisdictional claims in published maps and institutional affiliations.

Copyright: © 2021 by the authors. Licensee MDPI, Basel, Switzerland. This article is an open access article distributed under the terms and conditions of the Creative Commons Attribution (CC BY) license (https://creativecommons.org/licenses/by/4.0/).

Abstract: Recently the European Working Group on Sarcopenia in Older People (EWGSOP2) has updated diagnostic criteria for sarcopenia, which consist of one or more measures of muscle strength, muscle mass, and physical performance, plus an initial screening test called SARC-F. The main objective was to compare the number of cases of sarcopenia, using the different measurements and screening options. A cross-sectional study was conducted on Spanish older adults (n = 272, 72% women). Combining the different measures proposed by the steps described in the EWGSOP2 algorithm, 12 options were obtained (A–L). These options were studied in each of the three models: (1) using SARC-F as initial screening; (2) not using SARC-F; and (3) using SARC-CalF instead of SARC-F. A χ^2 independence test was statistically significant ($\chi^2(6) = 88.41$, $p < 0.001$), and the association between the algorithm used and the classification of sarcopenia was moderate (Cramer's V = 0.226). We conclude that the different EWGSOP2 measurement options imply case-finding differences in the studied population. Moreover, when applying the SARC-F, the number of people classified as sarcopenic decreases. Finally, when SARC-CalF is used as screening, case finding of sarcopenic people decreases. Thus, clinical settings should consider these outcomes, since these steps can make preventive and therapeutic interventions on sarcopenia vary widely.

Keywords: sarcopenia; older adults; diagnostic criteria; clinical

1. Introduction

The prevalence and impact of sarcopenia increase with age, and consequently, global aging of the population has turned sarcopenia into a public health concern of great priority both for clinicians and researchers [1]. Thus, the concept of sarcopenia has evolved in recent years at the same time that the number of scientific publications has increased in order to identify its possible causes and consequences [2–4].

Although there are different international teams which have published their guidelines or consensus for sarcopenia [5], the European Working Group on Sarcopenia in Older People of 2010 (EWGSOP) guideline has been one of the most widely used and has catalyzed research activity of sarcopenia worldwide [6–8]. In 2018, the Working Group updated the original definition (EWGSOP2), which since then considers low muscle strength as an essential characteristic of sarcopenia, uses detection of low muscle quantity or quality to confirm its diagnosis, and regards poor physical performance as confirmation of severe sarcopenia [7].

Therefore, in this recent definition (EWGSOP2), muscle strength is brought to the forefront of the diagnostic algorithm [9]. To measure muscle strength, handgrip strength or chair stand are recommended; for measuring muscle mass, two different options are given in order to adjust Appendicular Skeletal Muscle Mass (ASM) either by height squared, weight, or body mass index (BMI); finally, for physical performance, four assessment options are given: gait speed, the Short Physical Performance Battery (SPPB), the Timed-Up and Go test (TUG), and the 400 m walk [7]. Therefore, one or more measures of muscle strength, muscle mass, and/or physical performance together with gender-specific cut-off points for some of these measurements are needed for diagnosing sarcopenia [10,11]. From the clinical perspective, it has to be taken into account that these different options imply that the correct implementation of sarcopenia diagnosis in daily clinical practices requires many factors such as acquisition and financial costs of diagnostic measurement equipment, evaluator training and knowledge, and time constraints of diagnostic measures, among other factors [12]. The assessment in sarcopenia has become a challenge for healthcare professionals in order to identify those who may benefit from intervention [13], leading to a small percentage using diagnostic measures in clinical practice [12]. Therefore, while all different options of the definition are convenient and reliable [12,14], the impact of the different measurements on case finding of sarcopenia is to be elucidated and could help transfer the diagnosis of sarcopenia from research to the clinical context [12,14].

In addition, to facilitate the detection of sarcopenia, a screening test called SARC-F has been proposed to be carried out, before performing the measurements of strength and muscle mass, as indicative of the risk of sarcopenia [15]. SARC-F consists of five questions answered by the patients themselves, so it is a simple, practical, and easily applied screening tool for older adults and for the applicant. However, the use of SARC-F is not mandatory for healthcare professionals, except with screening purposes in high-risk patients [16]. Thus, EWGSOP2 recommends the SARC-F questionnaire as a way to obtain self-reports from patients with signs of sarcopenia and as a formal approach [16].

Moreover, although in previous studies conducted in community-dwelling older adults, SARC-F has shown very good specificity to diagnose sarcopenia, its sensitivity is low, which may be not desirable for a questionnaire aimed at screening purposes [17–20]. With the intention to solve this, SARC-CalF, which adds calf circumference (CC) to SARC-F, has been suggested as an option that may significantly increase the sensitivity of SARC-F [21]. If not only community-dwelling people are studied, but also institutionalized older adults are included, a broader population is characterized and therefore clinicians have more information about the use of these tools. Therefore, they should be validated in different populations and living settings [21], plus the new EWGSOP2 definition has to be taken into account.

It was hypothesized that although there are different measurement options for each step of the algorithm of the EWGSOP2 definition, no difference in case finding will be found in older adults, allowing healthcare professionals to use the most feasible in their daily clinical practice. We also hypothesized that by not using the SARC-F, case finding of sarcopenia could be increased. Moreover, it may be increased when using the SARC-CalF instead of the SARC-F in these populations.

Therefore, the aim of this study was to compare the number of cases of sarcopenia in older adults using the different measurement options of each step of the algorithm of the European Working Group on Sarcopenia in Older People 2018 (EWGSOP2). We also aimed to evaluate the impact of using SARC-F, SARC-CalF, or no screening on the case finding of sarcopenia in Spanish older adults living in the province of Valencia.

2. Experimental Section

2.1. Study Design

A multicenter cross-sectional study was carried out between January 2019 and February 2020 in institutionalized and community-dwelling older adults, living in the province of Valencia (Spain). This study was approved by the Ethics Committee for Human Research of the University of Valencia (H1542733812827) and was conducted in accordance with the Declaration of Helsinki. This research was registered in the ClinicalTrials.gov database (ID: NCT03832608). Before entering in the study, participants signed a written consent, briefed beforehand.

2.2. Participants

The sample included 272 adults aged 65 or older, living in the community ($n = 139$) or institutionalized in residential facilities ($n = 133$). Candidates were not included if they: (1) had edema which could interfere with the bioimpedance analysis (BIA); (2) had a cognitive impairment measured with the Mini-Mental State Examination (MMSE) < 18 points [22]; (3) were suffering from any acute or unstable chronic disease, or had a hospital admission in the last month.

2.3. Sarcopenia Definition

The algorithm of the EWGSOP2 was followed for case finding and diagnosing sarcopenia and determining its severity [7]. It included the SARC-F and the measurements of muscle strength, muscle quantity, and physical performance.

The SARC-F questionnaire is composed of five items questioning strength, assistance in walking, rise from a chair, stair climbing, and falls. It is scored between 0 and 2, and it allows identifying cases with a score of ≥ 4 points from a total of 12 points [15].

Muscle strength was measured by:

- Handgrip strength technique, with a Jamar Plus+ digital hand dynamometer (Patterson Medical, Sammons Preston, Bolingbrook, IL, USA) [23]. Cut-off points were gender-specific for low grip strength: <27 kg for men and <16 kg for women [24].
- Chair stand, in which participants had to stand up five times as quickly as possible from a chair without stopping, with arms folded across the chest. Time (in seconds) was used for the present analyses. The cut-off point for strength was >15 s for five rises for both men and women [25].

Muscle quantity as Appendicular Skeletal Muscle Mass (ASM) was measured with BIA using the Bodystat® 1500MDD (Bodystat Ltd., Douglas, UK). This device was calibrated previous to the measurements. Prior to the assessment, the following criteria were checked [26,27]: participants could not have done previous physical exercise; 2–3 h of fasting was needed, including alcohol or a large amount of water, and emptying their bladder; every metal piece was taken off; and the test was not implemented if they were wearing a pacemaker and/or had edema (diagnosed by the physician). When applying the BIA test (alternating sinusoidal electric current of 200 µA at 50 kHz), the patient was asked to lie in supine position, on a nonconductive surface, with no contact between the limbs. Electrodes were applied with an ipsilateral tetrapolar method, on previously cleaned skin. The electrodes of the upper limb were placed at the knuckles and wrist, and those of the lower limb were placed at the metatarsal head bones line and the anterior side of the ankle. ASM was calculated following Sergi's BIA equation: ASM (kg) = $-3.964 + (0.227 \times RI) + (0.095 \times weight) + (1.384 \times sex) + (0.064 \times Xc)$ [28]. The proposed ASM cut-offs were:

- ASM: low muscle mass was <20 kg for men and <15 kg for women [29].
- ASM Index (ASMI, defined as ASM/height squared): low muscle mass was <7.0 kg/m^2 for men and <5.5 kg/m^2 for women [7,8].

Physical performance of participants was measured by:

- Gait speed (m/s): participants were asked to walk along a 4 m corridor at usual speed and, if needed, using an aid [30], with <0.8 m/s being the cut-off for men and women [31,32].
- Short Physical Performance Battery (SPPB): this test assessed balance, gait, strength, and endurance. Participants were asked to stand with the feet together, semi-tandem, and tandem positions, the time they needed to walk 4 m was measured, and also the time to rise five times from sitting position [33], with ≤ 8 points being the cut-off for men and women [34].
- Timed-Up and Go test (TUG): participants were asked to rise from sitting position, walk a 3 m distance, turn around, walk back, and sit down, with ≥ 20 s being the cut-off for men and women [35].

Following these assessments, participants were classified according to the EWGSOP2 algorithm [7,8]: (1) they had probable sarcopenia with a score of ≥ 4 points SARC-F and low muscle strength (grip strength < 27 kg for men and <16 kg for women; or chair stand > 15 s); (2) they had confirmed sarcopenia when low quantity muscle was also detected (ASM < 20 kg for men and <15 kg for women; or ASMI <7.0 kg/m^2 for men and <5.5 kg/m^2 for women); and (3) they had severe sarcopenia, when low physical performance was added (gait speed < 0.8 m/s; SPPB $\leq$ 8 points; or TUG $\geq$ 20 s).

2.4. Additional Measurements

Anthropometric variables: Age and gender were registered; body weight (kg) was measured using a Tanita BC 601 (TANITA Ltd., Amsterdam, The Netherlands); height (cm) was assessed with a stadiometer SECA 213 (Seca Ltd., Hamburg, Germany); and finally, BMI (kg/m^2) was calculated.

SARC-CALF consists of the same five items as SARC-F which are scored the same [36] and adds the CC that was measured as the widest circumference of calf. The CC item is scored as 0 points when the participant had more than 31 cm circumference and as 10 points if it was less than or equal to 31 cm. A SARC-CalF $\geq$ 11 indicates positive screening for sarcopenia [37–39].

All the assessments were done on the same day for each participant, and different physiotherapists took these measurements for all the samples. Intraclass Correlation Coefficients (ICCs) were calculated to know the interrater reliability, and they ranged from 0.802 to 0.985, which may be considered very good reliability (values between 0.75 and 0.90 indicate good reliability; values over 0.90 show excellent reliability) [40].

2.5. Applied Models

Three models were applied: Model 1: using SARC-F as initial screening; Model 2: not using any initial screening; and Model 3: using SARC-CalF as initial screening instead of SARC-F. By combining the different measures proposed by the steps described in the EWGSOP2 algorithm (Find–Assess–Confirm–Severity), 12 options were obtained (A to L), and to each one of the three models, each of their twelve options was tested (Table 1).

Table 1. Description of the three models and their 12 options.

Name of Combination	Model *	Option	Muscle Strength Measurement	Muscle Quantity Measurement	Physical Performance Measurement
A1	1				
A2	2	A	Handgrip strength	ASMI	SPPB
A3	3				
B1	1				
B2	2	B	Handgrip strength	ASM	SPPB
B3	3				
C1	1				
C2	2	C	Handgrip strength	ASM	Gait speed
C3	3				
D1	1				
D2	2	D	Handgrip strength	ASMI	Gait speed
D3	3				
E1	1				
E2	2	E	Handgrip strength	ASM	TUG
E3	3				
F1	1				
F2	2	F	Handgrip strength	ASMI	TUG
F3	3				
G1	1				
G2	2	G	Chair stand	ASMI	SPPB
G3	3				
H1	1				
H2	2	H	Chair stand	ASM	SPPB
H3	3				
I1	1				
I2	2	I	Chair stand	ASM	Gait speed
I3	3				
J1	1				
J2	2	J	Chair stand	ASMI	Gait speed
J3	3				
K1	1				
K2	2	K	Chair stand	ASM	TUG
K3	3				
L1	1				
L2	2	L	Chair stand	ASMI	TUG
L3	3				

* Model 1: using SARC-F as initial screening; Model 2: not using any initial screening; and Model 3: using SARC-CalF instead of SARC-F.

2.6. Statistical Analyses

With descriptive purposes, means, standard deviations, and 95% confidence intervals (CI) for all variables were calculated. All statistical analyses were performed with R [41], also employing the packages vcd [42] and DescTools [43]. Descriptive statistics (proportions) of multinomial variables were performed [44] including 95% CI for the proportions of each category by the method of Glaz and Sison [45,46]. Chi-square tests of goodness-of-fit and independence were also performed together with their association measures (Pearson residuals and Cramer's V). The CI for V coefficient was bias-corrected [47]. Whenever multiple statistical tests were made, the Sidak correction was employed.

3. Results

3.1. Sample Characteristics

A total of 272 participants were included in this study. The age range for all the participants was 65–97 years, the mean age was 77.0 (8.7) years old, and according to setting, the mean was 72.3 and 81.9 years old for community dwelling and institutionalized participants, respectively. Seventy-two percent of participants (n = 197) were women (Table 2).

Table 2. Characteristics of the participants (n = 272) according to setting and gender: mean (standard deviation) and [95% confidence interval].

Variable	Community Dwelling (n = 139, 51.1%)				Institutionalized (n = 133, 48.9%)				
	Total	Men (n = 44, 31.7%)	Women (n = 95, 68.3%)	p-value	Total	Men (n = 31, 23.3%)	Women (n = 102, 76.7%)	p-Value
Anthropometrics								
Age (years)	72.3 (6.1) [71.2–73.3]	72.8 (6.32) [70.9–74.7]	72.0 (6.1) [70.8–73.3]	0.498	81.9 (8.4) [80.5–83.3]	78.2 (9.0) [74.9–81.5]	83.0 (7.9) [81.5–84.6]	0.005 *
Weight (kg)	71.6 (12.4) [69.5–73.7]	79.5 (10.5) [76.3–82.7]	67.9 (11.5) [65.6–70.3]	<0.001 †	66.6 (13.4) [64.4–69.0]	75.6 (12.5) [71.0–80.2]	63.9 (12.5) [61.5–66.4]	<0.001 †
Height (cm)	158.9 (7.8) [157.6–160.2]	166.5 (6.8) [164.4–168.6]	155.4 (5.3) [154.3–156.5]	<0.001 †	154.1 (9.1) [152.5–155.6]	164.9 (7.9) [162.0–167.8]	150.8 (6.5) [149.5–152.0]	<0.001 †
BMI (kg/m²)	28.3 (4.2) [27.6–29.0]	28.7 (3.7) [27.5–29.8]	28.1 (4.4) [27.2–29.0]	0.486	28.0 (4.9) [27.2–28.9]	27.8 (3.8) [26.4–29.2]	28.1 (5.2) [27.1–29.1]	0.075
Calf circumference	36.3 (3.2) [35.7–36.8]	37.5 (3.1) [36.6–38.5]	35.7 (3.0) [35.1–36.3]	0.001 *	33.4 (3.4) [32.8–34.0]	33.9 (3.0) [32.8–35.0]	33.3 (3.5) [32.6–34.0]	0.387
EWSGOP2 algorithm								
SARC-F (0–10 score)	0.7 (1.2) [0.5–0.9]	0.3 (0.6) [0.1–0.5]	0.9 (1.3) [0.7–1.2]	<0.001 †	3.9 (2.6) [3.5–4.4]	3.5 (2.8) [2.5–4.5]	4.0 (6.5) [3.5–4.5]	0.330
SARC-CalF (0–20 score)	0.9 (2.0) [0.6–1.3]	0.5 (1.6) [0.04–1.0]	1.1 (2.1) [0.7–1.6]	0.088	5.6 (5.1) [4.7–6.5]	4.8 (5.1) [2.9–6.7]	5.8 (5.2) [4.8–6.9]	0.338
Grip strength	28.4 (9.0) [26.9–29.9]	38.1 (8.4) [35.6–40.7]	23.8 (4.7) [22.9–24.8]	<0.001 †	18.8 (7.8) [17.4–20.1]	26.6 (9.8) [23.0–30.2]	16.4 (5.1) [15.4–17.4]	<0.001 †
Chair Stand	15.3 (13.0) [13.1–17.5]	11.4 (3.5) [10.4–12.5]	17.1 (15.2) [14.0–20.2]	0.001 *	31.2 (20.0) [27.8–34.7]	29.4 (19.2) [22.4–36.5]	31.8 (20.3) [27.8–35.8]	0.564
ASM (kg)	17.8 (4.0) [17.1–18.5]	22.3 (2.8) [21.4–23.2]	15.8 (2.5) [15.3–16.3]	<0.001 †	15.1 (3.5) [14.5–15.7]	19.5 (3.2) [18.3–20.7]	13.8 (2.3) [13.4–14.3]	<0.001 †
ASM/height² (kg/m²)	7.0 (1.1) [6.8–7.2]	8.1 (0.9) [7.8–8.3]	6.5 (0.9) [6.3–6.7]	<0.001 †	6.3 (1.0) [6.2–6.5]	7.2 (0.8) [6.8–7.5]	6.1 (0.9) [5.9–6.2]	<0.001 †
Gait speed (m/s)	1.1 (0.3) [1.1–1.2]	1.2 (0.2) [1.1–1.3]	1.1 (0.3) [1.0–1.1]	0.012 *	0.6 (0.3) [0.5–0.6]	0.6 (0.3) [0.5–0.7]	0.6 (0.3) [0.5–0.6]	0.576
SPPB (0–12 score)	10.4 (2.0) [10.1–10.8]	11.1 (1.1) [10.8–11.4]	10.4 (2.0) [9.6–10.6]	0.001 *	5.3 (3.0) [4.8–5.8]	6.1 (2.8) [5.1–7.2]	5.0 (3.0) [4.4–5.6]	0.064
TUG (s)	9.8 (3.3) [9.2–10.3]	9.1 (2.0) [8.5–9.7]	10.1 (3.7) [9.3–10.8]	0.044 *	26.9 (18.7) [23.6–30.1]	28.8 (24.1) [20.0–37.6]	26.3 (16.7) [23.0–29.6]	0.588

Abbreviations: BMI = Body Mass Index; ASM = Appendicular Skeletal Muscle Mass; SPPB = Short Physical Performance Battery; TUG = Timed-Up and Go test. p-value unpaired Student's t-test. * p < 0.05; † p < 0.001.

3.2. Analysis of the Models

For each of the three models, and each of their 12 options (A to L), 95% CI and each category of classification (no sarcopenia, probable sarcopenia, confirmed sarcopenia, and severe sarcopenia) were calculated. These CIs are presented in Figures 1–3.

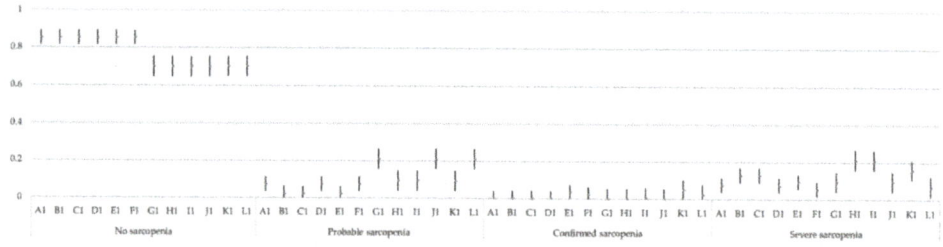

Figure 1. Multinomial 95% confidence intervals for the proportion of each category in the 12 options of Model 1.

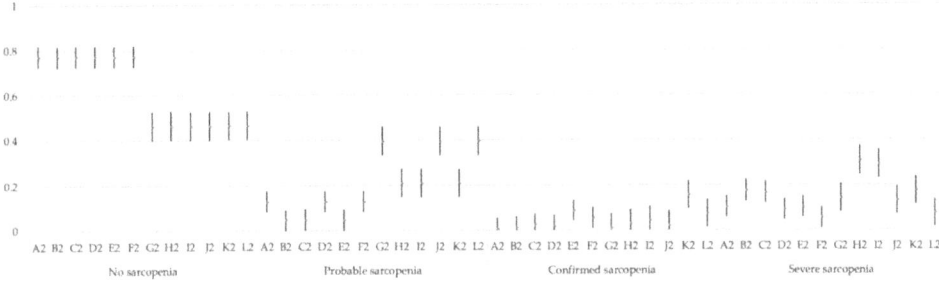

Figure 2. Multinomial 95% confidence intervals for the proportion of each category in the 12 options of Model 2.

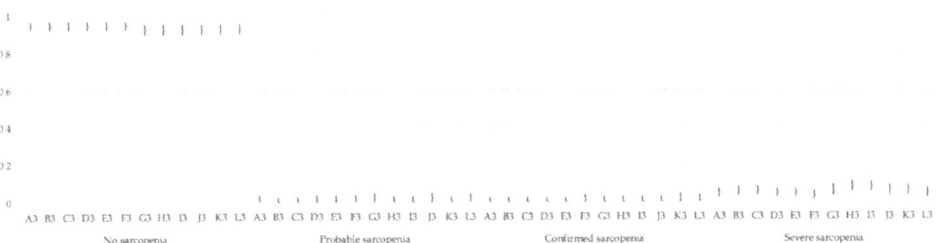

Figure 3. Multinomial 95% confidence intervals for the proportion of each category in the 12 options of Model 3.

Once these CIs were calculated, they were averaged for each model, and each of the 12 options (A to L) in each model was compared with a goodness-of-fit chi-square test with expected probabilities the average probabilities of each model. Therefore, the 12 tests within each model (algorithm) tested whether the classification of the different steps was statistically equal or different. Table 3 offers the results of all these chi-square tests. Regarding Model 1, all but two tests showed statistical significance, indicating that the different steps of the algorithm significantly affect the classification. Model 2 tests showed significant results in all cases, and therefore this supports that the different steps of the algorithm lead to different classifications. However, in Model 3, the results showed no statistical significance, and therefore for this algorithm, the different steps do not lead to significantly different classifications.

Table 3. Goodness-of-fit chi-square tests, probability level corrected with Sidak method.

Model 1	χ^2	df	p-Value	Model 2	χ^2	df	p-Value	Model 3	χ^2	df	p-Value
A1	10.45	3	>0.05	A2	30.43	3	<0.05	A3	1.64	3	>0.05
B1	21.47	3	<0.05	B2	48.49	3	<0.05	B3	3.12	3	>0.05
C1	21.47	3	<0.05	C2	44.05	3	<0.05	C3	3.12	3	>0.05
D1	10.45	3	>0.05	D2	27.92	3	<0.05	D3	1.64	3	>0.05
E1	31.86	3	<0.05	E2	57.01	3	<0.05	E3	8.39	3	>0.05
F1	10.45	3	<0.05	F2	34.16	3	<0.05	F3	8.12	3	>0.05
G1	37.98	3	<0.05	G2	72.80	3	<0.05	G3	4.35	3	>0.05
H1	26.07	3	<0.05	H2	56.71	3	<0.05	H3	5.78	3	>0.05
I1	22.79	3	<0.05	I2	46.70	3	<0.05	I3	5.78	3	>0.05
J1	37.98	3	<0.05	J2	69.28	3	<0.05	J3	4.35	3	>0.05
K1	41.36	3	<0.05	K2	90.20	3	<0.05	K3	14.45	3	<0.05
L1	42.65	3	<0.05	L2	81.24	3	<0.05	L3	9.56	3	>0.05

Notes: Model 1: using SARC-F; Model 2: not using any initial screening; Model 3: using SARC-CalF; p-values corrected with Sidak's correction.

A chi-square independence test was performed to compare the classifications into the different groups the three algorithms made. This chi-square was statistically significant (χ^2 (6) = 88.41, $p < 0.001$), and the association between the algorithm used and the classification of sarcopenia was moderate (Cramer's V = 0.226, 95% CI [0.177, 0.276]).

In addition, we have analyzed how each model on the whole is associated with severity levels. Figure 4 graphically presents the association based on the Pearson's residuals. It can be seen that Model 1 is not significantly associated with any classification as represented by the grey color. However, Model 2 is associated with the classification into the different groups of sarcopenia with a positive association (blue color) with the levels of severity, being higher with probable sarcopenia, and with negative association (red color) with nonsarcopenic older adults. On the contrary, Model 3 is associated positively (blue color) with no sarcopenia.

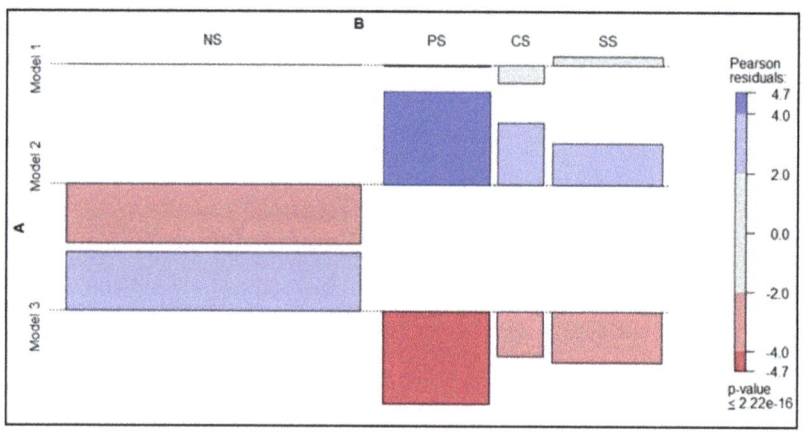

Figure 4. Association between the three models and the severity levels of sarcopenia (no sarcopenia (NS), probable sarcopenia (PS), confirmed sarcopenia (CS), and severe sarcopenia (SS)). Note: blue indicates positive association of row and column and red negative association.

4. Discussion

The present study showed that using the different measurement options for each step of the EWGSOP2 implied differences in case finding in the studied population. These differences have been analyzed in relation to each of the steps, describing which measurements detect more or less cases of sarcopenia. Moreover, our results indicate that when applying the SARC-F, case finding of sarcopenia decreases, thus by not applying it, more cases are found, especially among those with probable sarcopenia. Finally, when SARC-CalF is used as screening, the number of people classified as sarcopenic decreases.

To the best of our knowledge, this is the first study to analyze the different measurement options of the EWGSOP2 in Spanish older adults, and the fact that there are differences in case finding has important clinical consequences. Taking into account that sarcopenia is frequently not noticeable in earlier stages [48], detecting probable sarcopenia is of paramount importance in order to be able to start intervention. In Model 1, using SARC-F, and Model 2, using no screening, there are significant differences in case finding among most of the options. When analyzing these differences, it can globally be seen that those which use the chair stand for measuring muscle strength (G to L) are the ones that find more probable sarcopenic participants. This is interesting considering that previous research has highlighted that handgrip strength seems to be used widely for the measurement of muscle strength [13]. However, it requires the use of a calibrated handheld dynamometer under well-defined test conditions [23]. Therefore, commercial dynamometers are usually limited in clinical settings by the need to purchase specialized equipment, the relative expense, and the lack of trained staff [13]. In addition, sometimes measurement of grip is not possible due to hand disability, such as with patients who are suffering from advanced arthritis or stroke [7]. On the whole, these facts could explain why only a small percentage of healthcare professionals use diagnostic measures in clinical practice as stated before [12]. On the other hand, in previous research, the chair stand has been shown to be able to provide a valid tool for assessing lower body strength [49]. This is in line with our results, which seem to show chair stand can be a reliable method for case finding of probable sarcopenia in the studied population. From the clinical approach, detection of cases as early as possible is important considering that it is better to prevent the skeletal muscle mass depletion and loss of strength and function rather than trying to restore them when they have progressed [50]. Therefore, for clinical settings where a handgrip dynamometer is not always available, the chair stand could be used as an alternative assessment of muscle strength [13]. This way, preventive strategies together with treatment interventions could be implemented before the muscle deterioration occurs [50].

After detecting probable sarcopenia cases, the second step of the EWGSOP2 algorithm evaluates muscle quantity. The EWGSOP2 consensus presents cut-off points for both ASMI (kg/height squared) [51] and ASM (kg) [29] for use when calculating muscle mass. In relation to Model 1, when analyzing the different options, there are more cases of severe sarcopenia in those options that previously have confirmed it by using the ASM (kg) cut-off for muscle quantity (B1, C1, E1, H1, I1, K1). Considering that low muscle mass is highly related to disability and frailty in older adults [52], measuring muscle mass in a precise way is crucial for confirming sarcopenia in this population. There is an ongoing debate about the preferred adjustment for muscle mass indices and whether the same method can be used for all populations [7]. For our population, the results show the ASMI is a more restrictive cut-off, whereas with the ASM, more sarcopenic participants are detected and, consequently, more are classified as suffering severe sarcopenia. This could also explain why G1, J1, and L1 show more cases of probable sarcopenia, since they are using the ASMI and therefore more participants are not being confirmed with sarcopenia and stay as probable. Therefore, some participants could present low strength, however, their amount of muscle mass would still be within the EWGSOP2 criteria, preventing categorization in more advanced stages of the pathology, as similarly stated in previous research [53]. Although the most accurate way to define muscle mass remains uncertain [54], our results show ASMI is more restrictive for our population, classifying them mostly as probable, whereas they could have been classified as severe if the ASM had been used. Thus, methods used to define low lean mass can make preventive and therapeutic interventions on sarcopenia vary widely.

In relation to Model 2, with no initial screening, there are significant differences in case finding among all of the options. When analyzing them individually, again the same trend can be found in relation to muscle strength and muscle mass, that is, chair stand detects more probable sarcopenia (options G to L) and ASMI is more restrictive (A, D, F, G, J, L). In relation to physical performance, the options which confirm sarcopenia with the ASM and then classify its severity with the SPPB or gait speed (B, C, and G to J) are the ones which detect more cases of severe sarcopenia. Detection of low physical performance predicts adverse outcomes [7], so it becomes of paramount importance for the clinical approach. However, in older populations, physical performance is frequently difficult to measure due to acute illness or because of dementia, gait disorder, or a balance disorder [55–57], thus finding a safe and valid assessment becomes necessary. Gait speed is considered a quick and reliable test for sarcopenia, which is why it is widely used in practice [58]. Although the SPPB also predicts outcomes [34], it is a more time-consuming test to apply and therefore, it is more used in research than in clinical practice. Therefore, and considering our results, clinicians can rely on SPPB and gait speed to detect the severe cases, although the latter can be considered as a more approachable measurement in the clinical context.

Regarding the use or not of SARC-F, it was not implemented in Model 2, and more cases were found as probable, confirmed, or severe sarcopenia. Therefore, when using SARC-F for screening in our population, it is at the expense of missing cases who would have been at least in the category of probable sarcopenia, since more cases were detected in Model 2. Although the SARC-F has shown excellent specificity [15,17,18,59–61], it has shown some problems in relation to its low sensitivity [17,59], which means that there is a high risk of missed diagnosis of individuals who have sarcopenia. Moreover, as noted in the EWGSOP2 definition, in clinical settings, case finding should start when a patient has symptoms or signs of sarcopenia, and in these situations, further testing is recommended, the use of any screening tool not being mandatory [16]. This is in line with our results, which suggest SARC-F does not always detect possible cases of sarcopenia in our sample.

In relation to Model 3, which screens using the SARC-CalF, our results show case finding of sarcopenic people is not increased. Moreover, it is the model with which a lower amount of sarcopenic people are found. Although previous research has shown promising results regarding SARC-CalF, with a better sensitivity than SARC-F [21,39], this does not concur with our results. This may be explained by the cut-offs that have been used, since again different options are found in this regard [37], and should be addressed in future research. Moreover, the few participants that were detected as suffering from sarcopenia with any of the options of Model 3 were classified as severe sarcopenia, thus indicating they were highly impaired in their physical performance, which allows less options of recovery. From the clinical approach, if a sarcopenia screening test is used, it is expected to dismiss from further testing as many healthy individuals as possible but should also guarantee diagnosis of those who do have sarcopenia [39] in order to start the appropriate intervention, thus this may not be possible using the SARC-CalF in a population like ours.

Considering that from the three models, Model 2 has shown the highest positive associative probability in case finding of participants with sarcopenia, especially in probable and confirmed, this finding would allow clinicians to detect sarcopenia in earlier stages. This model has different options which have shown statistical differences and using one or other to detect the presence of sarcopenia can be time consuming and expensive and might require highly specialized equipment [50]. Moreover, selecting a way of diagnosing sarcopenia requires balancing the possible benefit of including functional and ASM measurements against the difficulties related to their inclusion [62]. Therefore, on the whole, those options of Model 2 which include the chair stand and use the ASM may be finding more cases of sarcopenia in its different classifications.

Limitations and Strengths

The main limitation of our study, common to other studies, is related to sample size. A larger sample size would be advisable, as well as studying case finding and implementing this model analysis in other populations besides the Spanish one to confirm our promising results. Another limitation is that the sample had a higher percentage of women, and although this is characteristic related to aged population in Spain, greater gender equality would be important in future research. Another interesting line to be implemented in the future could be analyzing how those older adults found to be sarcopenic in one model behave in the other models. However, this study offers the novelty of analyzing the different options of the EWGSOP2 to show the one that can find sarcopenia cases in an accurate way, which would promote an adequate and early intervention.

5. Conclusions

There are differences in case finding of sarcopenia in the studied Spanish older adults when the different measurement options for each step of the EWGSOP2 definition are applied. For muscle strength, the chair stand seems to be detecting more cases of probable sarcopenia, for muscle mass, ASM detects more confirmed and severe, and for physical performance, SPPB and gait speed seem to be reliable options. In addition, more sarcopenia cases are identified when no initial screening is used, therefore, in clinical practice, when a patient shows symptoms or signs of sarcopenia, a screening questionnaire may be surpassed and further testing is recommended to confirm sarcopenia. Thus, clinical settings should take into consideration that the methods used to define these steps can make preventive and therapeutic interventions on sarcopenia vary widely.

Author Contributions: Conceptualization, M.A.C.i.I., A.A.-G. and N.C.-S.; methodology, M.A.C.i.I., A.A.-G., N.C.-S., M.A.T.-C., M.B.-B., S.F. and T.S.-M.; formal analysis, J.M.T., M.A.C.i.I., A.A.-G. and N.C.-S.; investigation, M.A.C.i.I., A.A.-G., N.C.-S., M.A.T.-C., M.B.-B., S.F. and T.S.-M.; resources, M.A.C.i.I., A.A.-G. and N.C.-S.; data curation, M.A.C.i.I., A.A.-G., N.C.-S. and M.B.-B.; writing—original draft preparation, M.A.C.i.I., A.A.-G., N.C.-S. and J.M.T.; writing—review and editing, A.A.-G., M.A.C.i.I., N.C.-S., M.A.T.-C., M.B.-B., S.F., T.S.-M. and J.M.T.; project administration, M.A.C.i.I.; funding acquisition, M.A.C.i.I. All authors have read and agreed to the published version of the manuscript.

Funding: This research was funded by the Generalitat Valenciana (GV/2019/131) and by FEDER/Ministerio de Ciencia e Innovación—Agencia (RTI2018-093321-B-100).

Institutional Review Board Statement: The study was conducted according to the guidelines of the Declaration of Helsinki, and approved by the Ethics Committee for Human Research of the University of Valencia (protocol code H1542733812827 approved 18 December 2018).

Informed Consent Statement: Informed consent was obtained from all subjects involved in the study.

Acknowledgments: We gratefully acknowledge the participation of all community-dwelling participants as well as residents and staff of the residential facilities of La Saleta Care, Parque Luz Xirivella, Parque Luz Catarroja, El Mas Torrent, and especially Mary Martínez Martínez, the Technical Manager of La Saleta Care.

Conflicts of Interest: The authors declare no conflict of interest.

References

1. Tan, L.F.; Lim, Z.Y.; Choe, R.; Seetharaman, S.; Merchant, R. Screening for frailty and sarcopenia among older persons in medical outpatient clinics and its associations with healthcare burden. *J. Am. Med. Dir. Assoc.* **2017**, *18*, 583–587. [CrossRef]
2. Dennison, E.M.; Sayer, A.A.; Cooper, C. Epidemiology of sarcopenia and insight into possible therapeutic targets. *Nat. Rev. Rheumatol.* **2017**, *13*, 340–347. [CrossRef]
3. Marzetti, E.; Calvani, R.; Tosato, M.; Cesari, M.; di Bari, M.; Cherubini, A.; Collamati, A.; d'Angelo, E.; Pahor, M.; Bernabei, R.; et al. Sarcopenia: An overview. *Aging Clin. Exp. Res.* **2017**, *29*, 11–17. [CrossRef] [PubMed]
4. Norman, K.; Otten, L. Financial impact of sarcopenia or low muscle mass—A short review. *Clin. Nutr.* **2019**, *38*, 1489–1495. [CrossRef] [PubMed]
5. Dupuy, C.; Lauwers-Cances, V.; Guyonnet, S.; Gentil, C.; Abellan Van Kan, G.; Beauchet, O.; Schott, A.M.; Vellas, B.; Rolland, Y. Searching for a relevant definition of sarcopenia: Results from the cross-sectional EPIDOS study. *J. Cachexia Sarcopenia Muscle* **2015**, 144–154. [CrossRef]
6. Witham, M.D.; Stott, D.J. A new dawn for sarcopenia. *Age Ageing* **2019**, *48*, 2–3. [CrossRef] [PubMed]
7. Cruz-Jentoft, A.J.; Bahat, G.; Bauer, J.; Boirie, Y.; Bruyère, O.; Cederholm, T.; Cooper, C.; Landi, F.; Rolland, Y.; Sayer, A.A.; et al. Sarcopenia: Revised European consensus on definition and diagnosis. *Age Ageing* **2019**, *48*, 16–31. [CrossRef] [PubMed]
8. Cruz-Jentoft, A.J.; Bahat, G.; Bauer, J.; Boirie, Y.; Bruyère, O.; Cederholm, T.; Cooper, C.; Landi, F.; Rolland, Y.; Sayer, A.A.; et al. Sarcopenia: Revised European consensus on definition and diagnosis. *Age Ageing* **2019**, *48*, 601. [CrossRef]
9. Chew, J.; Yeo, A.; Yew, S.; Lim, J.P.; Tay, L.; Ding, Y.Y.; Lim, W.S. Muscle strength definitions matter: Prevalence of sarcopenia and predictive validity for adverse outcomes using the European working group on sarcopenia in older people 2 (EWGSOP2) criteria. *J. Nutr. Health Aging* **2020**, *24*, 614–618. [CrossRef]
10. Kim, H.; Hirano, H.; Edahiro, A.; Ohara, Y.; Watanabe, Y.; Kojima, N.; Kim, M.; Hosoi, E.; Yoshida, Y.; Yoshida, H.; et al. Sarcopenia: Prevalence and associated factors based on different suggested definitions in community-dwelling older adults. *Geriatr. Gerotol. Int.* **2016**, *16*, 110–122. [CrossRef]
11. Reijnierse, E.M.; Trappenburg, M.C.; Leter, M.J.; Blauw, G.J.; Sipilä, S.; Sillanpää, E.; Narici, M.V.; Hogrel, J.Y.; Butler-Browne, G.; McPhee, J.S.; et al. The impact of different diagnostic criteria on the prevalence of sarcopenia in healthy elderly participants and geriatric outpatients. *Gerontology* **2015**, *61*, 491–496. [CrossRef]
12. Reijnierse, E.M.; de van der Schueren, M.A.E.; Trappenburg, M.C.; Doves, M.; Meskers, C.G.M.; Maier, A.B. Lack of knowledge and availability of diagnostic equipment could hinder the diagnosis of sarcopenia and its management. *PLoS ONE* **2017**, *12*, e0185837. [CrossRef]
13. Beaudart, C.; McCloskey, E.; Bruyère, O.; Cesari, M.; Rolland, Y.; Rizzoli, R.; Araujo de Carvalho, I.; Thiyagarajan, J.A.; Bautmans, I.; Bertière, M.C.; et al. Sarcopenia in daily practice: Assessment and management. *BMC Geriatr.* **2016**, *16*, 170. [CrossRef]
14. Van Ancum, J.M.; Alcazar, J.; Meskers, C.G.M.; Rubaek Nielsen, B.; Suetta, C.; Maier, A.B. Impact of using the updated EWGSOP2 definition in diagnosing sarcopenia: A clinical perspective. *Arch. Gerontol. Geriatr.* **2020**, *90*, 104125. [CrossRef] [PubMed]
15. Malmstrom, T.K.; Miller, D.K.; Simonsick, E.M.; Ferrucci, L.; Morley, J.E. SARC-F: A symptom score to predict persons with sarcopenia at risk for poor functional outcomes. *J. Cachexia Sarcopenia Muscle* **2016**, *7*, 28–36. [CrossRef]
16. Bahat, G.; Cruz-Jentoft, A. Putting sarcopenia at the forefront of clinical practice. *Eur. J. Geriatr. Gerontol.* **2019**, *1*, 43–45. [CrossRef]

17. Woo, J.; Leung, J.; Morley, J.E. Validating the SARC-F: A suitable community screening tool for sarcopenia? *J. Am. Med. Dir. Assoc.* **2014**, *15*, 630–634. [CrossRef]
18. Parra-Rodríguez, L.; Szlejf, C.; García-González, A.I.; Malmstrom, T.K.; Cruz-Arenas, E.; Rosas-Carrasco, O. Cross-cultural adaptation and validation of the Spanish-language version of the SARC-F to assess sarcopenia in Mexican community-dwelling older adults. *J. Am. Med. Dir. Assoc.* **2016**, *17*, 1142–1146. [CrossRef]
19. Beaudart, C.; Locquet, M.; Bornheim, S.; Reginster, J.Y.; Bruyère, O. French translation and validation of the sarcopenia screening tool SARC-F. *Eur. Geriatr. Med.* **2018**, *9*, 29–37. [CrossRef]
20. Yang, M.; Hu, X.; Xie, L.; Zhang, L.; Zhou, J.; Lin, J.; Wang, Y.; Li, Y.; Han, Z.; Zhang, D.; et al. SARC-F for sarcopenia screening in community-dwelling older adults. Are 3 items enough? *Medicine* **2018**, *97*, e11726. [CrossRef]
21. Yang, M.; Hu, X.; Xie, L.; Zhang, L.; Zhou, J.; Lin, J.; Wang, Y.; Li, Y.; Han, Z.; Zhang, D.; et al. Screening sarcopenia in community-dwelling older adults: SARC-F vs SARC-F combined with calf circumference (SARC-CalF). *J. Am. Med. Dir. Assoc.* **2018**, *19*, 277.e1–277e8. [CrossRef]
22. Lobo, A.; Saz, P.; Marcos, G.; Día, J.L.; de la Cámara, C.; Ventura, T.; Morales Asín, F.; Pascual, L.F.; Montañés, J.A.; Aznar, S.; et al. Revalidación y normalización del Mini-Examen Cognoscitivo (primera versión en castellano del Mini-Mental Status Examination) en la población general geriátrica. *Med. Clin.* **1999**, *112*, 767–774.
23. Roberts, H.C.; Denison, H.J.; Martin, H.J.; Patel, H.P.; Syddall, H.; Cooper, C.; Sayer, A.A. A review of the measurement of grip strength in clinical and epidemiological studies: Towards a standardised approach. *Age Ageing* **2011**, *40*, 423–429. [CrossRef]
24. Dodds, R.M.; Syddall, H.E.; Cooper, R.; Benzeval, M.; Deary, I.J.; Dennison, E.M.; Der, G.; Gale, C.R.; Inskip, H.M.; Jagger, C.; et al. Grip strength across the life course: Normative data from twelve British studies. *PLoS ONE* **2014**, *9*, e113637. [CrossRef]
25. Cesari, M.; Kritchevsky, S.B.; Newman, A.B.; Simonsick, E.M.; Harris, T.B.; Penninx, B.W.; Brach, J.S.; Tylavsky, F.A.; Satterfield, S.; Bauer, D.C.; et al. Added value of physical performance measures in predicting adverse health-related events: Results from the health, aging and body composition study. *J. Am. Geriatr. Soc.* **2009**, *57*, 251–259. [CrossRef]
26. Bravo-José, P.; Moreno, E.; Espert, M.; Romeu, M.; Martínez, P.; Navarro, C. Prevalence of sarcopenia and associated factors in institutionalised older adult patients. *Clin. Nutr. ESPEN* **2018**, *27*, 113–119. [CrossRef]
27. Landi, F.; Liperoti, R.; Fusco, D.; Mastropaolo, S.; Quattrociocchi, D.; Proia, A.; Russo, A.; Bernabei, R.; Onder, G. Prevalence and Risk Factors of Sarcopenia Among Nursing Home Older Residents. *J. Gerontol. A Biol. Sci. Med. Sci.* **2012**, *67*, 48–55. [CrossRef] [PubMed]
28. Sergi, G.; de Rui, M.; Veronese, N.; Bolzetta, F.; Berton, L.; Carraro, G.; Bano, G.; Coin, A.; Manzato, E.; Perissinotto, E. Assessing appendicular skeletal muscle mass with bioelectrical impedance analysis in free-living Caucasian older adults. *Clin. Nutr.* **2015**, *34*, 667–673. [CrossRef]
29. Studenski, S.A.; Peters, K.W.; Alley, D.E.; Cawthon, P.M.; McLean, R.R.; Harris, T.B.; Ferrucci, L.; Guralnik, J.M.; Fragala, M.S.; Kenny, A.M.; et al. The FNIH sarcopenia project: Rationale, study description, conference recommendations, and final estimates. *J. Gerontol. A Biol. Sci. Med. Sci.* **2014**, *69*, 547–558. [CrossRef] [PubMed]
30. Working Group on Functional Outcome Measures for Clinical Trials. Functional outcomes for clinical trials in frail older persons: Time to be moving. *J. Gerontol. A Biol. Sci. Med. Sci.* **2008**, *63*, 160–164. [CrossRef]
31. Cruz-Jentoft, A.J.; Baeyens, J.P.; Bauer, J.M.; Boirie, Y.; Cederholm, T.; Landi, F.; Martin, F.C.; Michel, J.P.; Rolland, Y.; Schneider, S.M.; et al. European Working Group on Sarcopenia in Older People. Sarcopenia: European consensus on definition and diagnosis: Report of the European Working Group on Sarcopenia in Older People. *Age Ageing* **2010**, *39*, 412–414. [CrossRef] [PubMed]
32. Studenski, S.; Perera, S.; Patel, K. Gait speed and survival in older adults. *J. Am. Med. Assoc.* **2011**, *305*, 50–58. [CrossRef] [PubMed]
33. Guralnik, J.M.; Simonsick, E.M.; Ferrucci, L.; Glynn, R.J.; Berkman, L.F.; Blazer, D.G.; Scherr, P.A.; Wallace, R.B. A short physical performance battery assessing lower extremity function: Association with self-reported disability and prediction of mortality and nursing home admission. *J. Gerontol.* **1994**, *49*, M85–M94. [CrossRef]
34. Pavasini, R.; Guralnik, J.; Brown, J.C.; di Bari, M.; Cesari, M.; Landi, F.; Vaes, B.; Legrand, D.; Verghese, J.; Wang, C.; et al. Short physical performance battery and all-cause mortality: Systematic review and meta-analysis. *BMC Med.* **2016**, *14*, 215. [CrossRef]
35. Podsiadlo, D.; Richardson, S. The timed "Up & Go": A test of basic functional mobility for frail elderly persons. *J. Am. Geriatr. Soc.* **1991**, *39*, 142–148. [CrossRef]
36. Fu, X.; Tian, Z.; Thapa, S.; Sun, H.; Wen, S.; Xiong, H.; Yu, S. Comparing SARC-F with SARC-CalF for screening sarcopenia in advanced cancer patients. *Clin. Nutr.* **2020**, *39*, 3337–3345. [CrossRef] [PubMed]
37. Bahat, G.; Oren, M.M.; Yilmaz, O.; Kiliç, K.; Aydin, K.; Karan, M.A. Comparing SARC-F with SARC-CalF to screen sarcopenia in community living older adults. *J. Nutr. Health Aging* **2018**, *22*, 1034–1038. [CrossRef]
38. Kaiser, M.J.; Bauer, J.M.; Ramsch, C.; Uter, W.; Guigoz, Y.; Cederholm, T.; Thomas, D.R.; Anthony, P.; Charlton, K.E.; Maggio, M.; et al. MNA-International Group. Validation of the Mini Nutritional assessment short-form (MNA-SF): A practical tool for identification of nutritional status. *J. Nutr. Health Aging* **2009**, *13*, 782–788. [CrossRef] [PubMed]
39. Gonzalez Barbosa-Silva, T.; Baptista Menezes, A.M.; Moraes Bielemann, R.; Malmstrom, T.K.; Gonzalez, M.C. Enhancing SARC-F: Improving sarcopenia screening in the clinical practice. *J. Am. Med. Dir. Assoc.* **2016**, *17*, 1136–1141. [CrossRef]
40. Koo, T.K.; Li, M.Y. A guideline of selecting and reporting intraclass correlation coefficients for reliability research. *J. Chiropr. Med.* **2016**, *15*, 155–163. [CrossRef]

41. R Core Team. 2017 R: A Language and Environment for Statistical Computing. Available online: http://www.R-project.org/ (accessed on 21 November 2020).
42. Meyer, D.; Zeileis, A.; Hornik, K. VCD: Visualizing Categorical Data. R Package Version 1.4-8. 2020. Available online: https://cran.r-project.org/web/packages/vcd/vcd.pdf (accessed on 21 November 2020).
43. Signorell, A.; Aho, K.; Alfons, A.; Anderegg, N.; Aragon, T.; Arachchige, C.; Arppe, A.; Baddeley, A.; Barton, K.; Bolker, B.; et al. DescTools: Tools for Descriptive Statistics. R Package Version 0.99.38. 2020. Available online: https://cran.r-project.org/package=DescTools (accessed on 21 November 2020).
44. Agresti, A. *Introduction to Categorical Data Analysis*; John Wiley and Sons: New York, NY, USA, 1996.
45. Glaz, J.; Sison, C.P. Simultaneous confidence intervals for multinomial proportions. *J. Stat. Plan. Inference* **1999**, *82*, 251–262. [CrossRef]
46. Sison, C.P.; Glaz, J. Simultaneous confidence intervals and sample size determination for multinomial proportions. *J. Am. Stat. Assoc.* **1995**, *90*, 366–369. [CrossRef]
47. Bergsma, W.; Bergsma, W. A bias-correction for Cramer's V and Tschuprow's T. *J. Korean Stat. Soc.* **2013**, *42*, 323–328. [CrossRef]
48. Visvanathan, R.; Chapman, I. Preventing sarcopenia in older people. *Maturitas* **2010**, *66*, 383–388. [CrossRef]
49. Jones, C.J.; Rikli, R.E.; Beam, W.C. A 30-s chair-stand test as a measure of lower body strength in community-residing older adults. *Res. Q. Exerc. Sport* **1999**, *70*, 113–119. [CrossRef] [PubMed]
50. Yu, S.C.Y.; Khow, K.S.F.; Jadczak, A.D.; Visvanathan, R. Clinical screening tools for sarcopenia and its management. *Cur. Gerotol. Geriatr. Res.* **2016**, *2016*, 5978523. [CrossRef] [PubMed]
51. Gould, H.; Brennan, S.L.; Kotowicz, M.A.; Nicholson, G.C.; Pasco, J.A. Total and appendicular lean mass reference ranges for Australian men and women: The geelong osteoporosis study. *Calcif. Tissue Int.* **2014**, *94*, 363–372. [CrossRef] [PubMed]
52. Cawthon, P.M.; Peters, K.W.; Shardell, M.D.; McLean, R.R.; Dam, T.-T.L.; Kenny, A.M.; Fragala, M.S.; Harris, T.B.; Kiel, D.P.; Guralnik, J.M.; et al. Cutpoints for low appendicular lean mass that identify older adults with clinically significant weakness. *J. Gerontol. A Biol. Sci. Med. Sci.* **2014**, *69*, 567–575. [CrossRef]
53. Guillamón-Escudero, C.; Diago-Galmés, A.; Tenías-Burillo, J.M.; Soriano, J.M.; Fernández-Garrido, J.J. Prevalence of sarcopenia in community-dwelling older adults in Valencia, Spain. *Int. J. Environ. Res. Public Health* **2020**, *17*, 9130. [CrossRef] [PubMed]
54. Kim, K.M.; Jang, H.C.; Lim, S. Differences among skeletal muscle mass indices derived from height-, weight-, and body mass index-adjusted models in assessing sarcopenia. *Korean J. Intern. Med.* **2016**, *31*, 643–650. [CrossRef]
55. Coker, R.H.; Hays, N.P.; Williams, R.H.; Wolfe, R.R.; Evans, W.J. Bed rest promotes reductions in walking speed, functional parameters, and aerobic fitness in older, healthy adults. *J. Gerontol. A* **2014**, *70*, 91–96. [CrossRef]
56. Janssen, I.; Heymsfield, S.B.; Ross, R. Low relative skeletal muscle mass (sarcopenia) in older persons is associated with functional impairment and physical disability. *J. Am. Geriatr. Soc.* **2002**, *50*, 889–896. [CrossRef] [PubMed]
57. Kortebein, P.; Symons, T.B.; Ferrando, A.; Paddon-Jones, D.; Ronsen, O.; Protas, E.; Conger, S.; Lombeida, J.; Wolfe, R.; Evans, W.J. Functional impact of 10 days of bed rest in healthy older adults. *J. Gerontol. A Biol. Sci. Med. Sci.* **2008**, *63*, 1076–1081. [CrossRef] [PubMed]
58. Bruyère, O.; Beaudart, C.; Reginster, J.Y.; Buckinx, F.; Schoene, D.; Hirani, V.; Cooper, C.; Kanis, J.A.; Rizzoli, R.; McCloskey, E.; et al. Assessment of muscle mass, muscle strength and physical performance in clinical practice: An international survey. *Eur. Geriatr. Med.* **2016**, *7*, 243–246. [CrossRef]
59. Ida, S.; Murata, K.; Nakadachi, D.; Ishihara, Y.; Imataka, K.; Uchida, A.; Monguchi, K.; Kaneko, R.; Fujiwara, R.; Takahashi, H. Development of a Japanese version of the SARC-F for diabetic patients: An examination of reliability and validity. *Aging Clin. Exp. Res.* **2017**, *29*, 935–942. [CrossRef]
60. Wu, T.Y.; Liaw, C.K.; Chen, F.C.; Kuo, K.L.; Chie, W.C.; Yang, R.S. Sarcopenia screened with SARC-F questionnaire is associated with quality of life and 4-year mortality. *J. Am. Med. Dir. Assoc.* **2016**, *17*, 1129–1135. [CrossRef] [PubMed]
61. Yang, M.; Lu, J.; Jiang, J.; Zeng, Y.; Tang, H. Comparison of four sarcopenia screening tools in nursing home residents. *Aging Clin. Exp. Res.* **2019**, *31*, 1481–1489. [CrossRef]
62. Dawson-Hughes, B.; Bischoff-Ferrari, H. Considerations concerning the definition of sarcopenia. *Osteoporos. Int.* **2016**, *27*, 3139–3144. [CrossRef] [PubMed]

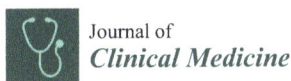 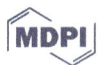

Journal of *Clinical Medicine*

Review

Diagnosis, Treatment and Prevention of Sarcopenia in Hip Fractured Patients: Where We Are and Where We Are Going: A Systematic Review

Gianluca Testa [1,*], Andrea Vescio [1], Danilo Zuccalà [1], Vincenzo Petrantoni [1], Mirko Amico [1], Giorgio Ivan Russo [2], Giuseppe Sessa [1] and Vito Pavone [1]

1. Department of General Surgery and Medical Surgical Specialties, Section of Orthopaedics and Traumatology, University Hospital Policlinico-San Marco, University of Catania, 95124 Catania, Italy; andreavescio88@gmail.com (A.V.); danilozuccala90@gmail.com (D.Z.); vpetrantoni1@gmail.com (V.P.); amico_mirko87@hotmail.com (M.A.); giusessa@unict.it (G.S.); vitopavone@hotmail.com (V.P.)
2. Department of General Surgery and Medical Surgical Specialties, Urology Section, University Hospital Policlinico-San Marco, University of Catania, 95124 Catania, Italy; giorgioivan.russo@unict.it
* Correspondence: gianpavel@hotmail.com

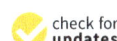

Received: 14 August 2020; Accepted: 15 September 2020; Published: 17 September 2020

Abstract: Background: Sarcopenia is defined as a progressive loss of muscle mass and muscle strength associated to increased adverse events, such as falls and hip fractures. The aim of this systematic review is to analyse diagnosis methods of sarcopenia in patients with hip fracture and evaluate prevention and treatment strategies described in literature. Methods: Three independent authors performed a systematic review of two electronic medical databases using the following inclusion criteria: Sarcopenia, hip fractures, diagnosis, treatment, and prevention with a minimum average of 6-months follow-up. Any evidence-level studies reporting clinical data and dealing with sarcopenia diagnosis, or the treatment and prevention in hip fracture-affected patients, were considered. Results: A total of 32 articles were found. After the first screening, we selected 19 articles eligible for full-text reading. Ultimately, following full-text reading, and checking of the reference list, seven articles were included. Conclusions: Sarcopenia diagnosis is challenging, as no standardized diagnostic and therapeutic protocols are present. The development of medical management programs is mandatory for good prevention. To ensure adequate resource provision, care models should be reviewed, and new welfare policies should be adopted in the future.

Keywords: sarcopenia; hip fracture; diagnosis; treatment; prevention; dual-energy X-ray absorptiometry; bisphosphonate; β-hydroxy-β-methylbutyrate; exercise intervention

1. Introduction

Sarcopenia-related falls and fractures play an important role in our society due to the increased average age of the population [1]. Hip fractures are becoming an evolving and more current problem, as well as one of the most serious medical and social concerns. Hip fractures result in enhanced mortality, perpetual physical morbidity and reduced activities of daily living (ADL) [2,3], with a decrease of the quality of life for caregivers and an increased economic impact on society and government spending [4–6]. Nowadays, the prevention of hip fractures is considered crucial for preserving an acceptable quality of life in older patients. For these reasons, the role of the muscles trophism and function is crucial to prevent traumas in older patients [1]. Ageing is inversely related to the mass and strength of skeletal muscles, and their loss accelerates after 65 years of age, leading to an increased risk of adverse outcomes [7]. For the last 30 years, a considerable effort has been made to understand the condition of sarcopenia, and several definitions have been proposed. Sarcopenia was first defined by

Rosenberg as an age-associated loss of skeletal muscle mass [8], but recently, it has been identified as a disease, and is included in the ICD-10 code (M62.84) [9]. Several disease descriptions were suggested during the last 20 years, but substantial operative variances are present concerning definitions, including nomenclature, the technique of assessment of lean mass, the technique of standardization of lean mass to body size, cut-points for weakness and cut-points for slowness [10]. One of the most accepted was described by the EWGSOP (European Working Group on Sarcopenia in Older Persons), updated in 2018 (EWGSOP2), considering sarcopenia as a "progressive loss of muscle mass and muscle strength, associated to an increased likelihood of adverse events, such as falls, fractures, physical disability and death" [7]. Several authors investigated the differences in sarcopenia cases, agreeing with EWGSOP1 and EWGSOP2 and noting substantial discordance and limited overlap of the definitions [11,12]. Nevertheless, the EWGSOP2 is crucial suggestion to evaluate a possible condition of sarcopenia by measuring the muscle strength, muscle mass and physical performance [13]. Aging is related to variations in body structure and uncontrolled weight loss. The progressive loss of skeletal muscle mass (SMM) and strength promotes functional and physical disability, leading to poor quality of life [7]. The body composition changes were reported in several studies [7,14,15]. Cruz-Jentoft et al. [7] showed a loss of muscle strength in older patients through measurement grip strength with a dynamometer. Hida et al. [14] demonstrated a greater sarcopenia prevalence and more diminished leg muscle mass in subjects following a hip fracture than uninjured subjects with the same age. The most efficient technique to date, dual energy X-ray absorptiometry (DXA), assesses lean mass [16]. Bioelectrical impedance analysis (BIA), CT, and MRI can be used in selected cases [16]. DXA has several advantages, including low cost, low irradiation exposure and easy availability and usability. However, the difficulty of performing this examination in patients with hip fracture or in subjects undergoing recent orthopaedic surgery, due to post-surgical pain and immobility, the use of machines with non-uniform calibrations between them and the lack of universally shared protocols, makes DXA not always reliable in the quantification of MM and in the instrumental diagnosis of sarcopenia [11,17]. No specific drugs have been approved for the treatment of sarcopenia and the literature lacks evidence [16]. Research activity is focused on developing new drugs for sarcopenia, although progress has not been straightforward. Initial interest in selective androgen receptor modulators is related to small phase I and II trials [18,19]. For these reasons, the interest in sarcopenia is rising in orthopaedic surgery, due to the high prevalence of older patients, especially those suffering for hip fractures [20], and sarcopenia could be considered as a hip fracture risk factor.

The aim of this systematic review was to analyse diagnosis methods of sarcopenia in patients with hip fracture and evaluate prevention and treatment strategies described in literature.

2. Experimental Section

2.1. Study Selection

From their date of inception to 19th March 2020, two independent authors (AV and GT) systematically reviewed the main web-based databases, Science Direct and PubMed, agreeing to the Preferred Reporting Items for systematic Reviews and Meta-Analyses (PRISMA) recommendations [19]. The research string used was "sarcopenia AND (diagnosis OR treatment OR prevention) AND (femoral neck fracture OR hip fracture)". In order to extract the number of patients, mean age at treatment, sex, type of treatment, follow-up, and year of the study a standard data entry form was used for each included original manuscript. Three independent reviewers (MA, PV and DZ) performed the quality evaluation of the studies. Discussing conflicts about data were resolved by consultation with a senior surgeon (VP).

2.2. Inclusion and Exclusion Criteria

Eligible studies for the present systematic review included sarcopenia diagnosis, treatment and prevention in hip-fractured patients. The original titles and abstracts examination were selected using the following inclusion criteria: Sarcopenia, hip fractures, diagnosis and treatment and prevention with a minimum average of 6-months follow-up in last 20 years. The exclusion criteria were: Patients' cohort with no sarcopenia diseases, less than 6 months of symptoms and no human trials. Each residual duplicate, articles related on other issues or with inadequate technical methodology and available abstract were ruled out.

2.3. Risk of Bias Assessment

According to the ROBINS-I tool for nonrandomized studies [21], a three-stage assessment of the studies included risk of bias assessment was performed. The first step involved the design of the systematic review, the next phase was the assessment of the ordinary bias discovered in these manuscripts and the final was about the total risk of bias. "Low risk" and "Moderate risk" studies were considered acceptable for the review. The assessment was separately performed by three authors (MA, PV and DZ). Any discrepancy was discussed with the senior investigator (VP) for the final decision. All the authors agreed on the result of every stage of the assessment.

3. Results

3.1. Included Studies

Thirty-two manuscripts were recovered. Twenty-four articles were chosen, following the exclusion of duplicates. At the end of the first screening, according to the selection criteria previously described, nine articles were chosen as eligible for full-text reading. Metanalysis or systematic reviews were eliminated from the study. Finally, after reading the complete articles and examining the reference list, we chose seven manuscripts comprised of randomized controlled human trials (hRCT), prospective and retrospective cohort or series studies, according to previously described criteria. A selection and screening method PRISMA [22] flowchart is provided in Figure 1.

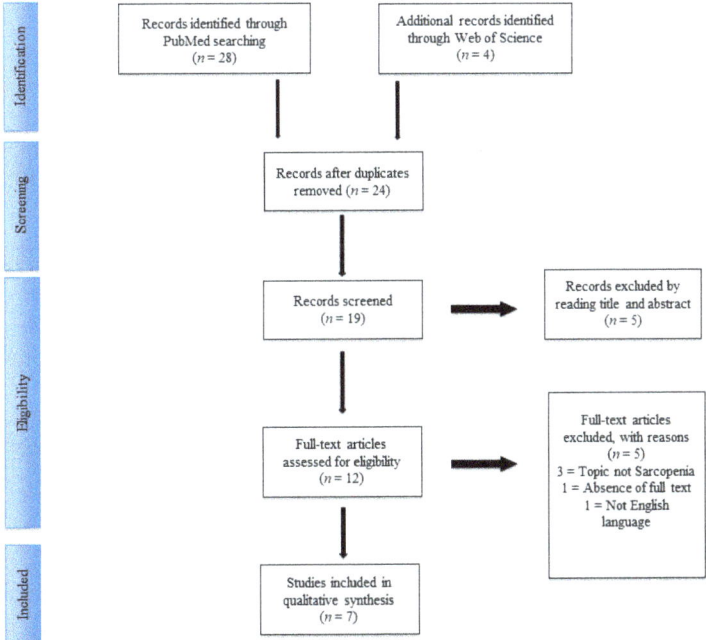

Figure 1. PRISMA (Preferred Reporting Items for Systematic Reviews and Meta-Analysis) flowchart.

3.2. The Diagnosis of Sarcopenia in Patients Affected by Hip Fracture

Kramer et al. [23] performed biopsies of vastus lateralis to assess the muscle changes. The sample was divided in to three groups: Healthy young women (HYW) (18–25 years), healthy older women (HEW) (>65 years) and older women (>65 years) affected by traumatic hip fracture (FEW). FEW Type 2 fibers (2.609 ± 185 μm^2) were noted significantly smaller compared to HEW (3.723 ± 322 μm^2; $p = 0.03$) and HYW (4.755 ± 335 μm^2; $p < 0.001$).

Hansen et al. [16] compared the Computed Tomography (CT) and dual-energy X-ray absorptiometry (DXA) efficiency in the assessment of midthigh muscle mass (SMM) and midthigh cross-sectional area (CSA) respectively, after a hip fracture with 12 months follow-up. The two measures were significantly linked to baseline ($r = 0.86$, $p < 0.001$). Ratios of midthigh fat to lean mass were comparably related (interclass correlation coefficient = 0.87, $p < 0.001$). Data of the change from baseline to follow-up showed a low correlation (interclass correlation coefficient = 0.87, $p = 0.019$). The assessment of muscle mass by DXA-derived midthigh slice has been shown to be reasonably accurate in comparison to a single-slice CT technique in this sample of frail older patients.

Villani et al. [24] evaluated the agreement degree between DXA and bioelectrical impedance spectroscopy (BIS) associated to corrected arm muscle area (CAMA). No significant changes ($p = 0.78$) were found when comparing fat-free mass (FFM) with BIS (FFMBIS) to FFM with DXA (FFMDXA) mean bias. Nevertheless, when included as an independent covariate, gender demonstrated an influence on variation in the mean bias over time ($p = 0.007$). The influence of BMI had no effect on change in the mean bias ($p = 0.19$). Similarly, no significant changes in the mean bias were observed between SMMDXA and SMMCAMA across each assessment time point ($p = 0.18$). At each assessment follow-up, both the techniques were observed overestimated SMM and FFM.

3.3. Treatment of Sarcopenia in Patients Affected by Hip Fracture

Flodin et al. [25] evaluated the efficacy of nutritional supplementation on body composition (BC), handgrip strength (HGS) and health-related quality of life (HRQoL) in 79 hip-fractured patients (mean age 79 ± 9 years). Patients were divided into a protein and bisphosphonate group (PB) group, bisphosphonate-only group (BO) and a control group (CG) with 12 months follow-up. All groups included the CG, received calcium and Vitamin D supplementation. No significant differences in changes of FFM Index, HGS and HRQoL were detected during the follow-up period between the groups.

Invernizzi et al. [26] assessed the essential amino acid supplementation (AAS) in hip-fractured patients. Thirty-two patients (sarcopenia-affected = 71.9%) underwent to a 2-month rehabilitative protocol combined with dietetic counselling. The AA group (16 subjects) had an AAS, while the NAA group did not receive AAS. According to Janssen criteria, both groups were divided in subgroups: Sarcopenic (Sac) and non-sarcopenic (No-Sac) patients. At 2 months follow-up, the Sac AA group ($n = 10$) obtained better significant results in the Iowa Level of Assistance scale (ILOA) and all the primary outcomes ($p < 0.017$) compared to Sac NAA cohort ($n = 13$). The No-Sac groups had similar results.

Malafarina et al. [27] investigated the effectiveness of β-hydroxy-β-methylbutyrate (HMB) oral NS on muscle mass and nutritional markers (BMI, proteins) in patients >65 years with hip fracture. Fifty-five patients (IG) received standard diet plus HMB NS and 52 patients (CG) received standard diet only. The authors used the EWGSOP criteria to diagnose sarcopenia and its prevalence among the entire population was 72%. The sarcopenia diagnostic markers were gait speed (GS), HGS and BC (assessed with BIA). Positive results were recorded in IG for grip work index ($p = 0.188$), muscle mass (MM) ($p = 0.031$) and appendicular lean mass (aLM) ($p = 0.020$). GS analysis did not show a significant difference ($p = 0.367$).

3.4. Prevention of Sarcopenia in Patients Affected by Hip Fracture

In a study by Ding-Cheng Chan et al. [28], 110 patients over 50 years of age with high-risk fracture underwent 3-month exercise interventions. According to different modalities of the exercise, the cohort were randomly divided into integrated care (IC) group and machine-based low extremities exercise (LEE) group. The authors observed a gain in limb mass in the entire cohort (1.13%, $p < 0.05$) with a significant change in the LEE group (1.13%, $p < 0.01$). Both groups obtained significant improvement in muscle strength measured with curl, press and leg extension, grip strength, gait speed, chair stand test and time up and go test. Improvements were seen in leg curl in the LEE group (29.78%, $p = 0.001$).

The most important results of the included articles were summarized (Table 1).

Table 1. Included studies summary. Dual-energy X-ray absorptiometry (DEXA); elderly women with a hip fracture (FEW); Dual-energy X-ray absorptiometry (DEXA); healthy young women (HYW); healthy elderly women (HEW); elderly women with a hip fracture (FEW); Dual-energy X-ray absorptiometry (DEXA); BIS (bioletrical impedance spectroscopy): corrected arm muscle area (CAMA); Fat-free mass (FFM) with BIS (FFMBIS); FFM with DXA (FFMDXA); handgrip strength (HGS) and health-related quality of life (HRQoL); Timed Up and Go test (TUG); Iowa Level of Assistance scale (ILOA); Mini Nutritional Assessment–Short Form (MNA-SF); Barthel index (BI); Functional Ambulation Categories (FAC).

Author	Sample	Intervention	Outcome Measures	Results	Limits of the Study
Kramer et al., 2017	15 HYW (age: 20.3 ± 0.4 years), 15 HEW (age: 78.8 ± 1.7 years), and 15 FEW (age: 82.3 ± 1.5 years)	Muscle biopsies and immunohistochemistry	Muscle fibre type distribution, myonuclear and satellite cell content	FEW resulted in atrophy of muscle fibres Type I and II, associated to a general deterioration in muscle fibres Type II size. Atrophy of Type II muscle fibre in these subjects is associated to a decrease in myonuclear content of Type II muscle fibre.	No measures of muscle mass and/or strength. No data about men
Hansen et al., 2007	30 patients over 60 years old with hip fractures affected in community living patients (not nursing houses, no dementia, no terminally ill)	DEXA-derived midthigh slice has been found to be reasonably accurate in comparison with a single-slice CT technique	Muscle mass and composition	Superior accessibility and simplicity of DEXA utilize. DEXA errors inherent suggest that it should be used to studying groups of patients rather than individuals and in longitudinal trials.	Patients with non-traumatic neck hip fracture
Villani et al., 2012	79 Patients with hip fracture, free in the community.	BIS; DEXA	FFM and SMM, and CAMA	BIS demonstrated sufficient agreement against DXA.	Predictive power and Repeatability
Flodin et al., 2015	79 patients divided in 3 groups: Group N (26 patients); Group B (28 patients); Group C (25 patients)	Group N: 40 g of protein and 600 kcal combined with risedronate and calcium 1 g and vit D 800 IE; Group B: Same of Group N + bisphosphonates alone once weekly for 12 months; Group C: Control. All groups received conventional rehabilitation	Body composition; HGS; HRQoL at 0, 6 and 12 months postoperatively	No considerable variation in baseline attributes was observed between the groups. There was a positive correlation between FFMI and aLMI, $r = 0.92$, $p < 0.01$.	Small number of study subjects. The use of different devices of DXA measurements inflict uncertainties on the validity of the results

Table 1. *Cont.*

Author	Sample	Intervention	Outcome Measures	Results	Limits of the Study
Invernizzi et al., 2018	32 patients over 65 years old divided in two groups: Sarcopenic and non-sarcopenic.	Physical exercise rehabilitative programme and received a dietetic counselling. One group was supplemented with two sachets of 4 g/day of essential amino acids.	HGS, TUG, ILOA, Nutritional assessment, HRQoL baseline (T0) and after 2 months of treatment (T1)	At T1 follow-up, statistically significant differences in all the outcomes ($p < 0.017$) in sarcopenic patient who received AA supplementation.	Small size, the use of BIA to calculate the SMI.
Malafarina et al., 2017	107 patients: Group control (CG), Group intervention (IG)	CG: standard diet (1500 kcal); IG: CG+oral nutritional supplementation (CaHMB 0.7 g/100 mL, 25(OH)D 227 IU/100 mL and 227 mg/100 mL of calcium). All patients received Physical therapy	Body composition, HGS, MNA-SF, BI, FAC	BMI and lean mass were constant in IG patients, while reduced in the CG. The vitamin D and proteins and concentration had improved more in the IG than in the CG. ADL recovery of was more frequent in the IG (68%) than in the CG (59%) ($p = 0.261$)	Patients received physiotherapy 5 days per week. No follow-up after discharge. Diagnostic criteria for sarcopenia.
Chan et al., 2018	110 participants divided in Integrated group (IG) and Low extremity group (LEG)	IC: 15 min warm-up + Resistance training (30 min) + Balance training (10 min) at least once a week for 12 weeks. LEG: 12-week machine based lower extremity resistance exercise twice per week (30 min each). All participants had received a lecture on prevention of osteoporosis, sarcopenia and fall-related injury	Body composition; Gait speed (m/s), chair stand test and timed up-and-go test. Hip and L-spine BMD.	Decrease in weight ($p < 0.01$) and limb fat ($p < 0.001$) were noted in IC group. In LLE group, Significant variations were detected in limb mass ($p < 0.01$). No variation in the cohorts regarding change on body composition. Significant enhancement in muscle strength in both the cohorts. After 3 months, significant improvement for leg strength but higher gain in LEE on leg curl performance ($p = 0.001$). BMD of L-spine improved but similar after 3 months.	BMD tests were not strictly performed on all participants.

4. Discussion

4.1. General Considerations and Key Findings

According to the review findings the diagnosis is still a challenge. The lack of an optimal instrumental tool for diagnosis in hip-fractured patients demonstrates the crucial role of physicians in these cases. The diagnosis is not instrumental data but the correct analysis of the clinical examination and patients' physical status evaluation in association with the results of the tool. At the same time, the nutritional supplementation and hip fracture prevention exercise program are mandatory to avoid the variances in body composition after midlife. Therefore, body composition evaluation is a crucial element for measuring health status in older adults.

The higher incidence of fractures, especially in the spinal column and femoral neck, is attributable to the condition of osteopenia or osteoporosis. Several authors have debated the correlation of bone mineral density (BMD) to muscle mass (MM). However, this association is controversial. Gillette-Guyonnet et al. [29] and Walsh et al. [30] claimed there was no muscle–bone relationship. On the other hand, Locquet et al. exhaustively explored the correlation between muscle and identified a subpopulation affected by the reduction in bone and muscle mass [31]. Moreover, Hirschfeld et al. suggested considering the two condition as a new pathologic disorder, where the subjects affected should be defined as "osteosarcopenic patients" [32]. The controversial findings should be explained by the different diagnosis protocols used. In fact, the sarcopenia diagnosis is often challenging, and there is not an instrumental method or standard algorithm commonly accepted for the evaluation. EWGSOP2 suggests combining clinical tests and instrumental investigations to evaluate the muscle strength, physical performance and muscle mass [11].

4.2. Sarcopenia Diagnosis in Hip-Fractured Patients

Determining grip strength is easy, inexpensive and routine in clinical practice. The evaluation requires calibrated handheld dynamometer use under well-definite exam circumstances with interpretive data from appropriate reference populations [11,33]. On the other hand, the technique measurements can be influenced by the examiner [33]. Similarly, the chair stand test (also called the chair rise test), aims to assess the quantity of time that the patient needs to rise five times from a seated position without using their arms [30]. The Gait Speed test is helpful in the evaluation of physical performance. The principles are the Short Physical Performance Battery (SPPB), and the Timed-Up and Go test (TUG), but the results can be influenced by patient compliance. The Gait Speed test is a rapid, secure and reliable test to assess sarcopenia by EWGSOP2 [11]. The patient walks for 4 m while the clinical staff records the walking speed using an electronic device or manually with a stopwatch. A Gait Speed of ≤0.8 m/s is a severe sarcopenia marker [34–36]. The SPPB is a complex test aimed to analyse gait speed using a balance test and a chair stand test. The highest score is 12 points, and a score of ≤8 points suggests inadequate physical performance. The TUG test assesses the taken time to rise from a standard chair, walk 3 m away, turn around, walk back and sit down again. A score of >20 s is indicative of poor physical performance [37].

Due to the reduced mobility in the hip-fractured patients, and consecutively, to the impossibility in performing the main tests used to assess the disease, the instrumental tools are important part of diagnosis, even if they can replace the clinical evaluation.

DXA is a more widely accessible tool to establish MM [38], and can be defined as total body SMM, as ASM or as muscle cross-sectional area of specific muscle groups [16]. New methods have been studied, including midthigh muscle measurement by CT or MRI, BIS, psoas muscle measurement with CT, the detection of specific biomarkers and other tests [16,24,25]. CT and MRI allow for a precise and detailed study of soft tissues and they offer reliable and universally shared data. On the other hand, these methods have a high cost and it is difficult to find institutes where it is possible to quickly perform them. Moreover, CT exposes patients to a high rate of irradiation [16,34]. Hansen et al. [16] compared SMM estimated by DXA to midthigh muscle CSA, determined by CT, in a group of older patients with hip fracture, observing a positive correlation between CT-determined midthigh muscle CSA and DXA-derived midthigh SMM. The assessment of MM and body composition by DXA-derived midthigh slice has been shown to be reasonably accurate in comparison to a single-slice CT technique in this sample of frail older patients [16].

BIS is another technique used to estimate SMM. The measurement is not a direct evaluation of MM, but an estimation on the whole-body electrical conductivity, through conversion equations [37]. BIS needs highly trained personnel, and the institutes where it can be performed are very difficult to find. Villani et al. [24] compared BIS associated to CAMA and DXA, noting BIS were reliable, but the difficulties in carrying out the examination and in the use of conversion equations led to DXA as the preferred reference technique. Muscle mass evaluation is not the only parameter that can be associated to sarcopenia. A low muscle quality is considered as one of the diagnosis criteria by EWGSOP [11]. Muscle quality is one of the main determinants of muscle function, depending on different factors (fibre composition, architecture, metabolism, intermuscular adipose tissue, fibrosis, motor unit activation) [39]. In particular, the decline of type II muscle fibres (II-MF) is responsible for muscle mass reduction [40].

Kramer et al. [22] performed vastus lateralis biopsies in different groups, confirming a significant II-MF atrophy in older women with hip fractures when compared to healthy older or young women. Since muscle atrophy is associated to loss of function, the author suggested that II-MF atrophy could lead to a higher risk of falls and consequent fractures. This study has some limits. There was no measure of strength and the sample was exclusively female, but the findings could be relevant to treat sarcopenia and to understand the II-MF atrophy causes. The histological diagnosis of sarcopenia could be a valuable way to understand physiopathology of sarcopenia in patients with hip fractures, even if it is not obviously suitable for routine diagnosis.

4.3. Sarcopenia Treatment in Hip-Fractured Patients

The treatment of sarcopenia in patients affected by hip fractures is a multidisciplinary challenge and, according to our findings, great attention should be given to nutritional status. Malnutrition is a highly prevalent condition in the geriatric population affected by this fracture [27]. Therefore, oral nutritional supplementation (ONS), in addition to rehabilitation programs, has become the subject of debate between different authors. Flodin et al. [25] investigated the effects of protein-rich supplementation and bisphosphonate on body composition, handgrip strength and quality of life in patients with hip fracture at 12-months follow-up. In a group, the combination of bisphosphonates and protein supplementation had no significant effects on handgrip strength (HGS), body composition and health-related quality of life (HRQoL). In another group, a positive effect of protein-rich supplementation and bisphosphonates on HGS and HRQoL was demonstrated.

Malafarina et al. [27] showed good results using oral nutritional supplementation with β-hydroxy-β-methylbutyrate (HMB). This approach improves MM, function and general nutritional status in hip-fractured patients [27]. HMB, a metabolite of leucine, has beneficial effect on MM and function in older people [41], but considering the lack of evidence focused on hip-fractured people, more investigations are needed in the treatment of sarcopenia with HMB in these patients. On the other hand, the role of a nutritional intervention without exercise for the treatment of sarcopenia is debated [41]. Although many studies have described good results in increasing protein intake in the older population [42,43], the timing and distribution is unclear [44].

4.4. Sarcopenia Prevention in Hip-Fractured Patients

Despite the few studies focused on sarcopenia prevention in our study, it could be considered the major area of research for future clinical activity and observational epidemiological trials [39] in order to identify and modify the sarcopenia risk factors. A midlife lifestyle approach could be more proper to limit the sarcopenia incidence [45].

Physical activity programs have been suggested as a relevant technique in reducing the risk of hip fracture in older patients [46,47]. In the study by Piastra et al. [47], data showed a significant improvement in MM, muscle mass index, and handgrip strength in muscle reinforcement training group, demonstrating that a muscle reinforcement program moved participants from a condition of moderate sarcopenia at baseline to a condition of normality. Ding-Cheng Chan et al. [28] evaluated effects of programs in community-dwelling older adults with high risk of fractures (> or =3% for hip fracture). The exercise authors clarified the lack of differences in the types of exercise to improve sarcopenia when compared an integrated care model to a lower extremity exercise model. However, several authors promoted rehabilitation protocols for hip-fractured patients, consisting of oral nutritional supplementation with proteins and amino acids and exercise programs [46,47]. Singh et al. [47] proposed a new rehabilitation protocol in the older with hip fracture after orthopaedic surgery. The 12-month rehabilitation program was characterized by a high-intensity progressive resistance training and a targeted treatment of balance, osteoporosis, nutrition, vitamin D and calcium, depression, home safety and social support. The authors showed a statistically significant reduction in mortality, nursing home hospitalization and disability, especially in those subjects with a systematic good health status.

A life course approach to prevention is paramount and offers chance to intervention when lifestyle changes, inspiring the increase of physical activity with immediate to lifelong advantages for skeletal muscle health [16].

4.5. Limits of the Study

The limits of the study are represented by the heterogenicity of the definition of sarcopenia and by the tools considered to assess the patient functional outcome. We extensively searched and identified all relevant last 20 years sarcopenia diagnosis-, treatment- and prevention-related articles. Therefore, risk of bias assessment showed moderate overall risk, which could influence our analysis. Moreover, in the diagnosis section, only instrumental tool evaluations without clinical assessment were detected.

5. Conclusions

Sarcopenia is a physiological condition and contributes to the increased risk of falls and hip fractures in the older population. However, the diagnosis of sarcopenia is challenging, especially in hip-fractured patients, and there are currently no standardised diagnostic and therapeutic protocols. The development of medical management programs is mandatory for good prevention. To ensure adequate resource provision, care models should be reviewed, and new welfare policies should be adopted in the future.

Author Contributions: Conceptualization, G.T., A.V. and V.P. (Vito Pavone); methodology, A.V.; software, M.A.; validation, G.T., V.P. (Vincenzo Petrantoni) and G.I.R.; formal analysis, A.V.; investigation, M.A., V.P. (Vincenzo Petrantoni) and D.Z.; resources, A.V.; data curation, G.T.; writing—original draft preparation, D.Z.; writing—review and editing, G.T. and A.V.; visualization, G.I.R.; supervision, G.S.; project administration, V.P. (Vito Pavone); funding acquisition, V.P. (Vito Pavone). All authors have read and agreed to the published version of the manuscript.

Funding: This research received no external funding.

Conflicts of Interest: The authors declare no conflict of interest. The author GT declares to be the Guest Editor of the Special Issue "Prevention and Treatment of Sarcopenia" of Journal of Clinical Medicine.

References

1. Auais, M.; Morin, S.; Nadeau, L.; Finch, L.; Mayo, N. Changes in frailty-related characteristics of the hip fracture population and their implications for healthcare services: Evidence from Quebec, Canada. *Osteoporos. Int.* **2013**, *24*, 2713–2724. [CrossRef]
2. Kitamura, S.; Hasegawa, Y.; Suzuki, S.; Sasaki, R.; Iwata, H.; Wingstrand, H.; Thorngren, K.G. Functional outcome after hip fracture in Japan. *Clin. Orthop. Relat. Res.* **1998**, *348*, 29–36. [CrossRef]

3. Cummings, S.R.; Melton, L.J. Epidemiology and outcomes of osteoporotic fractures. *Lancet* **2002**, *359*, 1761–1767. [CrossRef]
4. Marottoli, R.A.; Berkman, L.F.; Leo-Summers, L.; Cooney, L.M., Jr. Predictors of mortality and institutionalization after hip fracture: The New Haven EPESE cohort. Established Populations for Epidemiologic Studies of the Elderly. *Am. J. Public Health* **1994**, *84*, 1807–1812. [CrossRef]
5. Saltz, C.; Zimmerman, S.; Tompkins, C.; Harrington, D.; Magaziner, J. Stress among caregivers of hip fracture patients. *J. Gerontol. Soc. Work* **1998**, *30*, 167–181. [CrossRef]
6. Duclos, A.; Couray-Targe, S.; Randrianasolo, M.; Hedoux, S.; Couris, C.M.; Colin, C.; Schott, A.M. Burden of hip fracture on inpatient care: A before and after population-based study. *Osteoporos. Int.* **2009**, *21*, 1493–1501. [CrossRef] [PubMed]
7. Cruz-Jentoft, A.J.; Baeyens, J.P.; Bauer, J.M.; Boirie, Y.; Cederholm, T.; Landi, F.; Martin, F.C.; Michel, J.P.; Rolland, Y.; Schneider, S.M.; et al. Sarcopenia: European consensus on definition and diagnosis: Report of the European Working Group on sarcopenia in older people. *Age Ageing* **2010**, *39*, 412–423. [CrossRef] [PubMed]
8. Rosenberg, I.H. Sarcopenia: Origins and clinical relevance. *Clin. Geriatr. Med.* **2011**, *27*, 337–339. [CrossRef]
9. International Classification of Diseases 11th Revision (Version 04/2019). Foundation Id. Available online: http://id.who.int/icd/entity/1254324785 (accessed on 23 December 2019).
10. Cawthon, P.M. Recent progress in sarcopenia research: A focus on operationalizing a definition of sarcopenia. *Curr. Osteoporos. Rep.* **2018**, *16*, 730–737. [CrossRef]
11. Reiss, J.; Iglseder, B.; Alzner, R.; Mayr-Pirker, B.; Pirich, C.; Kässmann, H.; Kreutzer, M.; Dovjak, P.; Reiter, R. Consequences of applying the new EWGSOP2 guideline instead of the former EWGSOP guideline for sarcopenia case finding in older patients. *Age Ageing* **2019**, *48*, 719–724. [CrossRef]
12. Villani, A.; McClure, R.; Barrett, M.; Scott, D. Diagnostic differences and agreement between the original and revised European Working Group (EWGSOP) consensus definition for sarcopenia in community-dwelling older adults with type 2 diabetes mellitus. *Arch. Gerontol. Geriatr.* **2020**, *89*, 104081. [CrossRef]
13. Bruyère, O.; Beaudart, C.; Reginster, J.Y.; Buckinx, F.; Schoene, D.; Hirani, V.; Cooper, C.; Kanis, J.A.; Rizzoli, R.; Cederholm, T.; et al. Assessment of muscle mass, muscle strength and physical performance in clinical practice: An international survey. *Eur. Geriatr. Med.* **2016**, *7*, 243–246. [CrossRef]
14. Hida, T.; Ishiguro, N.; Shimokata, H.; Sakai, Y.; Matsui, Y.; Takemura, M.; Terabe, Y.; Harada, A. High prevalence of sarcopenia and reduced leg muscle mass in Japanese patients immediately after a hip fracture. *Geriatr. Gerontol. Int.* **2013**, *13*, 413–420. [CrossRef]
15. Gentil, P.; Lima, R.M.; Jacó de Oliveira, R.; Pereira, R.W.; Reis, V.M. Association between femoral neck bone density and lower limb fat-free mass in postmenopausal women. *J. Clin. Densitom.* **2007**, *10*, 174–178. [CrossRef] [PubMed]
16. Cruz-Jentoft, A.J.; Sayer, A.A. Sarcopenia. *Lancet* **2019**, *393*, 2636–2646. [CrossRef]
17. Hansen, R.D.; Williamson, D.A.; Finnegan, T.P.; Lloyd, B.D.; Grady, J.N.; Diamond, T.H.; Smith, E.U.; Stavrinos, T.M.; Thompson, M.W.; Gwinn, T.H.; et al. Estimation of thigh muscle cross-sectional area by dual-energy X-ray absorptiometry in frail elderly patients. *Am. J. Clin. Nutr.* **2007**, *86*, 952–958. [CrossRef]
18. Dalton, J.T.; Barnette, K.G.; Bohl, C.E.; Hancock, M.L.; Rodriguez, D.; Dodson, S.T.; Morton, R.A.; Steiner, M.S. The selective androgen receptor modulator GTx-024 (enobosarm) improves lean body mass and physical function in healthy elderly men and postmenopausal women: Results of a double-blind, placebo-controlled phase II trial. *J. Cachexia Sarcopenia Muscle* **2011**, *2*, 153–161. [CrossRef]
19. Papanicolaou, D.A.; Ather, S.N.; Zhu, H.; Zhou, Y.; Lutkiewicz, J.; Scott, B.B.; Chandler, J. A phase IIA randomized, placebo-controlled clinical trial to study the efficacy and safety of the selective androgen receptor modulator (SARM) MK-0773 in female participants with sarcopenia. *J. Nutr. Health Aging* **2013**, *17*, 533–543. [CrossRef]
20. Hong, W.; Cheng, Q.; Zhu, X.; Zhu, H.; Li, H.; Zhang, X.; Zheng, S.; Du, Y.; Tang, W.; Xue, S.; et al. Prevalence of Sarcopenia and Its Relationship with Sites of Fragility Fractures in Elderly Chinese Men and Women. *PLoS ONE* **2015**, *10*, e0138102. [CrossRef]
21. Moher, D.; Liberati, A.; Tetzlaff, J.; Altman, D.G.; PRISMA Group. Preferred reporting items for systematic reviews and meta-analyses: The PRISMA statement. *PLoS Med.* **2009**, *6*, e1000097. [CrossRef]

22. Sterne, J.A.; Hernán, M.A.; Reeves, B.C.; Savović, J.; Berkman, N.D.; Viswanathan, M.; Henry, D.; Altman, D.G.; Ansari, M.T.; Boutron, I.; et al. ROBINS-I: A tool for assessing risk of bias in non-randomised studies of interventions. *BMJ* **2016**, *355*, 4919. [CrossRef] [PubMed]
23. Kramer, I.F.; Snijders, T.; Smeets, J.; Leenders, M.; van Kranenburg, J.; den Hoed, M.; Verdijk, L.B.; Poeze, M.; van Loon, L. Extensive Type II Muscle Fiber Atrophy in Elderly Female Hip Fracture Patients. *J. Gerontol. A Biol. Sci. Med. Sci.* **2017**, *72*, 1369–1375. [CrossRef] [PubMed]
24. Villani, A.M.; Miller, M.; Cameron, I.D.; Kurrle, S.; Whitehead, C.; Crotty, M. Body composition in older community-dwelling adults with hip fracture: Portable field methods validated by dual-energy X-ray absorptiometry. *Br. J. Nutr.* **2013**, *109*, 1219–1229. [CrossRef]
25. Flodin, L.; Cederholm, T.; Sääf, M.; Samnegård, E.; Ekström, W.; Al-Ani, A.N.; Hedström, M. Effects of protein-rich nutritional supplementation and bisphosphonates on body composition, handgrip strength and health-related quality of life after hip fracture: A 12-month randomized controlled study. *BMC Geriatr.* **2015**, *15*, 149. [CrossRef]
26. Invernizzi, M.; de Sire, A.; D'Andrea, F.; Carrera, D.; Renò, F.; Migliaccio, S.; Iolascon, G.; Cisari, C. Effects of essential amino acid supplementation and rehabilitation on functioning in hip fracture patients: A pilot randomized controlled trial. *Aging Clin. Exp. Res.* **2019**, *31*, 1517–1524. [CrossRef]
27. Malafarina, V.; Uriz-Otano, F.; Malafarina, C.; Martinez, J.A.; Zulet, M.A. Effectiveness of nutritional supplementation on sarcopenia and recovery in hip fracture patients. A multi-centre randomized trial. *Maturitas* **2017**, *101*, 42–50. [CrossRef]
28. Chan, D.C.; Chang, C.B.; Han, D.S.; Hong, C.H.; Hwang, J.S.; Tsai, K.S.; Yang, R.S. Effects of exercise improves muscle strength and fat mass in patients with high fracture risk: A randomized control trial. *J. Formos. Med. Assoc.* **2018**, *117*, 572–582. [CrossRef]
29. Gillette-Guyonnet, S.; Nourhashemi, F.; Lauque, S.; Grandjean, H.; Vellas, B. Body composition and osteoporosis in elderly women. *Gerontology* **2000**, *46*, 189–193. [CrossRef]
30. Walsh, M.C.; Hunter, G.R.; Livingstone, M.B. Sarcopenia in premenopausal and postmenopausal women with osteopenia, osteoporosis and normal bone mineral density. *Osteoporos. Int.* **2006**, *17*, 61–67. [CrossRef]
31. Locquet, M.; Beaudart, C.; Bruyère, O.; Kanis, J.A.; Delandsheere, L.; Reginster, J.Y. Bone health assessment in older people with or without muscle health impairment. *Osteoporos. Int.* **2018**, *29*, 1057–1067. [CrossRef]
32. Hirschfeld, H.P.; Kinsella, R.; Duque, G. Osteosarcopenia: Where bone, muscle, and fat collide. *Osteoporos. Int.* **2018**, *28*, 2781–2790. [CrossRef]
33. Roberts, H.C.; Denison, H.J.; Martin, H.J.; Patel, H.P.; Syddall, H.; Cooper, C.; Sayer, A.A. A review of the measurement of grip strength in clinical and epidemiological studies: Towards a standardised approach. *Age Ageing* **2011**, *40*, 423–429. [CrossRef]
34. Beaudart, C.; McCloskey, E.; Bruyère, O.; Cesari, M.; Rolland, Y.; Rizzoli, R.; Araujo de Carvalho, I.; Amuthavalli Thiyagarajan, J.; Bautmans, I.; Bertière, M.C.; et al. Sarcopenia in daily practice: Assessment and management. *BMC Geriatr.* **2016**, *16*, 170. [CrossRef] [PubMed]
35. Maggio, M.; Ceda, G.P.; Ticinesi, A.; De Vita, F.; Gelmini, G.; Costantino, C.; Meschi, T.; Kressig, R.W.; Cesari, M.; Fabi, M.; et al. Instrumental and non-instrumental evaluation of 4-meter walking speed in older individuals. *PLoS ONE* **2016**, *11*, e0153583. [CrossRef] [PubMed]
36. Rydwik, E.; Bergland, A.; Forsén, L.; Frändin, K. Investigation into the reliability and validity of the measurement of elderly people's clinical walking speed: A systematic review. *Physiother. Theory Pract.* **2012**, *28*, 238–256. [CrossRef]
37. Podsiadlo, D.; Richardson, S. The timed 'Up & Go': A test of basic functional mobility for frail elderly persons. *J. Am. Geriatr. Soc.* **1991**, *39*, 142–148.
38. Treviño-Aguirre, E.; López-Teros, T.; Gutiérrez-Robledo, L.; Vandewoude, M.; Pérez-Zepeda, M. Availability and use of dual energy X-ray absorptiometry (DXA) and bio-impedance analysis (BIA) for the evaluation of sarcopenia by Belgian and Latin American geriatricians. *J. Cachexia Sarcopenia Muscle* **2014**, *5*, 79–81. [CrossRef]
39. McGregor, R.A.; Cameron-Smith, D.; Poppitt, S.D. It is not just muscle mass: A review of muscle quality, composition and metabolism during ageing as determinants of muscle function and mobility in later life. *Longev. Healthspan* **2014**, *3*, 9. [CrossRef]

40. Nilwik, R.; Snijders, T.; Leenders, M.; Groen, B.B.; van Kranenburg, J.; Verdijk, L.B.; van Loon, L.J. The decline in skeletal muscle mass with aging is mainly attributed to a reduction in type II muscle fiber size. *Exp. Gerontol.* **2013**, *48*, 492–498. [CrossRef]
41. Malafarina, V.; Reginster, J.Y.; Cabrerizo, S.; Bruyère, O.; Kanis, J.A.; Martinez, J.A.; Zulet, M.A. Nutritional Status and Nutritional Treatment Are Related to Outcomes and Mortality in Older Adults with Hip Fracture. *Nutrients* **2018**, *10*, 555. [CrossRef]
42. Bauer, J.; Biolo, G.; Cederholm, T.; Cesari, M.; Cruz-Jentoft, A.J.; Morley, J.E.; Phillips, S.; Sieber, C.; Stehle, P.; Teta, D.; et al. Evidence-based recommendations for optimal dietary protein intake in older people: A position paper from the PROT-AGE Study Group. *J. Am. Med. Dir. Assoc.* **2013**, *14*, 542–559. [CrossRef] [PubMed]
43. Deer, R.R.; Volpi, E. Protein intake and muscle function in older adults. *Curr. Opin. Clin. Nutr. Metab. Care* **2015**, *18*, 248–253. [CrossRef] [PubMed]
44. Dodds, R.; Kuh, D.; Aihie Sayer, A.; Cooper, R. Physical activity levels across adult life and grip strength in early old age: Updating findings from a British birth cohort. *Age Ageing* **2013**, *42*, 794–798. [CrossRef]
45. Landi, F.; Calvani, R.; Picca, A.; Marzetti, E. Beta-hydroxy-beta-methylbutyrate and sarcopenia: From biological plausibility to clinical evidence. *Curr. Opin. Clin. Nutr. Metab. Care* **2019**, *22*, 37–43. [CrossRef]
46. Piastra, G.; Perasso, L.; Lucarini, S.; Monacelli, F.; Bisio, A.; Ferrando, V.; Gallamini, M.; Faelli, E.; Ruggeri, P. Effects of Two Types of 9-Month Adapted Physical Activity Program on Muscle Mass, Muscle Strength, and Balance in Moderate Sarcopenic Older Women. *Biomed. Res. Int.* **2018**, *2018*, 5095673. [CrossRef]
47. Singh, N.A.; Quine, S.; Clemson, L.M.; Williams, E.J.; Williamson, D.A.; Stavrinos, T.M.; Grady, J.N.; Perry, T.J.; Lloyd, B.D.; Smith, E.U.; et al. Effects of High-Intensity Progressive Resistance Training and Targeted Multidisciplinary Treatment of Frailty on Mortality and Nursing Home Admissions After Hip Fracture: A Randomized Controlled Trial. *J. Am. Med. Dir. Assoc.* **2012**, *13*, 24–30. [CrossRef] [PubMed]

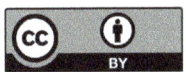

© 2020 by the authors. Licensee MDPI, Basel, Switzerland. This article is an open access article distributed under the terms and conditions of the Creative Commons Attribution (CC BY) license (http://creativecommons.org/licenses/by/4.0/).

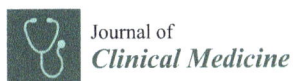 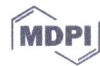

Review

Rehabilitation Strategies for Patients with Femoral Neck Fractures in Sarcopenia: A Narrative Review

Marianna Avola [1], Giulia Rita Agata Mangano [1], Gianluca Testa [2,*], Sebastiano Mangano [2], Andrea Vescio [2], Vito Pavone [2] and Michele Vecchio [1]

[1] Department of Biomedical and Biotechnological Sciences, Section of Pharmacology, University Hospital Policlinico-San Marco University of Catania, 95123 Catania, Italy; mariannaavola.md@gmail.com (M.A.); giuliarita.mangano@gmail.com (G.R.A.M.); michele.vecchio@unict.it (M.V.)

[2] Department of General Surgery and Medical Surgical Specialties, Section of Orthopaedics and Traumatology, University Hospital Policlinico-San Marco, University of Catania, 95123 Catania, Italy; sebymangano@hotmail.com (S.M.); andreavescio88@gmail.com (A.V.); vitopavone@hotmail.com (V.P.)

* Correspondence: gianpavel@hotmail.com

Received: 10 August 2020; Accepted: 26 September 2020; Published: 26 September 2020

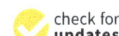

Abstract: Sarcopenia is defined as a syndrome characterized by progressive and generalized loss of skeletal muscle mass and strength. It has been identified as one of the most common comorbidities associated with femoral neck fracture (FNF). The aim of this review was to evaluate the impact of physical therapy on FNF patients' function and rehabilitation. The selected articles were randomized controlled trials (RCTs), published in the last 10 years. Seven full texts were eligible for this review: three examined the impact of conventional rehabilitation and nutritional supplementation, three evaluated the effects of rehabilitation protocols compared to new methods and a study explored the intervention with erythropoietin (EPO) in sarcopenic patients with FNF and its potential effects on postoperative rehabilitation. Physical activity and dietary supplementation are the basic tools of prevention and rehabilitation of sarcopenia in elderly patients after hip surgery. The most effective physical therapy seems to be exercise of progressive resistance. Occupational therapy should be included in sarcopenic patients for its importance in cognitive rehabilitation. Erythropoietin and bisphosphonates could represent medical therapy resources.

Keywords: sarcopenia; elderly; frailty; fractures; ageing fractures; complications; recovery; rehabilitation; nutritional supplements; physical therapy

1. Introduction

Sarcopenia is defined as a syndrome characterized by progressive and generalized loss of skeletal muscle mass and strength, with risk of adverse outcomes such as physical disability, poor quality of life and death. [1] Prevalence of sarcopenia varies among age groups, geographic regions and evaluated context. Estimated prevalence is 1% to 29% in community-dwelling older people, 14% to 33% in long-term care and 10% in acute hospital care populations [2,3]. Starting from 40 years of age, each ten years, healthy adults lose approximately 8% of their muscle mass. Moreover, between 40 and 70 years old, healthy adults lose an average of 24% of muscle, which accelerates to 15% per decade past the age of 70. [4] The diagnosis of sarcopenia should be based on concomitant presence of low muscle mass and low muscle function [4,5].

The European Working Group on Sarcopenia in Older People (EWGSOP) defined sarcopenia as an acute or chronic disease based on low levels three measured parameters: muscle strength, muscle quantity/quality and physical performance, as an indicator of its severity [1,6].

Early sarcopenia is characterized by size reduction in muscle. Gradually, it also occurs as a decrease in the quality of muscle tissue, which leads to loss of functionality and fragility [7,8]. The assessment of sarcopenia requires objective measurements of muscle strength and muscle mass. Several methods of evaluation for sarcopenia considered walking speed, the circumference of the calf, the analysis of bioimpedance, grip strength and DEXA imaging methods. However, none of these measurements are sufficiently sensitive or specific [8–10]. Sarcopenia has been identified as one of the most common comorbidities associated with femoral neck fracture (FNF) patients [11]. Among these different comorbidities, apart from Sarcopenia, protein-energy malnutrition has been reported in 20 to 85 % of cases, depending on age and gender [12,13]. Besides the age-related loss of muscle mass, trauma mechanism, and consequent associated immobilization, cause negative adjustment in body composition. Bed confinement, and the reduced mobility of hospitalized older patients, are associated with loss of muscle mass, muscle function and bone mineral density from the 10th day, and up to two months, after the fracture [13,14]. During the first year from fracture, about 5–6% of muscle mass may be lost [15,16]. It was reported that 28% of patients who were outpatients before hip fracture were unable to walk 12 months after surgery, while as many as 25–30% of patients were unable to return to their previous situation. [16–18].

Treatment of sarcopenia is mainly nonpharmacological. First, an adequate nutrition to ensure the intake of micronutrients and macronutrients is needed. Calories should be 24 to 36 kcal/kg per day; a minimum daily protein intake of 1.0 g/kg body weight, up to 1.5 g spread equally over three meals and maintenance of serum vitamin D levels to 100 nmol/L (40 ng/mL) from vitamin D–rich diet or vitamin D supplementation. Supplementation with creatine monohydrate, antioxidants, amino acid metabolites, omega-3 fatty acids and other compounds are being studied [3]. A crucial role is played by physical activity, especially resistance training, which is the key element for increasing muscle strength and physical performance. Currently, the strategy of combined nutrition supplementation and exercise appears encouraging in the management of sarcopenia.

The aim of this review is to evaluate the impact of rehabilitation with or without other interventions, including nutritional supplementation and pharmacological therapy, on indicators of sarcopenia for FNF (femoral neck fracture) patients.

2. Experimental Section

2.1. Literature Search Strategy

To find clinical trials involving the rehabilitation of sarcopenia and FNF, two authors (M.A, G.R.A.M.) searched in three medical databases (PubMed, Cochrane Library and PEDro) during the month of June 2020. The terms used for the research were sarcopenia and hip fracture and rehabilitation.

2.2. Selection Criteria

The selected articles had to be published in the last 10 years, written in the English language and had to be randomized controlled trials (RCT), observational studies or cases reports published in peer reviewed journals. The authors excluded articles written in other languages, studies with no results or subjects involved and reviews about the topic. Papers with no accessible data, or no available full texts, were also excluded. M.A. and G.R.A.M. selected the studies independently, resolving any discrepancies about the selection by discussion. The senior investigator (M.V.) was consulted to revise the selection process.

3. Results

3.1. Search Progress and Data Extraction

A total of 74 articles were selected based on their titles. Excluding doubles, 63 articles were screened upon their titles. At the end of this screening, 14 abstracts were selected and read independently by the two authors. Five abstracts were excluded: three were not trials, two were reviews and one did not assess sarcopenia in the subjects studied. The authors screened and read eight full texts, one of which was excluded, being a rehabilitation protocol without results on patients.

Every full text was examined, and characteristics of the study, study sample, type of rehabilitation and treatment, outcome measures and results were extracted from the full text and summarized in Table 1.

Table 1. Characteristics of examined studies.

Author	Study Type	Treatment	Type of Fracture	Sample Size	Outcome Measures	Results/Conclusions
Flodin et al. 2015	Randomized controlled study	40 g of protein and 600 kcal combined with risedronate and calcium 1 g and vit D 800 IE (group N); risedronate and calcium 1 g and vit D 800 IE (group B); calcium 1 g and vit D 800 IE (group C). All groups received conventional rehabilitation	Femoral neck or Trochanteric fracture	79 patients: 56 women (71 %), 23 men (29 %); Mean age 79 (SD 9, range 61-96 years)	Body composition, Hand grip strength (HGS), Health-related quality of life (HRQoL)	No differences among the groups regarding change in fat-free mass index (FFMI), HGS, or HRQoL. Intra-group analyses showed improvement of HGS between baseline and six months in the N group ($p = 0.04$). HRQoL decreased during the first year in the C and B groups ($p = 0.03$ and $p = 0.01$, respectively) but not in the nutritional supplementation N group ($p = 0.22$).
Invernizzi et al. 2018	Randomized controlled study	Two groups (A and B). Both groups performed a physical exercise rehabilitative program and received dietetic counseling; only group A was supplemented with two sachets of 4 g/day of essential amino acids.	Osteoporotic hip fracture	32 patients aged more than 65 years (mean aged 79.03 ± 7.80 years) divided in two groups. Patients in both groups were divided into sarcopenic and nonsarcopenic.	Hand grip strength test (HGS), Timed Up and Go test (TUG), Iowa Level of Assistance scale (ILOA), Nutritional assessment, Health-related quality of life (HRQoL). All the outcome measures were assessed at baseline (T0) and after two months of treatment (T1)	Sarcopenic patients in group A showed statistically significant differences in all the outcomes at T1 ($p < 0.017$), whereas sarcopenic patients in group B showed a significant reduction of ILOA only. In nonsarcopenic patients, no differences at T1 in all outcome measures.
Lim et al. 2018	Prospective Observational Study	FIRM (Fragility Fracture Integrated Rehabilitation Management)	Femoral neck, Intertrochanteric, or Subtrochanteric fracture.	68 patients; M = 15, F = 53 Sarcopenia ($n = 32$): Age 81.66 ± 7.49; Nonsarcopenia ($n = 36$): Age 79.81 ± 5.95	KOVAL, FAC, (primary) MMRI, BBS, MMSE, K-GDS, EQ-5D, K-MBI, K-IADL, K-FRAIL scale (secondary)	The primary outcomes improved significantly in both sarcopenic and nonsarcopenic patients. Mobility, balance, cognitive functioning and quality of life improved in both groups. K-IADL ($p = 0.029$) and K-FRAIL ($p = 0.023$) scores were significantly improved in only the nonsarcopenia group after rehabilitation.

Table 1. *Cont*.

Author	Study Type	Treatment	Type of Fracture	Sample Size	Outcome Measures	Results/Conclusions
Lim et al. 2019	Prospective Observational Study	FIRM (Fragility Fracture Integrated Rehabilitation Management)	Femoral neck, Intertrochanteric, or Subtrochanteric fracture.	80 patients; M = 18, F = 62 Sarcopenia (n = 35): Age 82.8 ± 7.5 Nonsarcopenia (n = 45): Age 79.7 ± 6.5	KOVAL, FAC, (primary) MMRI, BBS, MMSE, K-GDS, EQ-5D, K-MBI, K-IADL, K-FRAIL scale, HGS (secondary)	Koval and FAC scores improved over time ($p < 0.001$). The two groups did not differ in terms of the time course of improvement in Koval scores. There was no difference between the groups regarding the time course for improvement in FAC scores after discharge. All secondary functional outcomes, except for HGS, significantly improved over time in both the sarcopenia and nonsarcopenia groups, even though the functional status of the sarcopenia group was lower at both the three- and six month follow-up evaluations. However, the two groups did not differ significantly in terms of final functional status
Malafarina et al. 2017	Multicentre randomized trial	Standard diet (1500 kcal, 23.3% protein (87.4 g/day), 35.5% fat (59.3 g/day) and 41.2% carbo-hydrates (154.8 g/day) plus oral nutritional supplementation (ONS) enriched with CaHMB 0.7 g/100 mL, 25(OH)D 227 IU/100 mL and 227 mg/100 mL of calcium. (Intervention Group (IG); Standard diet only (Control group CG). All patients received Physical therapy	Various type of hip fracture	107 patients aged 65 years and over (mean age 85.4 ± 6.3, 74% female)	Body composition, Hand grip strength (HGS), Mini Nutritional Assessment—Short Form (MNA-SF), Barthel index (BI), Functional Ambulation Categories (FAC) score	BMI and lean mass were stable in IG patients, while decreased in the CG. The concentration of proteins and vitamin D increased more in the IG than in the CG. The recovery of ADL was more common in the IG (68%) than in the CG (59%) ($p = 0.261$)

Table 1. Cont.

Author	Study Type	Treatment	Type of Fracture	Sample Size	Outcome Measures	Results/Conclusions
Min-Kyun et al. 2020	Randomized Control Double-Blinded Trial	Antigravity Treadmill (Experimental Group) Conventional Rehabilitation (Control Group)	Femoral neck, Intertrochanteric or Subtrochanteric fracture.	38 Patients; M = 12, F = 26 65–90 years old;	KOVAL (primary), FAC, BBS, Korean version of MMSE, EQ-5D, K-MBI, HGS (secondary)	Higher and longer improvement in KOVAL, FAC score, BBS, EQ-5D, and K-MBI in experimental group. The comparison of change scores in BBS between the two groups revealed a between-group difference of 11.63 (95% CI: 5.85, 17.40; p for trend = 0.001), 9.00 (95% CI: 2.28, 15.71; p for trend = 0.006), and 11.05 (95% CI: 3.62, 18.48; p for trend = 0.006), respectively. In the EQ-5D and KMBI, the experimental group showed an improvement of 0.49 and 32.63 scores, respectively, compared with 0.23 and 16.00, respectively, by the control group in the three weeks. The comparison of change scores in EQ-5D and K-MBI between the two groups revealed a between-group difference of 0.25 (95% CI: 0.10, 0.41; p for trend = 0.005) and 16.63 (95% CI: 4.80, 28.45; p for trend = 0.009), respectively.
Zhang et al. 2020	Randomized Control Trial	Recombinant Human Erythropoietin	Femoral Intertrochanteric fracture	141 patients; M = 64 (mean age 76.21 years, SD 7.90 years), F = 77 (mean age 79.16 years, SD 6.65 years)	Handgrip strength, ASM (appendicular skeletal muscle) index and post-operative stay and infection	In females, the handgrip strength during week one (13.9 ± 3.327 kg) became significantly higher in the intervention group than in the control group (9.30 ± 2.812 kg), and the difference was statistically significant ($p < 0.05$). During week two (13.212 ± 3.071) and week four (14.742 ± 3.375), the handgrip strength was consistently higher in the intervention group than in the control group ($p \leq 0.05$).

Table 1. *Cont.*

Author	Study Type	Treatment	Type of Fracture	Sample Size	Outcome Measures	Results/Conclusions
						At the fourth week after EPO intervention, the ASM increment in the female and male intervention group (0.56 ± 0.43 kg.) was significantly higher than the ASM increment (0.24 ± 0.38 kg) in the control group over the fourth week.($p < 0.001$). Infection rate in intervention group was significantly inferior and hospitalization state was significantly shorter.

KOVAL = walking ability scale; FAC = Functional Ambulatory Category; MMRI = modified Rivermead mobility index; BBS = Berg Balance Scale; MMSE = Mini-Mental State Examination; K-GDS = Korean version of the geriatric depression scale; EQ-5D = Euro quality-of-life questionnaire 5-dimensional classification; K-MBI = Korean modified Barthel index; K-IADL = the Korean instrumental activity of daily living.

Upon the seven full texts eligible for this review, three examined the impact of conventional rehabilitation and nutritional supplementation, based on food richness of proteins and aminoacids, on patients affected by sarcopenia following FNF [16,19,20] Three papers evaluated the effects of rehabilitation protocols only, especially comparing new methods to conventional rehabilitation and evaluating the impact of sarcopenia on rehabilitation progress [21–23]. A study explored the intervention with erythropoietin (EPO) in sarcopenic patients with femoral intertrochanteric fractures and its potential effects on postoperative rehabilitation. [24]

3.2. Sarcopenia Diagnosis

Various definitions of sarcopenia have been developed by different international consensus panels, (the Asian Working Group on Sarcopenia (AWGS), the European Working Group on Sarcopenia in Older People (EWGSOP) and the Foundation of the National Institute of Health, International Working Group on Sarcopenia) each defining cut-off values from mobility limitation measures (appendicular skeletal mass index, grip strength and physical performance). In our review, the authors specifically used the diagnostic criteria included in the AWGS [21–25] and EWGSOP [1,16,19,20].

The EWGSOP defines sarcopenia when ASM is less than 20 kg for men and 15 kg for women, ASM/height^2 is less than 7.0 kg/m^2 for men and 5.0 kg/m^2 for women (muscle quantity), grip strength is less than 27 kg for men and 16 kg for women, chair stand > 15 s for five rises (muscle strength), gait speed is no more than 0.8 m/s, short Ppysical performance battery (SPPB) is less than 8 points, timed up and go (TUG) test is less than 20 s and 400 m walk test is completed in more than 6 min or not completed at all (physical performance) [1].

AWGS criteria include decreased handgrip strength (males < 28 kg, females < 18 kg), physical performance evaluated with gait speed ≤ 0.8 m/s or 5-time chair stand test: ≥12 s or short physical performance battery: ≤9, and loss of muscle mass, indexed by appendicular skeletal muscle mass (ASM) divided by height squared evaluated through dual-energy X-ray absorptiometry (M: <7.0 kg/m2, F: <5.4 kg/m^2) or bioelectrical impedance analysis (M: <7.0 kg/m^2, F: <5.7 kg/m^2) [25].

3.3. New Rehabilitation Protocols

In Study 1 (Table 1), the functional outcomes of a new integrated rehabilitation management (FIRM) were assessed in sarcopenic and nonsarcopenic inpatients [21]. Sixty-eight patients (32 Sarcopenic and 36 nonsarcopenic) who had undergone surgery for fragility FNF were included.

FIRM included intensive physical and occupational therapy, fall prevention education with discharge planning and referral to community-based care. After surgery, the patients stayed in hospital with 10 days of physical therapy with two sessions per day and four days of occupational therapy. Physical therapy consisted of weight bearing exercises, strengthening exercises, gait training and aerobic exercise, and functional training progressed gradually based on the individual's functional level. Occupational therapy aimed to train the patients in ADL (transfer, sit to stand, bed mobility, dressing, self-care retraining and using adaptive equipment).

The outcome measures used in the eligible studies were walking ability through two scales: the KOVAL walking ability scale [26] and the functional ambulatory category (FAC) [27]; general mobility; balance and fall risk; cognitive functioning; quality of life; mood; ADL; frailty and handgrip strength of the patients; modified Rivermead mobility index [28]; Berg balance scale [29]; MMSE [30]; Korean version of the geriatric depression scale [31]; the Euro quality-of-life questionnaire 5-dimensional classification [32]; the Korean modified Barthel index [33]; the Korean instrumental ADL [34] and the Korean version of the fatigue, resistance, ambulation, illnesses and loss of weight (FRAIL) scale [35]) at admission to the in-hospital rehabilitation unit and at discharge.

KOVAL and FAC were significantly improved in both sarcopenic and nonsarcopenic patients. Prefacture ambulatory functioning, rather than the presence of sarcopenia, was significantly correlated with short-term recovery of ambulatory functioning. Mobility, balance, cognitive functioning and quality of life improved in both groups, demonstrating the clinical effectiveness of FIRM in sarcopenic patients. In contrast, K-IADL ($p = 0.029$) and K-FRAIL ($p = 0.023$) scores were significantly improved in only the nonsarcopenia group after rehabilitation.

Limitations of this study were the short time after which the outcomes were evaluated (after two weeks of interventions) and the exclusion of several patients before the start of the treatment. The use of the sarcopenia classification itself may have affected the group allocation. Even though the results of Study 1 suggest that FIRM was effective for short-term functional recovery in older patients with or without sarcopenia who have suffered fragility hip fracture, further research comparing FIRM with conventional therapy is needed.

Study 2 (Table 1) [22] evaluated the FIRM program in a prospective observational investigation of 80 patients (35 Sarcopenic and 45 nonsarcopenic) older than 65 after FNF surgery. The author, unlike the previous study, ruled out gait speed from the diagnostic criteria for sarcopenia in the sample evaluated because this result could not be estimated before the fracture or surgery. The FIRM program was administered during two weeks of hospital stay after surgery. All functional outcomes (KOVAL, FAC, EQ-5D, K-IADL, and K-FRAIL) were assessed on admission for rehabilitation, at discharge, and at the three and six months follow-up visits after surgery (or with a telephone interview). In the considered sample, patients with sarcopenia had impairment in cognitive function in a significantly superior percentage than the nonsarcopenic group. Both groups had improvement in the primary outcome (KOVAL) and functional outcome (FAC score) after discharge. Other evaluations, excluded HGS, significantly improved in both groups with no significant difference. Even though sarcopenia was not a predictor of poorer results in ambulatory independence, at six months from surgery, the type of operation and high HGS (handgrip strength) were significantly correlated.

Study 2 [22] demonstrated that ambulation and functional outcomes were improved in patients with or without sarcopenia suffering from fragility after FNF surgery, due to a complete multidisciplinary rehabilitation. Limitations were caused by the assessment of sarcopenia in patients soon after the surgery, namely the time of follow-up that in fragile patients may have been longer, and the lack of a control group following conventional rehabilitation.

Study 3 [23] compared the efficacy of an antigravity treadmill (AGT) combined with conventional physical therapy, and physical therapy alone, in a double-blinded (to outcome) study. Selected patients were 65–90 years old, who had undergone surgery for FNF associated with sarcopenia, according to the AWGS recommendation [25]. Thirty-eight patients included in the primary analysis were treated. One group ($n = 19$) had only standardized rehabilitation treatment for 30 min per day for 10 days, the other ($n = 19$) received standardized treatment plus AGT for 20 min per day. Standardized therapy consisted in passive hip and knee mobilization, strengthening of the hip abductor and extensor muscles, transfer, and gait training on the floor and stairs.

The outcomes evaluated were the same as Studies 1 and 2 [21,22], except for the absence of the I-ADL measurement. The experimental group experienced higher and longer therapeutic effects, with improvement in all outcomes. However, in both groups, KOVAL and FAC scores were slightly improved and then decreased from 3 three to 6 months. This study provided evidence not only that AGT with CR is more effective than only CR for sarcopenic patients, but also that there is a strong association between muscle mass and bone mass, supporting the theory that muscle forces mediate mechanical loading effects on bones [36]. Limitations of Study 3 were the high amount of drop outs after hospital discharge, it was carried out in only one center, and the number of the sample was not sufficient to significantly represent subgroups with different cognitive function, hip fracture and hip operation type.

3.4. Nutritional Supplements and Physical Therapy

Study 4 (Table 1) [16] was a randomized controlled study evaluating the effects of combined therapy with bisphosphonate, protein-rich nutritional supplementation and conventional rehabilitation in 79 sarcopenic patients after FNF [16]. Measured parameters were body composition, hand grip strength (HGS) and health-related quality of life (HRQoL). Patients were randomized into three treatment groups. All patients received calcium 1 g and vitamin D 800 I.E. divided into two daily doses for 12 months. The nutritional supplementation group (protein + energy = N group, $n = 26$) received a 200 mL package twice daily, each containing 20 g of protein and 300 kcal. This supplement was given for the first six months after FNF, combined with 35 mg risedronate once weekly for 12 months. The second group (B, $n = 28$) received risedronate alone, 35 mg once weekly for 12 months. The controls (C, $n = 25$) received only calcium and vitamin D for 12 months. Treatment began as soon as the patients were medically stable after surgery, able to take orally administered medications and able to sit upright for one hour after intaking bisphosphonates.

Energy supplementation combined with bisphosphonate, vitamin D and calcium had no positive effect on hand-grip strength, HRQoL, or lean mass, when compared to administration of bisphosphonate along with vitamin D and calcium supplementation, or just vitamin D and calcium supplementation, after FNF. Protein and energy supplementation combined with conventional rehabilitation was not able to preserve lean mass after a hip fracture better than vitamin D and calcium alone or combined with bisphosphonates. There were no intergroup differences concerning effects on HGS or HRQoL, but intragroup improvement in HGS, and a positive effect on HRQoL, were seen in the nutritional supplementation group. A limitation of this study was the small sample size.

In Study 5 (Table 1) [19], 32 patients (23 Sarcopenic, nine nonsarcopenic) aged more than 65 years were enrolled three months after osteoporotic FNF and treated with total hip replacement. The authors evaluated the impact of a two months rehabilitative protocol, combined with dietetic counseling with or without essential aminoacid supplementation, on functioning. Patients were divided into two groups. Patients in group A ($n = 16$, 11 Sarcopenic, five nonsarcopenic) were treated for two months with essential aminoacid supplementation sachets of 4 g per day. Furthermore, patients performed a concomitant specific physical exercise rehabilitative program consisting of five sessions of 40 min each per week for two weeks with the supervision of an experienced physiotherapist, and received dietetic counseling. The physical activity included walking training, resistance and stretching exercises and balance exercises. After these two two weeks, all participants performed a home-based exercise protocol up to the end of the study period, two months from intervention. Patients in group B ($n = 16$, 12 Sarcopenic and four nonsarcopenic) performed the same physical exercise rehabilitative program as group A and received concomitant dietetic counseling alone, without essential amino acid supplementation.

Outcome measures were the hand grip strength test (HGS), physical performance, using the timed up and go test (TUG) [37], level of assistance measured by the Iowa level of assistance scale (ILOA) [38], nutritional assessment, with evaluation of daily caloric intake and daily protein intake, and the health-related quality of life (HRQoL) evaluation. All outcome measures were assessed at baseline (T0) and after two months of treatment (T1). Patients in both groups were divided into sarcopenic and nonsarcopenic patients. All patients in both groups showed statistically significant differences in all primary outcome measures (HGS, TUG, ILOA) at the T1 evaluation ($p < 0.017$). Sarcopenic patients in group A showed statistically significant differences in all primary outcomes (HGS, TUG, ILOA) at T1 ($p < 0.017$), whereas sarcopenic patients in group B showed a significant reduction of ILOA at the end of treatment. On the other hand, in nonsarcopenic patients, they found no differences at T1 in the TUG test and level of assistance test. In both groups, there were no differences at T1 in all other outcome measurements. Furthermore, there were no differences between groups in all outcome measuresments both at baseline and after two months of treatment.

Even though it was performed on a small sample size, data emerging from this study showed a good impact of this combined intervention on function and disability in hip fracture patients after two months of treatment. Essential amino acid supplementation induced considerable improvements in the sarcopenic subpopulation of the study.

Study 6 (Table 1) [20] was a multicentric randomized trial evaluating a nutritional supplement, enriched with β-hydroxy-β-methylbutyrate (HMB), calcium (Ca) and 25-hydroxy-vitamin D (25(OH)D) during rehabilitation therapy to improve muscle mass and, thereby, functional recovery. It included 107 sarcopenic patients aged more than 65 years old with FNF. There were 15 drop-outs during the study. This was the first study to evaluate the effects of HMB in sarcopenic patients with hip fractures. Patients in the intervention group (IG, $n = 49$) received a standard diet plus oral nutritional supplementation enriched with 0.7 g/100 mL of HMB, 227 IU/100 mL of 25(OH)D and 227 mg/100 mL of Ca, while those in the control group (CG, $n = 43$) received a standard diet only. Physical therapy was based on moving patients early, using technical aids, and rehabilitation of activities of daily living including exercises to strengthen the lower limbs, balance exercises and walking retraining in individual or group 50 minute sessions, once a day five days a week. Outcomes measured were gait speed, hand grip strength, appendicular lean mass (aLM, kg/height^2), nutritional assessment carried out by the Mini Nutritional Assessment-Short Form (MNA-SF) [39] and patients' functional situation using the Barthel index (BI) [40] and the functional ambulation categories (FAC) score [27].

The outcome variable was the difference between aLM upon discharge and aLM upon admission (Δ-aLM). BMI and aLM were stable in intervention group (IG) patients, whilst these parameters decreased in the control group (CG). The concentration of proteins ($p = 0.007$) and vitamin D ($p.001$) increased more in the IG than the CG. A positive effect of oral nutritional supplementation was reported on recovery of ADL. The recovery of ADL was more common in the intervention group (68%) than in the control group (59%) ($p = 0.261$).

This study had a number of limitations. Patients received rehabilitation five days a week. It would be interesting to see whether participation in a program of resistance exercises during the patients' stay at a rehabilitation center improved the functional results reported. The authors could not do any follow-up of patients after discharge to assess whether the benefits obtained were maintained. Furthermore, diagnostic criteria for sarcopenia proposed by the EWGSOP were difficult to apply in patients with hip fractures admitted to rehabilitation units, because most of the patients were unable to walk when they arrived. Despite these limitations, this research had some important strengths. Due to the characteristics of the patients included, this study could be representative of the geriatric population admitted to rehabilitation centers.

3.5. Other Treatments

Study 7 (Table 1) [24] assessed the effects of recombinant human erythropoietin (EPO), already used in in sarcopenic patients for perioperative recovery, in patients with femoral intertrochanteric fracture and sarcopenia, to investigate its potential benefits on postoperative rehabilitation. EPO, through the activation of the signaling cascades in hematopoietic cells, may stimulate proliferation and differentiation of skeletal muscle myoblasts, making the skeletal muscle a potential target [41,42].

The effects of EPO were analyzed in 141 sarcopenic patients older than 60 years with intertrochanteric femoral fracture, randomly divided in intervention and control groups and examined by sex. The intervention group ($n = 83$) received recombinant human erythropoietin via intravenous injection once per day for 10 days after surgery. All patients, including the control group ($n = 58$) received adequate nutrition and exercise for recovery. The outcomes evaluated were: handgrip strength, appendicular skeletal muscle (ASM) index and postoperative hospitalization and infection. The intervention group, especially in female patients, had significant improvement in handgrip strength during the first week after the surgery. The improvement was consistent in the following three weeks. Even the ASM index was improved, with a more important improvement, but not significant, in the intervention group. The rate of post-operative infection and length of hospitalization were significantly decreased in patients who received EPO intervention.

4. Discussion

In this review, we considered seven studies of older adults (>60 years) in which both rehabilitation and nutrition, alone or combined, were used to improve recovery after hip fracture surgery in terms of walking independence, muscle strength, mobility, live activity and fragility. The studies included participants with different degrees of general, cognitive and mobility functions, who had experienced different types of fracture and undergone various surgery methods. The rehabilitation and supplementation strategies, as well as study designs (duration and setting) were different.

The main finding was that sarcopenia, being a multifactor disease, needs a treatment that cannot rely on a single drug. The treatment should be a combination of methods including nutritional intervention, intervention of functional exercise and medications [24]. Physical inactivity was negatively linked to losses of muscle mass and strength, suggesting that increasing levels of physical activity should have protective effects. Also, muscle strength is a critical component of walking, and its decrease in the elderly contributed to a high prevalence of falls [6,43]. Furthermore, early ambulation after hip fracture had beneficial effects on functioning, readmission rate and multidisciplinary rehabilitation reducing the risk of poor outcomes, such as death and admission to nursing homes following FNF [44].

To strengthen muscle and physical function, progressive resistance exercise training is a commonly used tool [21–23]. Ambulatory independence is a crucial outcome to examine in patients after hip-surgery, and it must be evaluated before and after the surgery intervention and rehabilitation protocol. In Study 1 [21], it was found that ambulatory independence is more associated with individual ambulatory function before the fracture than in the presence of sarcopenia. However, Study 2 [22] considered poor ambulatory independence as predictive factor for worse results in the evaluated outcome.

Progressive resistance training, associated with occupational therapy, in the above-mentioned studies, resulted in important improvements in walking ability, strength and general mobility, especially in the short-term rehabilitation of sarcopenic patients. Occupational therapy may also have an important role in cognitive function. Cognitive function is a crucial factor, affecting the rehabilitation outcomes after FNF in patients. When occupational therapy was not involved, there was no significant difference in outcome measurements between the two groups at all follow-ups in K-MMSE [21,22].

Type and intensity of exercise is an important variable that significantly influences functional outcomes in FNF patients. Study 3 [23], compared the effects of antigravity treadmill rehabilitation with conventional rehabilitation and conventional rehabilitation alone, and which did not include progressive resistance training and was uncertain in terms of compliance, found an important and significant improvement in the ability to walk, ambulatory function, general mobility, balance and quality of life in the experimental group. The antigravity treadmill, in fact, allowed a task-specific repetitive approach, facilitating the practice of numerous complex gait cycles, which were not possible in the control group.

In the literature, less is reported about the role of diet in older age, although there is evidence that improvements in diet among older adults at risk of developing sarcopenia may have the potential both to prevent, or delay, age-related losses of muscle mass and function, as well as being potential management strategies for sarcopenic patients. However, existing evidence from nutrient supplementation studies is mixed [2,6].

In our review, the effects of provision of additional amino acids, protein, bisphosphonates, calcium, Vitamin D and HMB, in combination with a standardized diet and exercise training, were reported. The supplements differed in type, dose, frequency and delivery among the patients, as did the results and improvement in patients. The sample was somewhat evenly distributed in terms of age, sex and type of fracture. All three studies (Studies 4, 5 and 6) showed that supplemental nutrition improved functional results in patients with sarcopenic FNF. However, some findings must be discussed. Study 4 [16] did not confirm any hypothesis because the improvements were not significant between the different groups. However, in the nutritional supplementation group, analysis did show a positive effect on quality of life and handgrip strength. In the other two studies, significant improvement was seen in ADLs, in particular, and in HGS and walking ability in the intervention groups [19,20]. Moreover, Study 5 [19] found that sarcopenic patients with amino acid intake had important improvements in ADLs, compared to other groups. The same difference did not occur in the nonsarcopenic patients. The improvement disappeared after two months when the intake was suspended. This may prove the importance of amino-acid supplementation, especially in sarcopenic patients after hip surgery, beinmg maintained for a longer period in older adults.

As for medical therapy, no drugs are specifically designed for the treatment of sarcopenia. Testosterone, growth hormone and beta-adrenergic receptor agonists are commonly used to improve sarcopenia [45], but more research is needed because they do not always improve muscle function [46].

Study 7 [24] tried to include EPO as a drug to treat sarcopenia when used as a perioperative red blood cell mobilization drug in patients with FNF. The authors found that EPO improved the muscle strength of female patients with sarcopenia during the perioperative period, increased muscle mass of both women and men to a certain degree and significantly reduced the incidence of complications during the preoperative period. EPO may work as a new treatment option for patients with FNF in short-term postoperative rehabilitation.

5. Conclusions

Physical activity, in its various forms, and dietary supplementation, are the basic tools of prevention and rehabilitation of sarcopenia in elderly patients after hip surgery. Exercise training increases muscle mass in the elderly population with varying fragility and nutritional status, helping outpatient recovery, which is the primary outcome in these patients. The most effective physical therapy seems to be exercise of progressive resistance. However, occupational therapy should be included in sarcopenic patients for its importance in cognitive rehabilitation, especially in older adults, to help their return to normal daily activities. Nutritional support, combined with task-specific repetitive exercises, is supported by accumulating evidence for improving sarcopenia and preventing disability. Protein-rich dietary supplementation should primarily include amino acids for a long period in elderly patients. Treatment should include medical therapy, such as erythropoietin and bisphosphonates, which are increasingly important resources, even though they need further research for their validation.

Author Contributions: Conceptualization, G.R.A.M. and M.A.; methodology, M.A.; software, A.V.; validation, G.T., V.P. and M.V.; formal analysis, S.M.; investigation, G.R.A.M.; resources, M.A.; data curation, A.V.; writing—original draft preparation, G.R.A.M.; writing—review and editing, M.A.; visualization, A.V.; supervision, G.T.; project administration, M.V.; funding acquisition, V.P. All authors have read and agreed to the published version of the manuscript.

Funding: This research received no external funding.

Conflicts of Interest: The authors declare no conflict of interest.

References

1. Cruz-Jentoft, A.J.; Bahat, G.; Bauer, J.; Boirie, Y.; Bruyère, O.; Cederholm, T.; Cooper, C.; Landi, F.; Rolland, Y.; Sayer, A.A.; et al. Sarcopenia: Revised European consensus on definition and diagnosis. *Age Ageing* **2019**, *48*, 16–31. [CrossRef] [PubMed]
2. Cruz-Jentoft, A.J.; Landi, F.; Schneider, S.; Zúñiga, C.; Arai, H.; Boirie, Y.; Chen, L.-K.; Fielding, R.A.; Martin, F.C.; Michel, J.-P.; et al. Prevalence of and interventions for sarcopenia in ageing adults: A systematic review. Report of the International Sarcopenia Initiative (EWGSOP and IWGS). *Age Ageing* **2014**, *43*, 748–759. [CrossRef] [PubMed]
3. Woo, J. Sarcopenia. *Clin. Geriatr. Med.* **2017**, *33*, 305–314. [CrossRef]
4. Marzetti, E.; on behalf of the SPRINTT Consortium; Calvani, R.; Tosato, M.; Cesari, M.; Di Bari, M.; Cherubini, A.; Collamati, A.; D'Angelo, E.; Pahor, M.; et al. Sarcopenia: An overview. *Aging Clin. Exp. Res.* **2017**, *29*, 11–17. [CrossRef] [PubMed]
5. Goodpaster, B.H.; Park, S.W.; Harris, T.B.; Kritchevsky, S.B.; Nevitt, M.; Schwartz, A.V.; Simonsick, E.M.; Tylavsky, F.A.; Visser, M.; Newman, A.B.; et al. The Loss of Skeletal Muscle Strength, Mass, and Quality in Older Adults: The Health, Aging and Body Composition Study. *J. Gerontol. Ser. A Boil. Sci. Med. Sci.* **2006**, *61*, 1059–1064. [CrossRef]

6. Robinson, S.; Denison, H.; Cooper, C.; Sayer, A.A. Prevention and optimal management of sarcopenia: A review of combined exercise and nutrition interventions to improve muscle outcomes in older people. *Clin. Interv. Aging* **2015**, *10*, 859–869. [CrossRef]
7. Ryall, J.G.; Schertzer, J.D.; Lynch, G.S. Cellular and molecular mechanisms underlying age-related skeletal muscle wasting and weakness. *Biogerontology* **2008**, *9*, 213–228. [CrossRef]
8. Dhillon, R.J.; Hasni, S.A. Pathogenesis and Management of Sarcopenia. *Clin. Geriatr. Med.* **2017**, *33*, 17–26. [CrossRef]
9. Cesari, M.; Fielding, R.A.; Pahor, M.; Goodpaster, B.; Hellerstein, M.; Van Kan, G.A.; Anker, S.D.; Rutkove, S.; Vrijbloed, J.W.; Isaac, M.; et al. Biomarkers of sarcopenia in clinical trials-recommendations from the International Working Group on Sarcopenia. *J. Cachex Sarcopenia Muscle* **2012**, *3*, 181–190. [CrossRef]
10. Van Kan, G.A.; Cedarbaum, J.M.; Cesari, M.; Dahinden, P.; Fariello, R.G.; Fielding, R.A.; Goodpaster, B.H.; Hettwer, S.; Isaac, M.; Laurent, D.; et al. Sarcopenia: Biomarkers and imaging (International Conference on Sarcopenia research). *J. Nutr. Heal. Aging* **2011**, *15*, 834–846. [CrossRef]
11. Bell, J.J.; Bauer, J.; Capra, S.; Pulle, C.R. Barriers to nutritional intake in patients with acute hip fracture: Time to treat malnutrition as a disease and food as a medicine? *Can. J. Physiol. Pharm.* **2013**, *91*, 489–495. [CrossRef] [PubMed]
12. Di Monaco, M.; Castiglioni, C.; Vallero, F.; Di Monaco, R.; Tappero, R. Sarcopenia is more prevalent in men than in women after hip fracture: A cross-sectional study of 591 inpatients. *Arch. Gerontol. Geriatr.* **2012**, *55*, e48–e52. [CrossRef] [PubMed]
13. Hida, T.; Ishiguro, N.; Shimokata, H.; Sakai, Y.; Matsui, Y.; Takemura, M.; Terabe, Y.; Harada, A. High prevalence of sarcopenia and reduced leg muscle mass in Japanese patients immediately after a hip fracture. *Geriatr. Gerontol. Int.* **2012**, *13*, 413–420. [CrossRef] [PubMed]
14. Vellas, B.; Fielding, R.; Miller, R.; Rolland, Y.; Bhasin, S.; Magaziner, J.; Bischoff-Ferrari, H. Designing drug trials for sarcopenia in older adults with hip fracture—A task force from the international conference onfrailty and sarcopenia research (icfsr). *J. Frailty Aging* **2014**, *3*, 199–204. [PubMed]
15. Fox, K.M.; Magaziner, J.; Hawkes, W.G.; Yu-Yahiro, J.; Hebel, J.R.; Zimmerman, S.I.; Holder, L.; Michael, R. Loss of Bone Density and Lean Body Mass after Hip Fracture. *Osteoporos. Int.* **2000**, *11*, 31–35. [CrossRef] [PubMed]
16. Flodin, L.; Cederholm, T.; Sääf, M.; Samnegård, E.; Ekström, W.; Al-Ani, A.N.; Hedström, M. Effects of protein-rich nutritional supplementation and bisphosphonates on body composition, handgrip strength and health-related quality of life after hip fracture: A 12-month randomized controlled study. *BMC Geriatr.* **2015**, *15*, 149. [CrossRef]
17. Al-Ani, A.N.; Flodin, L.; Söderqvist, A.; Ackermann, P.W.; Samnegård, E.; Dalen, N.; Sääf, M.; Cederholm, T.; Hedström, M. Does Rehabilitation Matter in Patients With Femoral Neck Fracture and Cognitive Impairment? A Prospective Study of 246 Patients. *Arch. Phys. Med. Rehabil.* **2010**, *91*, 51–57. [CrossRef]
18. Samuelsson, B.; Hedström, M.I.; Ponzer, S.; Söderqvist, A.; Samnegård, E.; Thorngren, K.-G.; Cederholm, T.; Sääf, M.; Dalen, N. Gender differences and cognitive aspects on functional outcome after hip fracture–a 2 years' follow-up of 2,134 patients. *Age Ageing* **2009**, *38*, 686–692. [CrossRef]
19. Invernizzi, M.; De Sire, A.; D'Andrea, F.; Carrera, D.; Renò, F.; Migliaccio, S.; Iolascon, G.; Cisari, C. Effects of essential amino acid supplementation and rehabilitation on functioning in hip fracture patients: A pilot randomized controlled trial. *Aging Clin. Exp. Res.* **2018**, *31*, 1517–1524. [CrossRef]
20. Malafarina, V.; Uriz-Otano, F.; Malafarina, C.; Martínez, J.A.; Zulet, M.A. Effectiveness of nutritional supplementation on sarcopenia and recovery in hip fracture patients. A multi-centre randomized trial. *Maturitas* **2017**, *101*, 42–50. [CrossRef]
21. Lim, S.-K.; Lee, S.Y.; Beom, J.; Lim, J.-Y. Comparative outcomes of inpatient fragility fracture intensive rehabilitation management (FIRM) after hip fracture in sarcopenic and non-sarcopenic patients: A prospective observational study. *Eur. Geriatr. Med.* **2018**, *9*, 641–650. [CrossRef]
22. Lim, J.-Y.; Beom, J.; Lee, S.Y.; Lim, J.-Y. Functional Outcomes of Fragility Fracture Integrated Rehabilitation Management in Sarcopenic Patients after Hip Fracture Surgery and Predictors of Independent Ambulation. *J. Nutr. Heal. Aging* **2019**, *23*, 1034–1042. [CrossRef] [PubMed]
23. Oh, M.-K.; Yoo, J.-I.; Byun, H.; Chun, S.-W.; Lim, S.-K.; Jang, Y.J.; Lee, C.H. Efficacy of combined antigravity treadmill and conventional rehabilitation after hip fracture in patients with sarcopenia. *J. Gerontol. Ser. A Boil. Sci. Med. Sci.* **2020**, *158*. [CrossRef]

24. Zhang, Y.; Chen, L.; Wu, P.; Lang, J.; Chen, L. Intervention with erythropoietin in sarcopenic patients with femoral intertrochanteric fracture and its potential effects on postoperative rehabilitation. *Geriatr. Gerontol. Int.* **2019**, *20*, 150–155. [CrossRef] [PubMed]
25. Chen, L.-K.; Woo, J.; Assantachai, P.; Auyeung, T.-W.; Chou, M.-Y.; Iijima, K.; Jang, H.C.; Kang, L.; Kim, M.; Kim, S.; et al. Asian Working Group for Sarcopenia: 2019 Consensus Update on Sarcopenia Diagnosis and Treatment. *J. Am. Med. Dir. Assoc.* **2020**, *21*, 300–307.e2. [CrossRef] [PubMed]
26. Koval, K.J.; Skovron, M.L.; Aharonoff, G.B.; Meadows, S.E.; Zuckerman, J.D. Ambulatory ability after hip fracture. A prospective study in geriatric patients. *Clin. Orthop. Relat. Res.* **1995**, *310*, 150–159.
27. Collen, F.M.; Wade, D.T.; Bradshaw, C.M. Mobility after stroke: Reliability of measures of impairment and disability. *Int. Disabil. Stud.* **1990**, *12*, 6–9. [CrossRef]
28. Lennon, S.; Johnson, L. The modified Rivermead Mobility Index: Validity and reliability. *Disabil. Rehabil.* **2000**, *22*, 833–839. [CrossRef]
29. Downs, S.; Marquez, J.; Chiarelli, P. The Berg Balance Scale has high intra- and inter-rater reliability but absolute reliability varies across the scale: A systematic review. *J. Physiother.* **2013**, *59*, 93–99. [CrossRef]
30. Kim, T.H.; Jhoo, J.H.; Park, J.H.; Kim, J.L.; Ryu, S.H.; Moon, S.W.; Choo, I.H.; Lee, N.W.; Yoon, J.C.; Do, Y.J.; et al. Korean Version of Mini Mental Status Examination for Dementia Screening and Its' Short Form. *Psychiatry Investig.* **2010**, *7*, 102–108. [CrossRef]
31. Jung, I.K.; Kwak, D.I.; Joe, S.H.; Lee, H.S. A study of standardization of Korean Form of Geriatric Depression Scale (KGDS). *Korean J. Geriatr. Psychiatry* **1997**, *1*, 61–72.
32. Group, The EuroQol. EuroQol—A new facility for the measurement of health-related quality of life. *Health Policy* **1990**, *16*, 199–208. [CrossRef]
33. Lee, K.W.; Kim, S.B.; Lee, J.H.; Lee, S.J.; Yoo, S.W. Effect of Upper Extremity Robot-Assisted Exercise on Spasticity in Stroke Patients. *Ann. Rehabil. Med.* **2016**, *40*, 961–971. [CrossRef] [PubMed]
34. Song, M.; Lee, S.H.; Jahng, S.; Kim, S.-Y.; Kang, Y. Validation of the Korean-Everyday Cognition (K-ECog). *J. Korean Med. Sci.* **2019**, *34*, e67. [CrossRef]
35. Jung, H.-W.; Yoo, H.-J.; Park, S.-Y.; Kim, S.-W.; Choi, J.-Y.; Yoon, S.-J.; Kim, C.-H.; Kim, K.-I. The Korean version of the FRAIL scale: Clinical feasibility and validity of assessing the frailty status of Korean elderly. *Korean J. Intern. Med.* **2016**, *31*, 594–600. [CrossRef]
36. Binder, E.F.; Storandt, M.; Birge, S.J. The relation between psychometric test performance and physical performance in older adults. *J. Gerontol. Ser. A Boil. Sci. Med. Sci.* **1999**, *54*, M428–M432. [CrossRef]
37. Podsiadlo, D.; Richardson, S. The TiMed. "Up & Go": A Test of Basic Functional Mobility for Frail Elderly Persons. *J. Am. Geriatr. Soc.* **1991**, *39*, 142–148. [CrossRef]
38. Soh, S.-E.; Stuart, L.; Raymond, M.; Kimmel, L.A.; Holland, A. The validity, reliability, and responsiveness of the modified Iowa Level of Assistance scale in hospitalized older adults in subacute care. *Disabil. Rehabil.* **2017**, *40*, 2931–2937. [CrossRef]
39. Rubenstein, L.Z.; Harker, J.O.; Salva, A.; Guigoz, Y.; Vellas, B. Screening for undernutrition in geriatric practice: Developing the short-form mini-nutritional assessment (MNA-SF). *J. Gerontol. Ser. A Boil. Sci. Med. Sci.* **2001**, *56*, M366–M372. [CrossRef]
40. Mahoney, F.I.; Barthel, D.W. Functional evaluation: The Barthel Index: A simple index of independence useful in scoring improvement in the rehabilitation of the chronically ill. *Md. State Med. J.* **1965**, *14*, 61–65.
41. Ogilvie, M.; Yu, X.; Nicolas-Metral, V.; Pulido, S.M.; Liu, C.; Ruegg, U.T.; Noguchi, C.T. Erythropoietin Stimulates Proliferation and Interferes with Differentiation of Myoblasts. *J. Boil. Chem.* **2000**, *275*, 39754–39761. [CrossRef] [PubMed]
42. Lamon, S.; Russell, A.P. The role and regulation of erythropoietin (EPO) and its receptor in skeletal muscle: How much do we really know? *Front. Physiol.* **2013**, *4*, 176. [CrossRef] [PubMed]
43. Liu, C.-J.; Latham, N.K. Progressive resistance strength training for improving physical function in older adults. *Cochrane Database Syst. Rev.* **2009**, *2009*, 002759. [CrossRef] [PubMed]
44. Siu, A.L.; Penrod, J.D.; Boockvar, K.S.; Koval, K.; Strauss, E.; Morrison, R.S. Early Ambulation after Hip Fracture. *Arch. Intern. Med.* **2006**, *166*, 766–771. [CrossRef]

45. West, D.W.D.; Phillips, S.M. Anabolic Processes in Human Skeletal Muscle: Restoring the Identities of Growth Hormone and Testosterone. *Physician Sportsmed.* **2010**, *38*, 97–104. [CrossRef]
46. Studenski, S.; Peters, K.W.; Alley, D.E.; Cawthon, P.M.; McLean, R.R.; Harris, T.B.; Ferrucci, L.; Guralnik, J.M.; Fragala, M.S.; Kenny, A.M.; et al. The FNIH sarcopenia project: Rationale, study description, conference recommendations, and final estimates. *J. Gerontol. Ser. A Boil. Sci. Med. Sci.* **2014**, *69*, 547–558. [CrossRef]

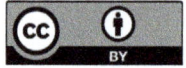

© 2020 by the authors. Licensee MDPI, Basel, Switzerland. This article is an open access article distributed under the terms and conditions of the Creative Commons Attribution (CC BY) license (http://creativecommons.org/licenses/by/4.0/).

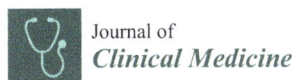

Review

Resistance Exercise, Electrical Muscle Stimulation, and Whole-Body Vibration in Older Adults: Systematic Review and Meta-Analysis of Randomized Controlled Trials

Nejc Šarabon [1,2,3,*], Žiga Kozinc [1,4], Stefan Löfler [5,6] and Christian Hofer [7]

1. Faculty of Health Sciences, University of Primorska, Polje 42, SI-6310 Izola, Slovenia; ziga.kozinc@fvz.upr.si
2. InnoRenew CoE, Human Health Department, Livade 6, SI6310 Izola, Slovenia
3. S2P, Science to practice, Ltd., Laboratory for Motor Control and Motor Behavior, Tehnološki Park 19, SI-1000 Ljubljana, Slovenia
4. Andrej Marušič Institute, University of Primorska, Muzejski Trg 2, SI-6000 Koper, Slovenia
5. Physiko- & Rheumatherapie, Institute for Physical Medicine and Rehabilitation, 3100 St. Pölten, Austria; stefan.loefler@rehabilitationresearch.eu
6. Centre of Active Ageing—Competence Centre for Health, Prevention and Active Ageing, 3100 St. Pölten, Austria
7. Ludwig Boltzmann Institute for Rehabilitation Research, 3100 St. Pölten, Austria; christian.hofer@rehabilitationresearch.eu
* Correspondence: nejc.sarabon@fvz.upr.si; Tel.: +386-5-662-64-66

Received: 31 July 2020; Accepted: 7 September 2020; Published: 8 September 2020

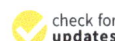

Abstract: It has been shown that resistance exercise (RT) is one of the most effective approaches to counteract the physical and functional changes associated with aging. This systematic review with meta-analysis compared the effects of RT, whole-body vibration (WBV), and electrical muscle stimulation (EMS) on muscle strength, body composition, and functional performance in older adults. A thorough literature review was conducted, and the analyses were limited to randomized controlled trials. In total, 63 studies were included in the meta-analysis (48 RT, 11 WBV, and 4 EMS). The results showed that RT and WBV are comparably effective for improving muscle strength, while the effects of EMS remains debated. RT interventions also improved some outcome measures related to functional performance, as well as the cross-sectional area of the quadriceps. Muscle mass was not significantly affected by RT. A limitation of the review is the smaller number of WBV and particularly EMS studies. For this reason, the effects of WBV and EMS could not be comprehensively compared to the effect of RT for all outcome measures. For the moment, RT or combinations of RT and WBV or EMS, is probably the most reliable way to improve muscle strength and functional performance, while the best approach to increase muscle mass in older adults remains open to further studies.

Keywords: sarcopenia; falls; elderly; resistance exercise; vibration; electrical stimulation

1. Introduction

With rising life expectancy and the increasing proportion of older adults in the population [1,2], effective interventions that promote lifelong well-being and health are more needed than ever before. There is no doubt that performing physical exercise is one of the most effective ways for older adults to maintain functional independence, maintain physical abilities, and reduce the risk of various diseases and injuries [3–7]. One of the most notable changes associated with aging is sarcopenia, which is characterized by a loss of muscle mass and other subsequent changes, such as reduced muscle strength and impaired functional ability [8]. Together with nutritional interventions, resistance exercise training

(RT) seems to be the most effective approach to prevent and treat sarcopenia [9–11]. Falls are also one of the major problems in the older adult population [12] and are thus given considerable attention in terms of prevention. It has been shown that the best way to prevent falls is by performing RT alone or in combination with other exercise types or other interventions [13,14]. Despite extensive research regarding the effects of resistance exercise on sarcopenia, fall risk, and general health of older adults, the recommendations for prescribing exercises in this population are still relatively vague and generic [3,11,15]. In contrast, previous studies have investigated several factors that are worth considering in order to maximize the effects of RT for older adults, such as intensity [16], speed of movement [17], and supervision of the training sessions [18]. Certain types of RT, such as speed-power training [19], are also increasingly being investigated as potentially superior to traditional resistance exercise.

Recent literature reviews have found numerous barriers, such as decreased physical ability, walking disability, lack of companionship, and lack of motivation, that are decreasing the participation of older adults in exercise programs [20,21]. For this reason, different methods to combat sarcopenia, prevent falls, and increase well-being in older adults should be considered as an alternative to RT. Recently, whole-body vibration (WBV) has been shown to improve postural balance [22] and muscle strength [23] and to reduce the likelihood of falls in older adults [24]. WBV is therefore a possible alternative to RT; however, direct comparisons between the effects of RT and WBV are lacking. Roelants et al., reported similar improvements in knee extension strength, jumping performance, and speed of movement after 12 and 24 weeks of RT and WBV interventions in older women [25]. Similarly, Bogaerts et al., showed comparable effects of WBV and RT on muscle mass and muscle strength in older men [26]. Another promising alternative to RT is electrical muscle stimulation (EMS) [27–31]. EMS has been shown to improve functional performance of aging muscles [27,31] and to counteract muscle decline in old age [30]. Moreover, EMS has been appreciated as a convenient intervention for older adults with lower physical abilities or low motivation to exercise [32].

Although many positive effects of RT, WBV, and EMS in older adults have been consistently demonstrated, it is not entirely clear which interventions should be prioritized for the best health benefits. Moreover, studies often follow only a limited set of outcome measures, making comparisons between interventions difficult. Therefore, the objective of this work was to provide a comprehensive systematic review with meta-analysis of high-quality studies that assessed the effects of RT, WBV, or ES in older adults. To obtain a broad overview of these effects, we included studies that assessed various outcome measures, including muscle strength, body composition, and muscle morphology, and the outcomes of functional performance tests. In addition, the aim of this review was to examine the effects of several independent variables, pertaining to the intervention programs, such as (but not limited to) intervention duration, weekly frequency, volume, intensity, supervision, and compliance. We hypothesized that RT, WBV, and EMS will have similar effects on body composition, muscle strength, and functional performance.

2. Materials and Methods

2.1. Inclusion Criteria

Study inclusion criteria were structured according to PICOS tool [33]:

- Population (P): Male or female older adults. The criterion for inclusion was mean sample age $\geq$ 65.0 years. Patients with sarcopenia were included if they met this criterion (age $\geq$ 65.0 years); however, sarcopenia was not an inclusion criterion.
- Intervention (I): RT, EMS, or WBW interventional programs of any duration. Studies exploring multimodal interventional programs (e.g., RT programs combined with stretching exercise) were excluded.

- Comparisons (C): Control groups, receiving no intervention or placebo intervention. Groups that received cognitive training or other non-physical interventions were also accepted as control groups. Studies in which control groups received any type of exercise, vibration intervention, electrical stimulation, or nutritional supplementation were excluded.
- Outcomes (O): (a) Muscular strength or power, not limited to type of testing or body part; (b) body composition and muscle architecture (including body fat, fat free mass, muscle mass, regional muscle mass, skeletal muscle mass, cross-sectional muscle area, circumference measures, and sarcopenia index) and (c) functional mobility outcomes (timed up-and-go test, stepping tests, sit-stand tests, functional reach tests, etc.).
- Study design (S): Only randomized controlled trials (RCT) that included at least one intervention group (RT, EMS, or WBV) and control group.

2.2. Search Strategy

Multiple databases of scientific literature (PubMed, Cochrane Central Register of Controlled Trials, PEDro, and ScienceDirect) were searched in May 2020 without regard to the date of publication. For the databases that enable using Boolean search operators, we used the following combination of search key words: (sarcopenia OR muscle atrophy OR muscle wasting) and (training OR exercise OR vibration OR electrical stimulation OR electrostimulation OR magnetic stimulation OR vibration training OR physical therapy) and (strength OR power OR muscle mass OR muscle diameter) and (elderly OR older OR older adults OR ageing OR age-related). Otherwise, we used several reduced combinations of key words, including, but not limited to resistance exercise older adults, vibration training elderly, electrical stimulation elderly and older adults sarcopenia intervention. Additionally, reference lists of several review articles describing interventions for older adults were carefully scrutinized. Finally, we carefully reviewed reference lists of all articles that were already retrieved through the database search and were published within the last 4 years. The database search was performed independently by two authors (N.Š. and Ž.K.). Two reviewers (N.Š. and S.L.) also screened the titles and the abstracts independently. Potentially relevant articles were screened in full text, followed by additional screening for their eligibility by the additional reviewers.

2.3. Data Extraction

The data extraction was carried out independently by two authors (Ž.K. and C.H.) and disagreements were resolved through consultation with other authors. The extracted data included: (a) baseline and post-intervention means and standard deviations for all eligible outcome measures for interventional and control groups; (b) baseline demographics of participants (gender, age, body height, body mass, body mass index); (c) intervention characteristics (target body area (upper, lower or whole-body), duration of the intervention, number of sessions per week, volume (number of exercises, sets, and repetitions), breaks between exercises and sets, supervision, and progression of exercise difficulty). For studies examining RT, we also extracted the type of load used (bodyweight, machine, elastics, weights, etc.) and intensity as a percentage of 1-maximum repetition (1RM) or subjective measures, such as the Borg scale. For EMS studies, we further extracted the stimulation frequency and amplitude, the stimulated body parts, pulse shapes, and breaks between repetitions or sets. For WBV studies, we additionally extracted the amplitude and the frequency that was used during training. Data were carefully entered into Microsoft Excel 2016 (Microsoft, Redmond, WA, USA). If the data were presented in a graphical rather than tabular form, we used Adobe Illustrator Software (version CS5, Adobe Inc., San Jose, CA, USA) to accurately determine the means and standard deviations. In case of missing data, the corresponding author of the respective articles was contacted by e-mail. If no response was received after 21 days, the author was contacted again. If the author did not reply to the second inquiry, the data was considered irretrievable.

2.4. Assessment of Study Quality

Two authors (Ž.K. and N.Š.) evaluated the quality of the studies using the PEDro tool [34], which assesses study quality based on a ten-level scale. Potential disagreements between ratings were resolved by consulting the other authors. Studies scoring from 9–10 were considered as "excellent," 6–8 as "good," 4–5 as "fair," and less than 4 as "poor" quality. The PEDro scale was chosen because it was developed specifically to assess the quality of randomized controlled trial studies evaluating physical therapist interventions [34].

2.5. Data Analysis and Synthesis

The main data analyses were carried out in Review Manager (Version 5.3, Copenhagen: The Nordic Cochrane Centre, The Cochrane Collaboration, 2014, London, UK). Before the results were entered into the meta-analytical model, the pre-post differences and pooled standard deviations were calculated according to the following formula $SD = \sqrt{[(SD_{pre}^2 + SD_{post}^2) - (2 \times r \times SD_{pre} \times SD_{post})]}$. The correction value (r), which represents the pre-test–post-test correlation of outcome measures, was conservatively set at 0.75. It should be noted that a change in the correction value in the range between 0.5 and 0.9 had little effect on the pooled SD and would not change the outcomes of the meta-analyses. For the meta-analyses, the inverse variance method for continuous outcomes with a random-effects model was used. The pooled effect sizes were expressed as mean difference (MD) where possible, which allows the effect size to be expressed in units of measurement. Where this was not possible due to the heterogeneity of the outcome variables (e.g., muscle strength reported in kg, N, Nm, N/kg, and Nm/kg), the effect sizes were expressed as standardized mean difference (SMD). For MD and SMD, the respective 95% confidence intervals were also calculated and reported.

Basic analysis compared the effects of the RT, EMS, and WBV interventions. Further subgroup analyses were conducted where possible (depending on the number of studies reporting a given outcome) based on several independent variables, related to the characteristics of the interventions (e.g., weekly number of sessions). Some outcomes did not appear in EMS and WBV studies and were thereby only analyzed in view of RT studies. Statistical heterogeneity among studies was determined by calculating the I2 statistics. According to Cochrane guidelines, the I2 statistics of 0% to 40% might not be important, 30% to 60% may represent moderate heterogeneity, 50% to 90% may represent substantial heterogeneity, and 75% to 100% indicates considerable heterogeneity [35]. The threshold for statistical significance was set at $p \leq 0.05$ for the main effect size and the subgroup difference tests.

Sensitivity analysis was performed when deemed necessary i.e., by examining the effect of exclusion of certain studies from the analyses (e.g., studies that could have included subsets of previous studies, studies with very low compliance, studies that did not report intensity, studies with and without elderly with sarcopenia, etc.). The sensitivity analyses showed no or very little effect on the main results (SMD changes = 0.01–0.10), except where noted and reported in the results.

3. Results

3.1. Summary of Search Results

The results of the search steps are summarized in Figure 1. The search resulted in 64 studies in total, 48 of which included RT interventions (55 intervention groups in total), 12 included WBV interventions (14 intervention groups in total) and 4 included EMS interventions (4 intervention groups in total). A table encompassing all the details regarding the participants, interventions and outcomes of individual studies is included in Supplementary data 1.

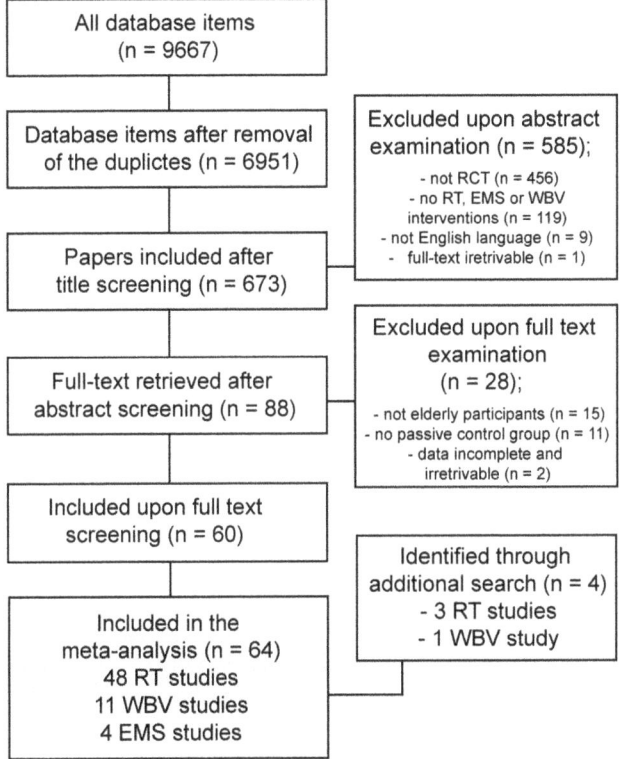

Figure 1. Summary of search results. RT—resistance training; WBV—whole-body vibration; EMS—electrical muscle stimulation.

3.2. Study Quality Assessment

The PEDro scale scores indicated overall fair to good quality of the RT studies (mean = 5.25 ± 1.26; median = 5.0; range = 2–8) and WBV studies (mean = 5.41 ± 1.24; median = 5.5; range = 4–7). Studies exploring EMS were all rated as good (mean = 6.52 ± 1.03; median = 6.0; range = 6–8). The most common items that almost all studies failed to satisfy were blinding of the subjects, therapists and assessors.

3.3. Participant Data and Intervention Characteristics

In total, there were 2017 participants (1158 in intervention groups and 1026 in control groups) in the RT studies, 606 in WBV studies (325 in intervention groups and 284 in control groups), and 192 in the EMS studies (99 in intervention groups and 93 in control groups). Across all studies, the pooled participant age was 73.5 ± 4.8 years (range of means: 65–92 years), the pooled participant body mass was 65.8 ± 10.33 kg (range of means: 40.5–101.8 kg), and the pooled body mass index was 26.39 ± 3.77 kg/m^2 (range of means: 18.8–36.7 kg/m^2). In total, 36 included participants of both genders, 24 studies included only females, and 4 studies included only males. In 16 RT studies, sarcopenia was listed as an inclusion criterion. In 47 studies, the interventions were supervised, while the interventions in the remaining studies were not supervised ($n = 9$) or the information regarding the supervision was missing ($n = 7$). The most typical duration of the interventions was 12 weeks ($n = 28$), while 12 interventions were shorter (4 interventions lasted 5–6 weeks, and 8 interventions lasted 8–11 weeks) and 23 interventions were longer (12 interventions lasted 13–24 weeks, and 11 interventions lasted 25 weeks or more). Most interventions included either 2 ($n = 23$) or 3 ($n = 32$) sessions per week, while 5 interventions were performed once per week and 3 interventions were performed 4–5 times per week. Only 4 WBV and 19 RT studies reported adherence to the intervention program, with mean values of 90 ± 3% and 84 ± 9%, respectively.

Across the RT studies, 14 intervention programs used machines, 6 used free weights, 5 used elastic resistance, 4 implemented bodyweight exercises, 1 used weighted tai-chi exercises, and 1 used isoinertial exercises on a flywheel device. The remaining 17 studies used mixed approaches (5 combined bodyweight and elastic exercise, 2 combined free weights and bodyweight exercises, 3 combined free weights and machines, and 7 used more three or four types of load). RT interventions included either full body workout ($n = 32$) or focused on the lower limb muscles ($n = 16$), while no interventions focused only on the trunk or the upper limbs. Most often ($n = 29$), the intervention included a combination of single-joint and multi-joint exercises; however, some interventions included predominantly single-joint ($n = 12$) or multi-joint ($n = 7$) exercises. The volume of exercise varied substantially between studies, with the number of exercises ranging from 1 to 12 (mean: 5.9 ± 2.9), the number of sets ranging from 1 to 5 (mean: 2.7 ± 0.8), and number of repetitions within sets ranging from 7 to 25 (mean: 11.0 ± 3.5). Intensity was set as percentage of 1-repetition-maximum in 27 studies (mean: 66.2 ± 15.3%; range: 20–80%) or using the 6–20 Borg scale for assessment of the rate of perceived exertion in 10 studies (all studies used 13 as the target value). One study determined the intensity as percentage of maximal heart rate (set between 60 and 80%). The remaining 12 studies did not report the intensity of the exercise. Breaks between sets were reported in 11 studies and ranged from 30 s to 150 s (mean: 100 ± 45 s). Breaks between exercises were only reported in 5 studies (range: 90–180 s).

In WBV studies, the number of exercises ranged from 1 to 9 (mean: 3.8 ± 3.1) and the number of sets ranged from 1 to 10 (mean: 3.5 ± 2.7). With the exception of 1 study, which used highly varying vibration frequency (27–114 Hz), the frequencies used ranged from 20 to 60 Hz (mean: 35.7 ± 10.1 Hz). The amplitude of the vibration ranged from 2 to 6 mm (mean: 3.8 ± 1.4 mm). Breaks between sets ranged from 30 to 180 s (mean: 75 ± 53.8 s).

Finally, 3 EMS studies targeted full body (all used stimulation frequency of 85 Hz, impulse width at 350 µs, moderate intensity (subjectively determined) and lasted 20 min per session), while 1 study stimulated only the lower limbs (frequency: 100 Hz; amplitude: 40–120 mA; impulse width: 400 µs).

3.4. Effects of RT and WBV on Muscle Strength

Knee extension strength was by far the most common outcome across studies and was reported in 2 EMS studies with 2 intervention groups [36,37], 6 WBW studies with 8 intervention groups [25,26,38–42], and 26 RT studies with 29 intervention groups [25,43–67]. In total, 5 studies measured isokinetic strength (1 study at 30°/s, 3 studies at 60°/s and 1 study sat 90°/s), and the rest measured isometric strength. Figure 2 displays the main analysis, comparing the effect of WBV, RT, and EMS on knee strength. Due to substantial discrepancy between the studies in terms of units of reporting, only the SMD could be computed.

There was a statistically significant increase in knee extension strength in the intervention groups across all studies compared to control groups (SMD = 1.12 (0.86–1.37); $p < 0.001$; $I^2 = 83\%$). Both WBV interventions (SMD = 0.97 (0.34–1.59); $p = 0.00$; $I^2 = 90\%$) and RT interventions (SMD = 1.24 (0.96–1.52); $p < 0.001$; $I^2 = 79\%$) improved knee extension strength, while EMS did not (SMD = −0.08 (−1.08–0.91); $p = 0.88$; $I^2 = 81\%$). RT appeared superior to WBV; however, the difference between intervention types was not statistically significant ($p = 0.32$). For WBV, the subgroup analysis was performed for intervention duration and indicated that interventions longer than 24 weeks have a higher effect (SMD = 1.61 (0.35–2.87) than interventions lasting up to 12 weeks (SMD = 0.55 (0.21–0.88) or interventions lasting 13–24 weeks (SMD = 0.55 (−0.29–1.40)), although the subgroup test showed that this difference was not statistically significant ($p = 0.28$). Within the RT studies, most interventions lasted 12 weeks (17/26 studies). Subgroup analyses showed no effect of intervention duration on knee strength increases (SMD = 0.94–1.26 across subgroups). The effect of RT was the highest in studies with participants aged > 80 years (SMD = 1.76 (1.01–2.52), lower in the < 70-year-old subgroup (SMD =

1.17 (0.73–1.61) and the lowest in the 70–80-year-old subgroup (SMD = 0.95 (0.65–1.25)) ($p = 0.14$ for subgroup differences). The effect was comparable in studies using predominantly single-joint (SMD = 1.38 (0.70–2.07), predominantly multi-joint (SMD = 1.12 (0.33–1.90)), or a combination of single- and multi-joint exercises (SMD = 1.27 (0.91–1.62)) ($p = 0.88$ for subgroup differences). No differences between studies were found ($p = 0.68$) based on the type of resistance, though there was a trend for higher effect of interventions based on machine training (SMD = 1.36 (0.97–1.75)) and free weights (SMD = 1.33 (0.37–2.29)) compared to elastic resistance (SMD = 0.91 (0.20–1.63)) and approaches that combined multiple types of resistance (SMD = 0.98 (0.49–1.47)). Finally, studies were grouped according to number of sessions per week and no differences were found between interventions performed ≤2 times per week (SMD = 1.30 (0.92–1.68)) and ≥3 times per week (SMD = 1.15 (0.75–1.55)) ($p = 0.59$ for subgroup differences).

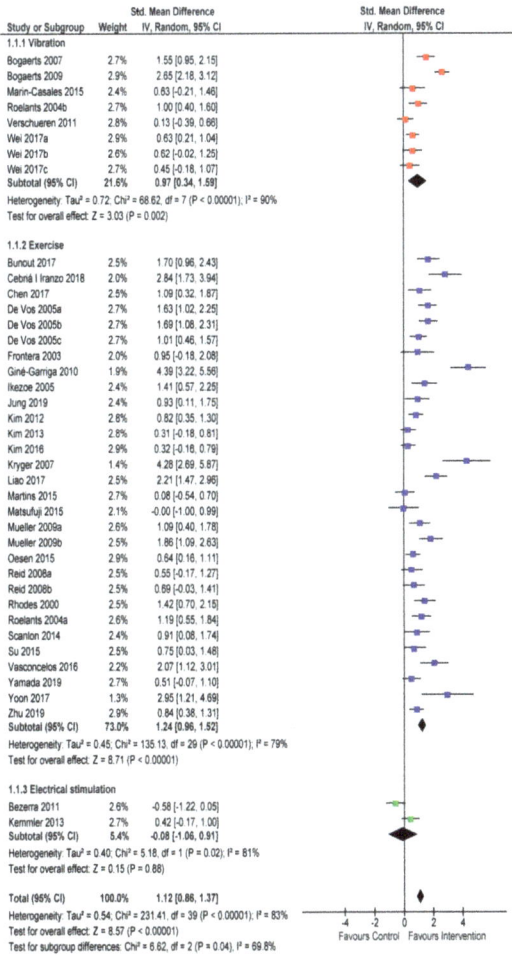

Figure 2. Effects of whole-body vibration, resistance exercise, and electrical muscle stimulation interventions on knee extension strength.

Sensitivity analysis was performed to examine the effect of certain concerns regarding the studies. Since it was not entirely clear if Bogaerts et al. (2007 and 2009, see Figure 2, top section) reported the data for entirely different sample in the two studies, we excluded the study with smaller sample size. The pooled effect of WBV was decreased from 0.97 to 0.88; however, it was still statistically significant

(p = 0.01). Furthermore, 4 WBV studies included in this analysis involved some component (lunges, squats) of RT. Therefore, it is unclear if this RT component contributed to the overall improvements. Removing these studies from the analysis yields a lower overall effect (SMD = 0.59 (0.30–0.87), which is statistically still significant (p = 0.03); however, with this reduction in studies, the subgroup analyses indicate statistically significant difference (p = 0.001) between RT and WBV, indicating the superiority of RT compared to WBV without any RT components. Additionally, we repeated the analysis with exclusion of RT studies on sarcopenia patients (SMD increased from 1.24 to 1.34) and vice versa (SMD dropped to 1.01). Therefore, a slight tendency for larger effect in healthy older adults was indicated. A final sensitivity analysis was performed for type of measurement. Removing the studies that measured isokinetic strength increased the main effect slightly (from 1.24 to 1.33). However, the studies with isokinetic measurements also had large and statistically significant pooled effect (SMD = 0.88; p < 0.001), which suggest isokinetic and isometric strength both substantially increased with RT.

Leg press strength was reported in 5 RT studies (8 interventional groups) [46,60,61,68,69]. There was a statistically significant increase in intervention groups across studies (SMD = 1.45 (0.85–2.06); p < 0.001; I^2 = 83%) (Figure 3). Interventions performed 3 times per week tended to have a larger effect (SMD = 1.98 (0.50–3.45)) than interventions performed 2 times per week (SMD = 1.12 (0.78–1.47)), but the subgroup difference was not statistically significant (p = 0.27 for subgroup differences). Two RT studies reported back extensor strength [45,70] and showed a statistically significant increase (MD = 7.97 kg (3.07–12.88 kg); p < 0.001; I^2 = 0.0%) (Figure 3). Three RT studies [71–73] reported a composite score for strength (i.e., sum of several strength tasks). There was a statistically significant improvement in intervention groups (SMD = 3.55 (2.28–4.83); p < 0.001; I^2 = 90%) (Figure 3). Grip strength was reported in 19 RT studies [44,45,49,52,53,55,56,59,61,65,67,69,70,74–79]. There was a mean increase of 1.48 kg (0.26–2–23 kg; p < 0.001) across studies with pre-post mean differences ranging from −1.00 to 5.70 kg.

3.5. Effects of RT on Body Composition

Muscle mass was reported in 7 RT studies (8 intervention groups) [45,52,70,71,74,78,80]. Compared to control groups, there was not a statistically significant increase in muscles mass in intervention groups across studies (MD = 0.60 kg (−0.18–1.37 kg); p = 0.13; I^2 = 83%) (Figure 4). There were no differences between interventions performed 2 times a week (MD = 0.60 kg (−1.01–2.22 kg)) and 3 times a week (MD = 0.68 kg (0.23–1.14 kg)) (p = 0.93 for subgroup differences). Appendicular muscle mass was reported in 7 RT studies [51–53,65,70,80–82]. The pooled effect showed no change after RT interventions compared to control groups (MD = 0.01 kg (−0.26–0.28 kg); p = 0.92; I^2 = 8%) (Figure 4). Lower-limb muscle mass was reported in 8 RT studies [51–53,55,56,67,80,82], with an overall small and statistically non-significant increase (MD = 0.18 kg (−0.11—0.47 kg); p = 0.22; I^2 = 45%) (Figure 4). No statistically significant differences were shown between interventions performed 3 times per week (MD = 0.55 kg (−0.44–1.55 kg)) compared to interventions performed 2 times per week (MD = 0.10 kg (−0.10–0.31 kg)) (p = 0.39 for subgroup differences). Upper limb muscle mass was reported in 5 RT studies [53,56,67,80,82], and the pooled effect was negligible (MD = 0.01 kg (−0.11–0.13 kg); p = 0.84; I^2 = 0%) (Figure 4).

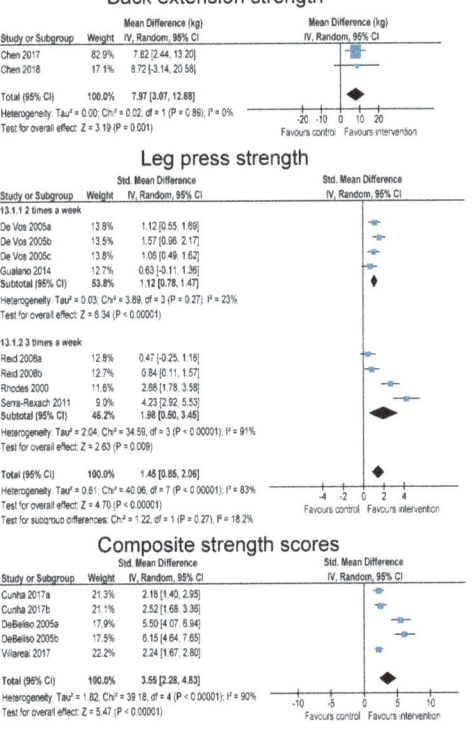

Figure 3. Effect of resistance exercise interventions on back extension, leg press, and composite strength scores.

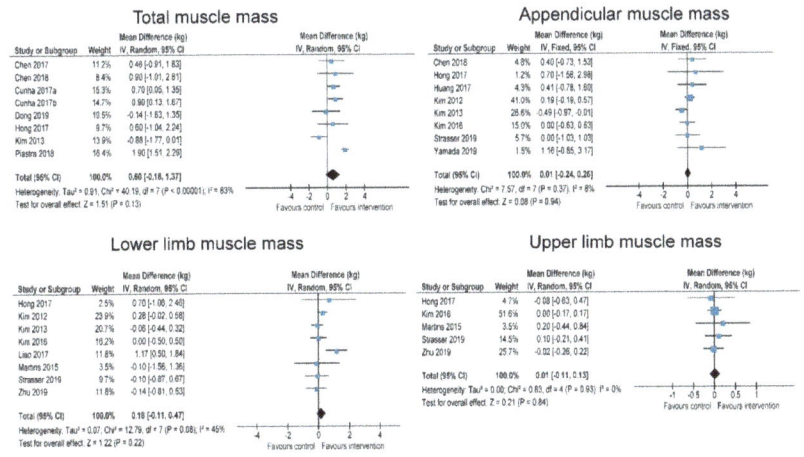

Figure 4. Effect of resistance exercise interventions on muscle mass.

Fat-free mass was recorded in 2 WBV [39,83], 7 RT [55,62,73–76,81], and 1 EMS studies [84], with a very small and statistically non-significant reduction across studies (MD = −0.27 kg (−0.84–0.31 kg); $p = 0.46$; $I^2 = 0\%$). The pooled effect of the two WBV studies showed a slight increase (MD = 0.53 kg (−1.75–2.81 kg); $p = 0.15$), as did one EMS study (MD = 0.61 kg (−0.81–2.03 kg); $p = 0.40$), while there was a small and statistically non-significant decrease across RT interventions (MD = −0.60 kg

(−1.28–0.09 kg); $p = 0.09$). The differences between WBV, RT, and EMS were not statistically significant ($p = 0.25$).

Body fat mass was reported in 2 WBV [39,41] and 14 RT (16 intervention groups) studies [45,50,53,55,58,62,70,71,73,74,76,80,81,85], with a statistically significant decrease overall (SMD = −0.65 (−1.09−−0.21); $p < 0.001$; $I^2 = 86\%$). For the purposes of MD calculation, three studies (4 intervention groups) [45,58,74] that reported body mass in kg instead of the percentage of body weight were removed and the analysis was repeated. SMD slightly increased (SMD = −0.74) and MD calculation showed a mean reduction of body fat mass percentage of −1.99% (−3.75−−0.22%).

Nine RT studies [44,50,67,70,74,77,78,82] and one EMS study [86] also reported the sarcopenia index (sometimes termed skeletal muscle index) (Figure 5). Mainly (7 studies), the index was computed as the ratio of appendicular skeletal muscle mass and the square body height. However, since two studies did not report the exact calculation of the index, we opted for SMD in order analyses to be conservative. There was a moderate, but statistically non-significant improvement across all studies (SMD = 0.65 (−0.02–1.32); $p = 0.06$; $I^2 = 90\%$). Subgroup analyses favored RT interventions, performed 2 times weekly ($p = 0.008$); this is being heavily influenced by one RT study that showed substantial improvement (SMD = 3.44). Most of the studies showed very small negative or very small positive effects, while the pooled effect was heavily influenced by the aforementioned study. Furthermore, 3 WBV studies [42,87,88] (5 intervention groups) and 3 RT studies [47,62,66] reported the quadriceps muscle (or individual heads of quadriceps muscle) cross-sectional area. In order to obtain a sufficient number of studies for meaningful comparison, these results were compared together and expressed as SMD. Overall, there was a statistically significant effect of interventions (SMD = 0.29 (0.03–0.55); $p = 0.03$; $I^2 = 0\%$) (Figure 5). Subgroup differences showed no differences between RT (SMD = 0.61 (0.04–1.18)) and WBV (SMD = 0.20 (−0.09–0.49) ($p = 0.21$ for subgroup differences). For the RT studies (all reported the cross-sectional area for the full quadriceps muscle), the MD was 1.80 (0.51–3.09) cm^2. One RT study [57] reported thigh circumference, with no effect of the intervention (MD = −0.10 cm (−2.55–2.35 cm); $p = 0.94$; I^2 not applicable).

Two RT studies [58,89] reported the percentage of type I fibers, with small and statistically non-significant pooled effect (MD = 0.14% (−1.38–1.66%); $p = 0.86$; $I^2 = 0\%$). The same two studies reported the percentage of type IIa fibers, showing slight but statistical non-significant increase (MD = 1.03% (−0.43–2.48%); $p = 0.17$; $I^2 = 11\%$). Finally, one RT study [58] reported a statistically significant increase in the percentage of type IIx fibers (MD = 2.42% (1.96–2.88); $p < 0.001$; I^2 not applicable).

3.6. Effects of RT and WBV on Body Functional Performance

The results on functional performance are summarized in Figure 6. The timed up-and-go test was performed in 2 WBV [87,88] and 6 RT studies [52,55,69,75,90]. Overall, there were no differences between intervention and control groups across all studies (MD = −0.12 s (−1.36–1.12 s); $p = 0.85$; $I^2 = 93\%$). There were also no differences between the WBV and RT (MD = 0.20 and −0.08 s, respectively; $p = 0.89$ for subgroup differences). The 30-s sit-stand test was performed in 6 RT studies [55,59,68,76,80,85], with an overall improvement of 2.68 repetitions (1.90–3.47 repetitions, $p < 0.001$; $I^2 = 0.50\%$). There was no difference between interventions performed 2 times per week (MD = 2.85 (1.16–4.54 repetitions)) and 3 times per week (MD = 2.73 (2.07–3.39 repetitions)) ($p = 0.90$ for subgroup differences). The 5-repetition sit-stand test was recorded in 4 RT studies [65,67,75,76], and there was a significant improvement (i.e., decreased time to complete the test) across all studies (MD = −2.36 s (−3.9−−0.82 s); $p = 0.003$; $I^2 = 83\%$).

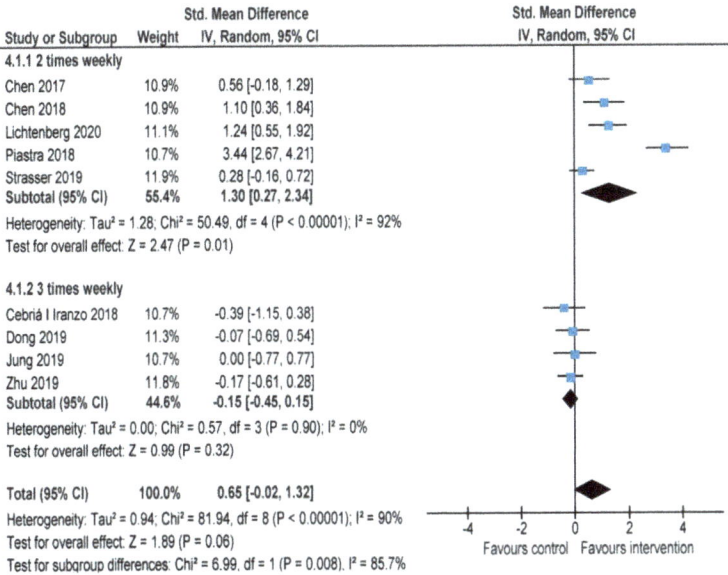
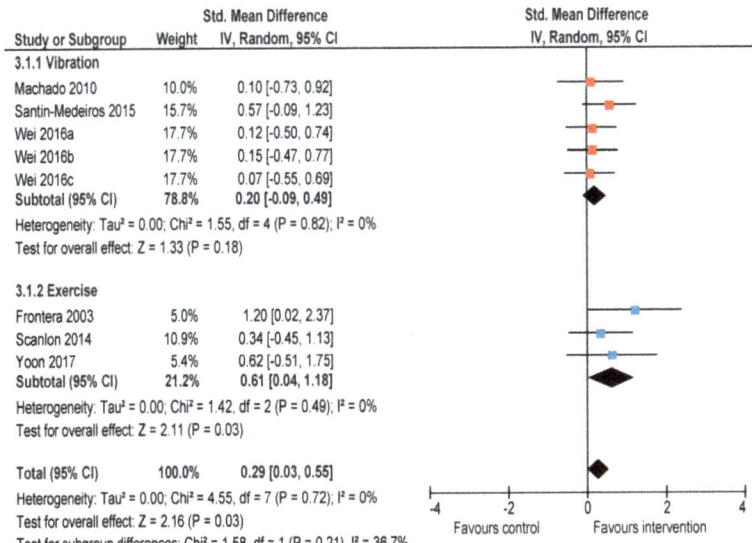

Figure 5. Effects of whole-body vibration and resistance exercise on sarcopenia index and quadriceps cross-sectional area.

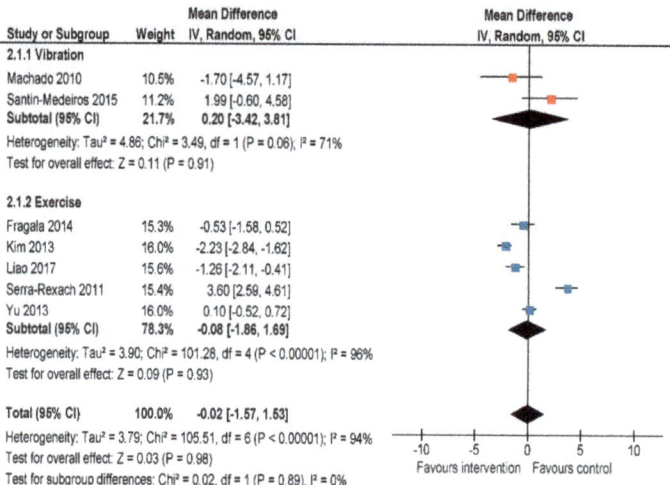
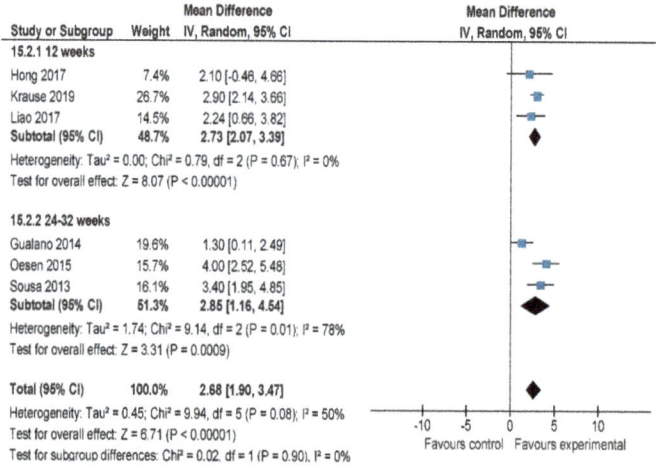
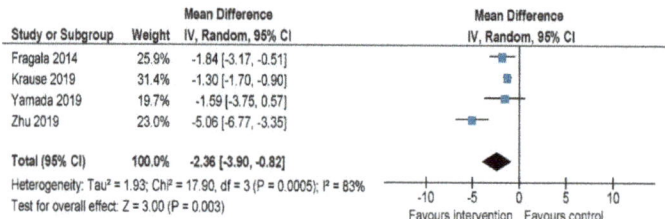

Figure 6. Effects of whole-body vibration and resistance exercise on functional mobility tests.

4. Discussion

The purpose of this systematic review with meta-analysis was to investigate the effects of RT, WBV, and EMS interventions on muscle strength, body composition, and functional performance in older adults. It included randomized controlled trials involving at least one intervention group (RT, EMS, or WBV) and a control group were included. In total, 64 studies were included in the meta-analysis (48 RT studies, 12 WBV studies, and 4 EMS studies). The main findings of the present systematic reviews are: (1) knee extension strength was improved by RT and WBV, but not ES; (2) the remaining strength outcomes were only assessed in RT studies and significant positive effects were observed; (3) the effects of RT on body composition were small, while the effects of WBV and EMS are unclear due to the small number of studies; (4) there were small effects on sarcopenia index, while quadriceps cross-sectional area was improved in RT studies, but not WBV studies; (5) functional performance was improved by RT interventions, though not in all tests. Overall, the RT interventions proved to be effective for improving muscle strength, muscle cross-sectional area and functional performance, while the effects on body composition were small or non-existent. WBV seems to be comparably effective for improving muscle strength, but not muscle cross-sectional area. A major limitation of the review is the smaller number of WBV and particularly EMS studies. Comparisons between the different intervention types were therefore limited and were not possible for several outcome measures. Subgroup analyses revealed that some of the independent variables (duration of intervention, weekly frequency, type of resistance in RT studies, and age of participants) might have influenced the results; however, these findings were not statistically significant and cannot be conclusively confirmed.

The positive effects of RT, WBV, and EMS in older adults have been reported numerous times [9–11,13,14,19,22,23,25,26,30,31,91–93]. In this review, we included only randomized controlled trials that included at least one group that did not receive any interventions (control group). While the positive effects of RT were clearly demonstrated, the effects of WBV, and in particular EMS, were smaller or absent. Individual studies that directly compared RT and WBV have shown similar effects of the two interventions related to muscle strength and power outcomes [25,26]. In a non-controlled single-group study, improvements in muscle strength and power and functional performance were also observed after 9 weeks of WBV [94]. While the present review showed improvements in muscle strength after WBV interventions, only 2 WBV studies that assessed functional performance were included. Therefore, the effects of WBV on functional performance remain unclear. Since improvements in functional performance are often observed in parallel with increases in muscle strength [92,95,96] and muscle power [97], it can be expected that WBV will also increase functional performance. In addition to increases on muscle strength and possible improvements in functional performance after WBV, previous research also showed positive effects of WBV on postural balance [22], cardiovascular outcomes [98] and possibly muscle activation [99] in older adults. Overall, we can recommend the prescription of WBV to older adults, but it cannot be guaranteed that WBV will produce comparable effects to RT in view of all outcomes relevant to health and well-being.

EMS has been used extensively in people who cannot engage in normal physical activity and has been shown to produce somewhat similar responses to exercise at the muscular level [100]. In this review, a very limited amount of randomized controlled trials has been identified to investigate the effects of EMS in older adults. Our analyses could not confirm or indicate any effects of EMS interventions. EMS has previously been shown to be effective in counteracting muscle weakness in advanced disease [101] and sarcopenia in older adults [30,32], and even to provide additive effects in terms of morphological outcomes when combined with RT in healthy adults [102]. However, the effect of EMS on functional performance of the older adults are less consistent [103]. Nevertheless, the above-mentioned promising results should be re-evaluated in randomized controlled trials to strengthen the findings and enable better comparison to RT and WBV. Based on the results of this and previous research [92], the use of EMS should be encouraged when performing physical activities is not possible or older adults are not motivated to perform it.

Across all interventions, the improvements in muscle strength were much more evident than improvements in muscle mass. It is known that improvements in strength due to neural adaptations occur much earlier before a meaningful increase in muscle mass is seen [104]. While most of the interventions in the present review lasted 12 weeks or longer, improvements in muscle mass could nonetheless be expected. It is possible that muscle mass measurements are not reliable enough to detect the effect of the interventions. Alternatively, the cross-sectional area of the quadriceps was statistically significantly increased across RT studies in this review. Moreover, a previous review also reported notable increases in the cross-sectional area of thigh muscles (+2.31 cm^2) in older adults aged >75 years [105]. Interestingly, the latter review reported such effects for WBV, while the pooled effects of the WBV studies in our review were small.

The results on functional performance were different across outcome measures. Neither WBV, RT nor EMS improved the performance of the timed up-and-go test. Conversely, the sit-stand performance was significantly improved by RT interventions (an increase of 2.68 repetitions in 30-s sit-stand task and a decrease of 2.36 s in the 5-repetition sit-stand task time). It should be noted that the results regarding functional performance were significantly influenced by the heterogeneity of the studies. In particular, the timed up-and-go test performance was substantially improved (−1.77 s) in one study and reduced even more in the second study (+1.99 s). Similarly, most RT studies showed improvements in this test, but one study [69] showed a large reduction (+3.6 s), which led to a negligible pooled effect. This particular study was conducted on very old participants (> 90 years) and included a short-term resistance exercise program, based on light to moderate loads. If this study is excluded from the analysis, the pooled effect size would show statistically significant positive improvements (MD = −0.93 s; $p < 0.001$).

The secondary aim of this paper was to determine the independent variables, related to the interventions, that can influence the magnitude of the outcomes. Most of the subgroup analyses that could be conducted as the number of studies was sufficient, showed no such statistically significant effects. There were statistically non-significant trends for lower limb muscle mass and leg press strength to be improved more with a higher (≥3) weekly session frequency. The literature in the field of sports science [106,107] suggests that weekly frequency is not an independent factor for improvements in muscle strength and muscle mass. A recent meta-analysis suggested that similar is true for older adults [108], although a minimum of 2 sessions per week is typically recommended. Our results also indicated a potentially higher effect of interventions based on machine training and free weights, compared to elastic resistance and approaches combining several types of resistance. In the general population, the effect of elastic resistance appears to be essentially the same as machine-based resistance and free weights [109]. Note that our observation on lesser effects of elastic resistance compared to machines and free weights is limited to knee extension strength and that the difference between the effect of elastic resistance (SMD = 0.91) and machine-based resistance (SMD = 1.36) and free weights (SMD = 1.33) was not statistically significant ($p = 0.68$). Therefore, it is probably appropriate to include elastic resistance in RT programs for older adults.

The first limitation of this systematic review with meta-analysis is the inclusion of only randomized controlled trials. While this was done to compile only high-quality evidence, important findings from studies with different designs were omitted. In particular, the number of EMS studies was very small. It should be emphasized that the lack of reported effects of EMS in the review is partly due to the lack of randomized controlled trials and not necessarily because the EMS is not effective. Furthermore, a major limitation of the review is the high heterogeneity of the studies, which precluded more subgroup analyses and is potentially a major confounding factor. Partially, we investigated this issue with several sensitivity analyses which showed that the results were not heavily influenced by certain factors, such as type of measurements (for knee strength), presence of sarcopenia (though somewhat smaller effects were observed in elderly sarcopenia patients), and adherence to studies. Because there are several factors that can influence response to resistance exercise (in particular, the characteristics of the intervention in addition to those mentioned above), we did our best to perform subgroup analyses to exclude or confirm several factors, such as exercise frequency, intervention duration, and resistance exercise type. Nevertheless, some of the variability between the interventions could not be accounted for. Therefore, we strongly emphasize that these results should be viewed with high caution. Future studies and practitioners should not use the numbers we obtained as a standalone guideline, but rather view our analyses as an exploration of general trends in the field of interventions for older adults.

5. Conclusions

This paper reviewed RCT studies that examined the effects of RT, WBV, and EMS on muscle strength, body composition, and functional performance of older adults. It was found that RT and WBV are effective for increasing muscle strength, while the data was very limited for EMS. RT interventions also improve functional performance and increase muscle-cross sectional area but have no effect on muscle mass. Further studies exploring the effect of WBV and in particular of EMS are needed for better comparison with RT. For the time being, EMS can be recommended for people that are unable to perform RT or WBV. Otherwise, RT or a combination of RT and WBV or EMS is probably the most efficient way to improve muscle strength and functional performance, while the best approach to increase muscle mass in older adults still needs to be determined by further studies. Due to the several limitations of this review, we urge the readers to view the results with caution.

Supplementary Materials: The following are available online at http://www.mdpi.com/2077-0383/9/9/2902/s1, Supplementary data 1: Detailed data regarding study outcomes, interventions and participants.

Author Contributions: Conceptualization, N.S. and Ž.K.; methodology, N.Š., Ž.K., S.L., C.H.; software, Ž.K.; formal analysis, N.Š., Ž.K., S.L., C.H.; investigation, N.Š., Ž.K., S.L., C.H.; resources, N.S., S.L.; data curation, N.Š., Ž.K., S.L., C.H.; writing—original draft preparation, N.Š., Ž.K.; writing—review and editing, S.L., C.H.; visualization, N.Š, Ž.K.; supervision, N.S.; project administration, N.Š. funding acquisition, S.L. All authors have read and agreed to the published version of the manuscript.

Funding: The study was supported by Institute for Physical Medicine and Rehabilitation, Physiko- & Rheumatherapie GmbH.

Acknowledgments: We want to acknowledge the support of the European Regional Development Fund and Physiko- and Rheumatherapie institute through the Centre of Active Ageing project in the Interreg Slovakia-Austria cross-border cooperation program (partners: Faculty for Physical Education and Sports, Comenius University in Bratislava: Institute for Physical Medicine and Rehabilitation, Physiko- & Rheumatherapie GmbH). Authors NS and ZK acknowledge the European Commission for funding the InnoRenew CoE project (Grant Agreement 739574) under the Horizon2020 Widespread-Teaming program.

Conflicts of Interest: The authors declare no conflict of interest.

References

1. Cheng, X.; Yang, Y.; Schwebel, D.C.; Liu, Z.; Li, L.; Cheng, P.; Ning, P.; Hu, G. Population ageing and mortality during 1990–2017: A global decomposition analysis. *PLoS Med.* **2020**, *17*, e1003138. [CrossRef] [PubMed]
2. Lutz, W.; Sanderson, W.; Scherbov, S. The coming acceleration of global population ageing. *Nature* **2008**, *451*, 716–719. [CrossRef] [PubMed]
3. Galloza, J.; Castillo, B.; Micheo, W. Benefits of Exercise in the Older Population. *Phys. Med. Rehabil. Clin. N. Am.* **2017**, *28*, 659–669. [CrossRef] [PubMed]
4. De Labra, C.; Guimaraes-Pinheiro, C.; Maseda, A.; Lorenzo, T.; Millán-Calenti, J.C. Effects of physical exercise interventions in frail older adults: A systematic review of randomized controlled trials. *BMC Geriatr.* **2015**, *15*, 154. [CrossRef] [PubMed]
5. Lopez, P.; Pinto, R.S.; Radaelli, R.; Rech, A.; Grazioli, R.; Izquierdo, M.; Cadore, E.L. Benefits of resistance training in physically frail elderly: A systematic review. *Aging Clin. Exp. Res.* **2018**, *30*, 889–899. [CrossRef] [PubMed]
6. Barreto, P.D.S.; Rolland, Y.; Vellas, B.; Maltais, M. Association of Long-term Exercise Training with Risk of Falls, Fractures, Hospitalizations, and Mortality in Older Adults: A Systematic Review and Meta-analysis. *JAMA Intern. Med.* **2019**, *179*, 394–405. [CrossRef]
7. Cvecka, J.; Tirpakova, V.; Sedliak, M.; Kern, H.; Mayr, W.; Hamar, D. Physical activity in elderly. *Eur. J. Transl. Myol.* **2015**, *25*, 249–252. [CrossRef]

8. Cruz-Jentoft, A.J.; Bahat, G.; Bauer, J.; Boirie, Y.; Bruyère, O.; Cederholm, T.; Cooper, C.; Landi, F.; Rolland, Y.; Sayer, A.A.; et al. Sarcopenia: Revised European consensus on definition and diagnosis. *Age Ageing* **2019**, *48*, 16–31. [CrossRef]
9. Phu, S.; Boersma, D.; Duque, G. Exercise and Sarcopenia. *J. Clin. Densitom.* **2015**, *18*, 488–492. [CrossRef]
10. Landi, F.; Marzetti, E.; Martone, A.M.; Bernabei, R.; Onder, G. Exercise as a remedy for sarcopenia. *Curr. Opin. Clin. Nutr. Metab. Care* **2014**, *17*, 25–31. [CrossRef]
11. Marzetti, E.; Calvani, R.; Tosato, M.; Cesari, M.; Di Bari, M.; Cherubini, A.; Broccatelli, M.; Savera, G.; D'Elia, M.; Pahor, M.; et al. Physical activity and exercise as countermeasures to physical frailty and sarcopenia. *Aging Clin. Exp. Res.* **2017**, *29*, 35–42. [CrossRef] [PubMed]
12. Cuevas-Trisan, R. Balance Problems and Fall Risks in the Elderly. *Phys. Med. Rehabil. Clin. N. Am.* **2017**, *28*, 727–737. [CrossRef] [PubMed]
13. Tricco, A.C.; Thomas, S.M.; Veroniki, A.A.; Hamid, J.S.; Cogo, E.; Strifler, L.; Khan, P.A.; Robson, R.; Sibley, K.M.; MacDonald, H.; et al. Comparisons of interventions for preventing falls in older adults: A systematic review and meta-analysis. *JAMA J. Am. Med. Assoc.* **2017**, *318*, 1687–1699. [CrossRef] [PubMed]
14. Sherrington, C.; Michaleff, Z.A.; Fairhall, N.; Paul, S.S.; Tiedemann, A.; Whitney, J.; Cumming, R.G.; Herbert, R.D.; Close, J.C.T.; Lord, S.R. Exercise to prevent falls in older adults: An updated systematic review and meta-analysis. *Br. J. Sports Med.* **2017**, *51*, 1749–1757. [CrossRef]
15. Aguirre, L.E.; Villareal, D.T. Physical Exercise as Therapy for Frailty. *Nestle Nutr. Inst. Workshop Ser.* **2015**, *83*, 83–92. [CrossRef]
16. Csapo, R.; Alegre, L.M. Effects of resistance training with moderate vs heavy loads on muscle mass and strength in the elderly: A meta-analysis. *Scand. J. Med. Sci. Sports* **2016**, *26*, 995–1006. [CrossRef]
17. Watanabe, Y.; Tanimoto, M.; Oba, N.; Sanada, K.; Miyachi, M.; Ishii, N. Effect of resistance training using bodyweight in the elderly: Comparison of resistance exercise movement between slow and normal speed movement. *Geriatr. Gerontol. Int.* **2015**, *15*, 1270–1277. [CrossRef]
18. Lacroix, A.; Hortobágyi, T.; Beurskens, R.; Granacher, U. Effects of Supervised vs. Unsupervised Training Programs on Balance and Muscle Strength in Older Adults: A Systematic Review and Meta-Analysis. *Sports Med.* **2017**, *47*, 2341–2361. [CrossRef]
19. Šarabon, N.; Smajla, D.; Kozinc, Ž.; Kern, H. Speed-power based training in the elderly and its potential for daily movement function enhancement. *Eur. J. Transl. Myol.* **2020**, *30*, 8898. [CrossRef]
20. Yarmohammadi, S.; Saadati, H.M.; Ghaffari, M.; Ramezankhani, A. A systematic review of barriers and motivators to physical activity in elderly adults in Iran and worldwide. *Epidemiol. Health* **2019**, *41*, e2019049. [CrossRef]
21. Freiberger, E.; Kemmler, W.; Siegrist, M.; Sieber, C. Frailty und Trainingsinterventionen: Evidenz und Barrieren für Bewegungsprogramme. *Z. Gerontol. Geriatr.* **2016**, *49*, 606–611. [CrossRef] [PubMed]
22. Rogan, S.; Taeymans, J.; Radlinger, L.; Naepflin, S.; Ruppen, S.; Bruelhart, Y.; Hilfiker, R. Effects of whole-body vibration on postural control in elderly: An update of a systematic review and meta-analysis. *Arch. Gerontol. Geriatr.* **2017**, *73*, 95–112. [CrossRef] [PubMed]
23. Rogan, S.; de Bruin, E.D.; Radlinger, L.; Joehr, C.; Wyss, C.; Stuck, N.J.; Bruelhart, Y.; de Bie, R.A.; Hilfiker, R. Effects of whole-body vibration on proxies of muscle strength in old adults: A systematic review and meta-analysis on the role of physical capacity level. *Eur. Rev. Aging Phys. Act.* **2015**, *12*, 12. [CrossRef] [PubMed]
24. Jepsen, D.B.; Thomsen, K.; Hansen, S.; Jørgensen, N.R.; Masud, T.; Ryg, J. Effect of whole-body vibration exercise in preventing falls and fractures: A systematic review and meta-analysis. *BMJ Open* **2017**, *7*, e018342. [CrossRef]
25. Roelants, M.; Delecluse, C.; Verschueren, S.M. Whole-body-vibration training increases knee-extension strength and speed of movement in older women. *J. Am. Geriatr. Soc.* **2004**, *52*, 901–908. [CrossRef]
26. Bogaerts, A.; Delecluse, C.; Claessens, A.; Coudyzer, W.; Boonen, S.; Verschueren, S. Impact of Whole-Body Vibration Training Versus Fitness Training on Muscle Strength and Muscle Mass in Older Men: A 1-Year Randomized Controlled Trial. *J. Gerontol. Ser. A* **2007**, *62*, 630–635. [CrossRef]
27. Mayr, W. Neuromuscular electrical stimulation for mobility support of elderly. *Eur. J. Transl. Myol.* **2015**, *25*, 263–268. [CrossRef]
28. Pette, D.; Vrbová, G. The contribution of neuromuscular stimulation in elucidating muscle plasticity revisited. *Eur. J. Transl. Myol.* **2017**, *27*, 33–39. [CrossRef]

29. Taylor, M.J.; Schils, S.; Ruys, A.J. Home FES: An exploratory review. *Eur. J. Transl. Myol.* **2019**, *29*, 283–292. [CrossRef]
30. Kern, H.; Barberi, L.; Löfler, S.; Sbardella, S.; Burggraf, S.; Fruhmann, H.; Carraro, U.; Mosole, S.; Sarabon, N.; Vogelauer, M.; et al. Electrical stimulation (ES) counteracts muscle decline in seniors. *Front. Aging Neurosci.* **2014**, *6*. [CrossRef]
31. Zampieri, S.; Mosole, S.; Löfler, S.; Fruhmann, H.; Burggraf, S.; Cvečka, J.; Hamar, D.; Sedliak, M.; Tirptakova, V.; Šarabon, N.; et al. Physical exercise in Aging: Nine weeks of leg press or electrical stimulation training in 70 years old sedentary elderly people. *Eur. J. Transl. Myol.* **2015**, *25*, 237–242. [CrossRef] [PubMed]
32. O'Connor, D.; Brennan, L.; Caulfield, B. The use of neuromuscular electrical stimulation (NMES) for managing the complications of ageing related to reduced exercise participation. *Maturitas* **2018**, *113*, 13–20. [CrossRef] [PubMed]
33. Methley, A.M.; Campbell, S.; Chew-Graham, C.; McNally, R.; Cheraghi-Sohi, S. PICO, PICOS and SPIDER: A comparison study of specificity and sensitivity in three search tools for qualitative systematic reviews. *BMC Health Serv. Res.* **2014**, *14*, 579. [CrossRef] [PubMed]
34. Maher, C.G.; Sherrington, C.; Herbert, R.D.; Moseley, A.M.; Elkins, M. Reliability of the PEDro Scale for Rating Quality of Randomized Controlled Trials. *Phys. Ther.* **2003**, *83*, 713–721. [CrossRef]
35. Higgins, J.P.T.; Green, S. Cochrane Handbook for Systematic Reviews of Interventions|Cochrane Training. Available online: https://training.cochrane.org/handbook/current (accessed on 15 May 2020).
36. Kemmler, W.; von Stengel, S. Whole-body electromyostimulation as a means to impact muscle mass and abdominal body fat in lean, sedentary, older female adults: Subanalysis of the TEST-III trial. *Clin. Interv. Aging* **2013**, *8*, 1353–1364. [CrossRef]
37. Bezerra, P.; Zhou, S.; Crowley, Z.; Davie, A.; Baglin, R. Effects of electromyostimulation on knee extensors and flexors strength and steadiness in older adults. *J. Mot. Behav.* **2011**, *43*, 413–421. [CrossRef]
38. Bogaerts, A.C.; Delecluse, C.; Claessens, A.L.; Troosters, T.; Boonen, S.; Verschueren, S.M. Effects of whole body vibration training on cardiorespiratory fitness and muscle strength in older individuals (a 1-year randomised controlled trial). *Age Ageing* **2009**, *38*. [CrossRef]
39. Marín-Cascales, E.; Rubio-Arias, J.A.; Romero-Arenas, S.; Alcaraz, P.E. Effect of 12 weeks of whole-body vibration versus multi-component training in post-menopausal women. *Rejuvenation Res.* **2015**, *18*, 508–516. [CrossRef]
40. Verschueren, S.M.; Bogaerts, A.; Delecluse, C.; Claessens, A.L.; Haentjens, P.; Vanderschueren, D.; Boonen, S. The effects of whole-body vibration training and vitamin D supplementation on muscle strength, muscle mass, and bone density in institutionalized elderly women: A 6-month randomized, controlled trial. *J. Bone Miner. Res.* **2011**, *26*, 42–49. [CrossRef]
41. Zheng, A.; Sakari, R.; Cheng, S.M.; Hietikko, A.; Moilanen, P.; Timonen, J.; Fagerlund, K.M.; Kärkkäinen, M.; Alèn, M.; Cheng, S. Effects of a low-frequency sound wave therapy programme on functional capacity, blood circulation and bone metabolism in frail old men and women. *Clin. Rehabil.* **2009**, *23*, 897–908. [CrossRef]
42. Wei, N.; Pang, M.Y.C.; Ng, S.S.M.; Ng, G.Y.F. Optimal frequency/time combination of whole-body vibration training for improving muscle size and strength of people with age-related muscle loss (sarcopenia): A randomized controlled trial. *Geriatr. Gerontol. Int.* **2017**, *17*, 1412–1420. [CrossRef] [PubMed]
43. Bunout, D.; Barrera, G.; de la Maza, P.; Avendaño, M.; Gattas, V.; Petermann, M.; Hirsch, S. The impact of nutritional supplementation and resistance training on the health functioning of free-living Chilean elders: Results of 18 months of follow-up. *J. Nutr.* **2001**, *131*, 2441S–2446S. [CrossRef] [PubMed]
44. Iranzo, M.A.C.; Balasch-Bernat, M.; Tortosa-Chuliá, M.; Balasch-Parisi, S. Effects of resistance training of peripheral muscles versus respiratory muscles in older adults with sarcopenia who are institutionalized: A randomized controlled trial. *J. Aging Phys. Act.* **2018**, *26*, 637–646. [CrossRef] [PubMed]
45. Chen, H.T.; Chung, Y.C.; Chen, Y.J.; Ho, S.Y.; Wu, H.J. Effects of Different Types of Exercise on Body Composition, Muscle Strength, and IGF-1 in the Elderly with Sarcopenic Obesity. *J. Am. Geriatr. Soc.* **2017**, *65*, 827–832. [CrossRef] [PubMed]
46. De Vos, N.J.; Singh, N.A.; Ross, D.A.; Stavrinos, T.M.; Orr, R.; Singh, M.A.F. Optimal load for increasing muscle power during explosive resistance training in older adults. *J. Gerontol. Ser. A* **2005**, *60*, 638–647. [CrossRef] [PubMed]
47. Frontera, W.R.; Hughes, V.A.; Krivickas, L.S.; Kim, S.K.; Foldvari, M.; Roubenoff, R. Strength training in older women: Early and late changes in whole muscle and single cells. *Muscle Nerve* **2003**, *28*, 601–608. [CrossRef]

48. Giné-Garriga, M.; Guerra, M.; Pagès, E.; Manini, T.M.; Jiménez, R.; Unnithan, V.B. The effect of functional circuit training on physical frailty in frail older adults: A randomized controlled trial. *J. Aging Phys. Act.* **2010**, *18*, 401–424. [CrossRef]
49. Ikezoe, T.; Tsutou, A.; Asakawa, Y.; Tsuboyama, T. Low Intensity Training for Frail Elderly Women: Long-term Effects on Motor Function and Mobility. *J. Phys. Ther. Sci.* **2005**, *17*, 43–49. [CrossRef]
50. Jung, W.S.; Kim, Y.Y.; Park, H.Y. Circuit Training Improvements in Korean Women with Sarcopenia. *Percept. Mot. Skills* **2019**, *126*, 828–842. [CrossRef]
51. Kim, H.K.; Suzuki, T.; Saito, K.; Yoshida, H.; Kobayashi, H.; Kato, H.; Katayama, M. Effects of exercise and amino acid supplementation on body composition and physical function in community-dwelling elderly Japanese sarcopenic women: A randomized controlled trial. *J. Am. Geriatr. Soc.* **2012**, *60*, 16–23. [CrossRef]
52. Kim, H.; Suzuki, T.; Saito, K.; Yoshida, H.; Kojima, N.; Kim, M.; Sudo, M.; Yamashiro, Y.; Tokimitsu, I. Effects of exercise and tea catechins on muscle mass, strength and walking ability in community-dwelling elderly Japanese sarcopenic women: A randomized controlled trial. *Geriatr. Gerontol. Int.* **2013**, *13*, 458–465. [CrossRef]
53. Kim, H.; Kim, M.; Kojima, N.; Fujino, K.; Hosoi, E.; Kobayashi, H.; Somekawa, S.; Niki, Y.; Yamashiro, Y.; Yoshida, H. Exercise and Nutritional Supplementation on Community-Dwelling Elderly Japanese Women With Sarcopenic Obesity: A Randomized Controlled Trial. *J. Am. Med. Dir. Assoc.* **2016**, *17*, 1011–1019. [CrossRef] [PubMed]
54. Kryger, A.I.; Andersen, J.L. Resistance training in the oldest old: Consequences for muscle strength, fiber types, fiber size, and MHC isoforms. *Scand. J. Med. Sci. Sports* **2007**, *17*, 422–430. [CrossRef] [PubMed]
55. De Liao, C.; Tsauo, J.Y.; Lin, L.F.; Huang, S.W.; Ku, J.W.; Chou, L.C.; Liou, T.H. Effects of elastic resistance exercise on body composition and physical capacity in older women with sarcopenic obesity. *Medicine* **2017**, *96*, e7115. [CrossRef]
56. Martins, W.R.; Safons, M.P.; Bottaro, M.; Blasczyk, J.C.; Diniz, L.R.; Fonseca, R.M.C.; Bonini-Rocha, A.C.; De Oliveira, R.J. Effects of short term elastic resistance training on muscle mass and strength in untrained older adults: A randomized clinical trial. *BMC Geriatr.* **2015**, *15*, 99. [CrossRef]
57. Matsufuji, S.; Shoji, T.; Yano, Y.; Tsujimoto, Y.; Kishimoto, H.; Tabata, T.; Emoto, M.; Inaba, M. Effect of Chair Stand Exercise on Activity of Daily Living: A Randomized Controlled Trial in Hemodialysis Patients. *J. Ren. Nutr.* **2015**, *25*, 17–24. [CrossRef] [PubMed]
58. Mueller, M.; Breil, F.A.; Vogt, M.; Steiner, R.; Klossner, S.; Hoppeler, H.; Däpp, C.; Lippuner, K.; Popp, A. Different response to eccentric and concentric training in older men and women. *Eur. J. Appl. Physiol.* **2009**, *107*, 145–153. [CrossRef]
59. Oesen, S.; Halper, B.; Hofmann, M.; Jandrasits, W.; Franzke, B.; Strasser, E.M.; Graf, A.; Tschan, H.; Bachl, N.; Quittan, M.; et al. Effects of elastic band resistance training and nutritional supplementation on physical performance of institutionalised elderly—A randomized controlled trial. *Exp. Gerontol.* **2015**, *72*, 99–108. [CrossRef]
60. Reid, K.F.; Callahan, D.M.; Carabello, R.J.; Phillips, E.M.; Frontera, W.R.; Fielding, R.A. Lower extremity power training in elderly subjects with mobility limitations: A randomized controlled trial. *Aging Clin. Exp. Res.* **2008**, *20*, 337–343. [CrossRef]
61. Rhodes, E.C.; Martin, A.D.; Taunton, J.E.; Donnelly, M.; Warren, J.; Elliot, J. Effects of one year of resistance training on the relation between muscular strength and bone density in elderly women. *Br. J. Sports Med.* **2000**, *34*, 18–22. [CrossRef]
62. Scanlon, T.C.; Fragala, M.S.; Stout, J.R.; Emerson, N.S.; Beyer, K.S.; Oliveira, L.P.; Hoffman, J.R. Muscle architecture and strength: Adaptations to short-term resistance training in older adults. *Muscle Nerve* **2014**, *49*, 584–592. [CrossRef]
63. Su, Z.; Zhao, J.; Wang, N.; Chen, Y.; Guo, Y.; Tian, Y. Effects of weighted tai chi on leg strength of older adults. *J. Am. Geriatr. Soc.* **2015**, *63*, 2208–2210. [CrossRef] [PubMed]
64. Vasconcelos, K.S.S.; Dias, J.M.D.; Araújo, M.C.; Pinheiro, A.C.; Moreira, B.S.; Dias, R.C. Effects of a progressive resistance exercise program with high-speed component on the physical function of older women with sarcopenic obesity: A randomized controlled trial. *Brazilian J. Phys. Ther.* **2016**, *20*, 432–440. [CrossRef]
65. Yamada, M.; Kimura, Y.; Ishiyama, D.; Nishio, N.; Otobe, Y.; Tanaka, T.; Ohji, S.; Koyama, S.; Sato, A.; Suzuki, M.; et al. Synergistic effect of bodyweight resistance exercise and protein supplementation on

skeletal muscle in sarcopenic or dynapenic older adults. *Geriatr. Gerontol. Int.* **2019**, *19*, 429–437. [CrossRef] [PubMed]

66. Yoon, S.J.; Lee, M.J.; Lee, H.M.; Lee, J.S. Effect of low-intensity resistance training with heat stress on the HSP72, anabolic hormones, muscle size, and strength in elderly women. *Aging Clin. Exp. Res.* **2017**, *29*, 977–984. [CrossRef] [PubMed]

67. Zhu, L.Y.; Chan, R.; Kwok, T.; Cheng, K.C.C.; Ha, A.; Woo, J. Effects of exercise and nutrition supplementation in community-dwelling older Chinese people with sarcopenia: A randomized controlled trial. *Age Ageing* **2019**, *48*, 220–228. [CrossRef] [PubMed]

68. Gualano, B.; Macedo, A.R.; Alves, C.R.R.; Roschel, H.; Benatti, F.B.; Takayama, L.; de Sá Pinto, A.L.; Lima, F.R.; Pereira, R.M.R. Creatine supplementation and resistance training in vulnerable older women: A randomized double-blind placebo-controlled clinical trial. *Exp. Gerontol.* **2014**, *53*, 7–15. [CrossRef]

69. Serra-Rexach, J.A.; Bustamante-Ara, N.; Hierro Villarán, M.; González Gil, P.; Sanz Ibáñez, M.J.; Blanco Sanz, N.; Ortega Santamaría, V.; Gutiérrez Sanz, N.; Marín Prada, A.B.; Gallardo, C.; et al. Short-term, light- to moderate-intensity exercise training improves leg muscle strength in the oldest old: A randomized controlled trial. *J. Am. Geriatr. Soc.* **2011**, *59*, 594–602. [CrossRef]

70. Chen, H.T.; Wu, H.J.; Chen, Y.J.; Ho, S.Y.; Chung, Y.C. Effects of 8-week kettlebell training on body composition, muscle strength, pulmonary function, and chronic low-grade inflammation in elderly women with sarcopenia. *Exp. Gerontol.* **2018**, *112*, 112–118. [CrossRef]

71. Cunha, P.M.; Ribeiro, A.S.; Tomeleri, C.M.; Schoenfeld, B.J.; Silva, A.M.; Souza, M.F.; Nascimento, M.A.; Sardinha, L.B.; Cyrino, E.S. The effects of resistance training volume on osteosarcopenic obesity in older women. *J. Sports Sci.* **2018**, *36*, 1564–1571. [CrossRef]

72. DeBeliso, M.; Harris, C.; Spitzer-Gibson, T.; Adams, K.J. A comparison of periodised and fixed repetition training protocol on strength in older adults. *J. Sci. Med. Sport* **2005**, *8*, 190–199. [CrossRef]

73. Villareal, D.T.; Aguirre, L.; Gurney, A.B.; Waters, D.L.; Sinacore, D.R.; Colombo, E.; Armamento-Villareal, R.; Qualls, C. Aerobic or Resistance Exercise, or Both, in Dieting Obese Older Adults. *N. Engl. J. Med.* **2017**, *376*, 1943–1955. [CrossRef] [PubMed]

74. Dong, Z.J.; Zhang, H.L.; Yin, L.X. Effects of intradialytic resistance exercise on systemic inflammation in maintenance hemodialysis patients with sarcopenia: A randomized controlled trial. *Int. Urol. Nephrol.* **2019**, *51*, 1415–1424. [CrossRef] [PubMed]

75. Fragala, M.S.; Fukuda, D.H.; Stout, J.R.; Townsend, J.R.; Emerson, N.S.; Boone, C.H.; Beyer, K.S.; Oliveira, L.P.; Hoffman, J.R. Muscle quality index improves with resistance exercise training in older adults. *Exp. Gerontol.* **2014**, *53*, 1–6. [CrossRef] [PubMed]

76. Krause, M.; Crognale, D.; Cogan, K.; Contarelli, S.; Egan, B.; Newsholme, P.; De Vito, G. The effects of a combined bodyweight-based and elastic bands resistance training, with or without protein supplementation, on muscle mass, signaling and heat shock response in healthy older people. *Exp. Gerontol.* **2019**, *115*, 104–113. [CrossRef] [PubMed]

77. Lichtenberg, T.; Von Stengel, S.; Sieber, C.; Kemmler, W. The favorable effects of a high-intensity resistance training on sarcopenia in older community-dwelling men with osteosarcopenia: The randomized controlled frost study. *Clin. Interv. Aging* **2019**, *14*, 2173–2186. [CrossRef]

78. Piastra, G.; Perasso, L.; Lucarini, S.; Monacelli, F.; Bisio, A.; Ferrando, V.; Gallamini, M.; Faelli, E.; Ruggeri, P. Effects of Two Types of 9-Month Adapted Physical Activity Program on Muscle Mass, Muscle Strength, and Balance in Moderate Sarcopenic Older Women. *BioMed Res. Int.* **2018**, *2018*, 5095673. [CrossRef]

79. Tsuzuku, S.; Kajioka, T.; Sakakibara, H.; Shimaoka, K. Slow movement resistance training using body weight improves muscle mass in the elderly: A randomized controlled trial. *Scand. J. Med. Sci. Sports* **2018**, *28*, 1339–1344. [CrossRef]

80. Hong, J.; Kim, J.; Kim, S.W.; Kong, H.J. Effects of home-based tele-exercise on sarcopenia among community-dwelling elderly adults: Body composition and functional fitness. *Exp. Gerontol.* **2017**, *87*, 33–39. [CrossRef]

81. Huang, S.W.; Ku, J.W.; Lin, L.F.; Liao, C.D.; Chou, L.C.; Liou, T.H. Body composition influenced by progressive elastic band resistance exercise of sarcopenic obesity elderly women: A pilot randomized controlled trial. *Eur. J. Phys. Rehabil. Med.* **2017**, *53*, 556–563. [CrossRef]

82. Strasser, E.M.; Hofmann, M.; Franzke, B.; Schober-Halper, B.; Oesen, S.; Jandrasits, W.; Graf, A.; Praschak, M.; Horvath-Mechtler, B.; Krammer, C.; et al. Strength training increases skeletal muscle quality but not muscle

mass in old institutionalized adults: A randomized, multi-arm parallel and controlled intervention study. *Eur. J. Phys. Rehabil. Med.* **2018**, *54*, 921–933. [CrossRef] [PubMed]
83. Gómez-Cabello, A.; González-Agüero, A.; Ara, I.; Casajús, J.A.; Vicente-Rodríguez, G. Efectos de una intervención de vibración corporal total sobre la masa magra en personas ancianas. *Nutr. Hosp.* **2013**, *28*, 1255–1258. [CrossRef] [PubMed]
84. Kemmler, W.; Bebenek, M.; Engelke, K.; Von Stengel, S. Impact of whole-body electromyostimulation on body composition in elderly women at risk for sarcopenia: The Training and ElectroStimulation Trial (TEST-III). *Age (Omaha)* **2014**, *36*, 395–406. [CrossRef] [PubMed]
85. Sousa, N.; Mendes, R.; Abrantes, C.; Sampaio, J.; Oliveira, J. Is once-weekly resistance training enough to prevent sarcopenia? *J. Am. Geriatr. Soc.* **2013**, *61*, 1423–1424. [CrossRef]
86. Kemmler, W.; Teschler, M.; Weissenfels, A.; Bebenek, M.; von Stengel, S.; Kohl, M.; Freiberger, E.; Goisser, S.; Jakob, F.; Sieber, C.; et al. Whole-body electromyostimulation to fight sarcopenic obesity in community-dwelling older women at risk. Resultsof the randomized controlled FORMOsA-sarcopenic obesity study. *Osteoporos. Int.* **2016**, *27*, 3261–3270. [CrossRef] [PubMed]
87. Machado, A.; García-López, D.; González-Gallego, J.; Garatachea, N. Whole-body vibration training increases muscle strength and mass in older women: A randomized-controlled trial. *Scand. J. Med. Sci. Sports* **2010**, *20*, 200–207. [CrossRef]
88. Santin-Medeiros, F.; Rey-López, J.P.; Santos-Lozano, A.; Cristi-Montero, C.S.; Vallejo, N.G. Effects of Eight Months of Whole-Body Vibration Training on the Muscle Mass and Functional Capacity of Elderly Women. *J. Strength Cond. Res.* **2015**, *29*, 1863–1869. [CrossRef]
89. Strandberg, E.; Ponsot, E.; Piehl-Aulin, K.; Falk, G.; Kadi, F. Resistance training alone or combined with N-3 PUFA-rich diet in older women: Effects on muscle Fiber hypertrophy. *J. Gerontol. Ser. A* **2019**, *74*, 489–494. [CrossRef]
90. Yu, W.; An, C.; Kang, H. Effects of resistance exercise using Thera-band on balance of elderly adults: A randomized controlled trial. *J. Phys. Ther. Sci.* **2013**, *25*, 1471–1473. [CrossRef]
91. Carraro, U.; Gava, K.; Baba, A.; Marcante, A.; Piccione, F. To contrast and reverse skeletal muscle atrophy by full-body in-bed gym, a mandatory lifestyle for older olds and borderline mobility-impaired persons. In *Advances in Experimental Medicine and Biology*; Springer: New York, NY, USA, 2018; Volume 1088, pp. 549–560.
92. Sajer, S.; Guardiero, G.S.; Scicchitano, B.M. Myokines in home-based functional electrical stimulation-induced recovery of skeletal muscle in elderly and permanent denervation. *Eur. J. Transl. Myol.* **2018**, *28*, 337–345. [CrossRef]
93. Oreská, Ľ.; Slobodová, L.; Vajda, M.; Kaplánová, A.; Tirpáková, V.; Cvečka, J.; Buzgó, G.; Ukropec, J.; Ukropcová, B.; Sedliak, M. The effectiveness of two different multimodal training modes on physical performance in elderly. *Eur. J. Transl. Myol.* **2020**, *30*, 8920. [CrossRef]
94. Cristi, C.; Collado, P.S.; Márquez, S.; Garatachea, N.; Cuevas, M.J. Whole-body vibration training increases physical fitness measures without alteration of inflammatory markers in older adults. *Eur. J. Sport Sci.* **2014**, *14*, 611–619. [CrossRef] [PubMed]
95. Mazini Filho, M.L.; Aidar, F.J.; Gama De Matos, D.; Costa Moreira, O.; Patrocínio De Oliveira, C.E.; Rezende De Oliveira Venturini, G.; Magalhäes Curty, V.; Menezes Touguinha, H.; Caputo Ferreira, M.E. Circuit strength training improves muscle strength, functional performance and anthropometric indicators in sedentary elderly women. *J. Sports Med. Phys. Fitness* **2018**, *58*, 1029–1036. [CrossRef] [PubMed]
96. Lima, A.B.; de Souza Bezerra, E.; da Rosa Orssatto, L.B.; de Paiva Vieira, E.; Picanço, L.A.A.; dos Santos, J.O.L. Functional resistance training can increase strength, knee torque ratio, and functional performance in elderly women. *J. Exerc. Rehabil.* **2018**, *14*, 654–659. [CrossRef]
97. Bean, J.F.; Kiely, D.K.; Larose, S.; Goldstein, R.; Frontera, W.R.; Leveille, S.G. Are changes in leg power responsible for clinically meaningful improvements in mobility in older adults? *J. Am. Geriatr. Soc.* **2010**, *58*, 2363–2368. [CrossRef] [PubMed]
98. Licurci, M.D.; de Almeida Fagundes, A.; Arisawa, E.A. Acute effects of whole body vibration on heart rate variability in elderly people. *J. Bodyw. Mov. Ther.* **2018**, *22*, 618–621. [CrossRef]
99. Wei, N.; Ng, G.Y.F. The effect of whole body vibration training on quadriceps voluntary activation level of people with age-related muscle loss (sarcopenia): A randomized pilot study. *BMC Geriatr.* **2018**, *18*, 240. [CrossRef]

100. Barberi, L.; Scicchitano, B.M.; Musarò, A. Molecular and cellular mechanisms of muscle aging and sarcopenia and effects of electrical stimulation in seniors. *Eur. J. Transl. Myol.* **2015**, *25*, 231. [CrossRef]
101. Jones, S.; Man, W.D.C.; Gao, W.; Higginson, I.J.; Wilcock, A.; Maddocks, M. Neuromuscular electrical stimulation for muscle weakness in adults with advanced disease. *Cochrane Database Syst. Rev.* **2016**, *2016*, CD009419. [CrossRef]
102. Evangelista, A.; Teixeira, C.; Barros, B.M.; de Azevedo, J.; Paunksnis, M.; Souza, C.; Wadhi, T.; Rica, R.; Braz, T.V.; Bocalini, D. Does Whole-Body Electrical Muscle Stimulation Combined With Strength Training Promote Morphofunctional Alterations? *Clinics* **2019**, *74*, e1334. [CrossRef]
103. Langeard, A.; Bigot, L.; Chastan, N.; Gauthier, A. Does neuromuscular electrical stimulation training of the lower limb have functional effects on the elderly?: A systematic review. *Exp. Gerontol.* **2017**, *91*, 88–98. [CrossRef] [PubMed]
104. Hughes, D.C.; Ellefsen, S.; Baar, K. Adaptations to endurance and strength training. *Cold Spring Harb. Perspect. Med.* **2018**, *8*, a029769. [CrossRef] [PubMed]
105. Stewart, V.H.; Saunders, D.H.; Greig, C.A. Responsiveness of muscle size and strength to physical training in very elderly people: A systematic review. *Scand. J. Med. Sci. Sports* **2014**, *24*, e1–e10. [CrossRef] [PubMed]
106. Schoenfeld, B.J.; Ogborn, D.; Krieger, J.W. Effects of Resistance Training Frequency on Measures of Muscle Hypertrophy: A Systematic Review and Meta-Analysis. *Sports Med.* **2016**, *46*, 1689–1697. [CrossRef]
107. Ralston, G.W.; Kilgore, L.; Wyatt, F.B.; Buchan, D.; Baker, J.S. Weekly Training Frequency Effects on Strength Gain: A Meta-Analysis. *Sports Med. Open* **2018**, *4*, 36. [CrossRef]
108. Grgic, J.; Schoenfeld, B.J.; Davies, T.B.; Lazinica, B.; Krieger, J.W.; Pedisic, Z. Effect of Resistance Training Frequency on Gains in Muscular Strength: A Systematic Review and Meta-Analysis. *Sports Med.* **2018**, *48*, 1207–1220. [CrossRef]
109. Lopes, J.S.S.; Machado, A.F.; Micheletti, J.K.; de Almeida, A.C.; Cavina, A.P.; Pastre, C.M. Effects of training with elastic resistance versus conventional resistance on muscular strength: A systematic review and meta-analysis. *SAGE Open Med.* **2019**, *7*, 205031211983111. [CrossRef]

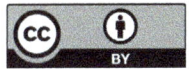

© 2020 by the authors. Licensee MDPI, Basel, Switzerland. This article is an open access article distributed under the terms and conditions of the Creative Commons Attribution (CC BY) license (http://creativecommons.org/licenses/by/4.0/).

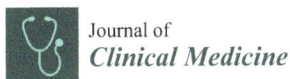

Article

Effect of Aerobic Exercise Training and Deconditioning on Oxidative Capacity and Muscle Mitochondrial Enzyme Machinery in Young and Elderly Individuals

Andreas Mæchel Fritzen [1,2,*], Søren Peter Andersen [1], Khaled Abdul Nasser Qadri [1], Frank D. Thøgersen [1], Thomas Krag [1], Mette C. Ørngreen [1], John Vissing [1] and Tina D. Jeppesen [1]

[1] Department of Neurology, Copenhagen Neuromuscular Center, Rigshospitalet, DK-2100 Copenhagen, Denmark; ggspa@greve-gym.dk (S.P.A.); khaled_qadri@hotmail.com (K.A.N.Q.); frank.thogersen@gmail.com (F.D.T.); thomas.krag@regionh.dk (T.K.); mette.cathrine.oerngreen.01@regionh.dk (M.C.Ø.); john.vissing@regionh.dk (J.V.); tina@dysgaard.dk (T.D.J.)
[2] Molecular Physiology Group, Department of Nutrition, Exercise, and Sports, Faculty of Science, University of Copenhagen, DK-2100 Copenhagen, Denmark
* Correspondence: amfritzen@nexs.ku.dk; Tel.: +45-4263-3359

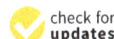

Received: 31 August 2020; Accepted: 23 September 2020; Published: 26 September 2020

Abstract: Mitochondrial dysfunction is thought to be involved in age-related loss of muscle mass and function (sarcopenia). Since the degree of physical activity is vital for skeletal muscle mitochondrial function and content, the aim of this study was to investigate the effect of 6 weeks of aerobic exercise training and 8 weeks of deconditioning on functional parameters of aerobic capacity and markers of muscle mitochondrial function in elderly compared to young individuals. In 11 healthy, elderly (80 ± 4 years old) and 10 healthy, young (24 ± 3 years old) volunteers, aerobic training improved maximal oxygen consumption rate by 13%, maximal workload by 34%, endurance capacity by 2.4-fold and exercise economy by 12% in the elderly to the same extent as in young individuals. This evidence was accompanied by a similar training-induced increase in muscle citrate synthase (CS) (31%) and mitochondrial complex I–IV activities (51–163%) in elderly and young individuals. After 8 weeks of deconditioning, endurance capacity (−20%), and enzyme activity of CS (−18%) and complex I (−40%), III (−25%), and IV (−26%) decreased in the elderly to a larger extent than in young individuals. In conclusion, we found that elderly have a physiological normal ability to improve aerobic capacity and mitochondrial function with aerobic training compared to young individuals, but had a faster decline in endurance performance and muscle mitochondrial enzyme activity after deconditioning, suggesting an age-related issue in maintaining oxidative metabolism.

Keywords: aerobic exercise training; mitochondria; sarcopenia; endurance; deconditioning; skeletal muscle; elderly

1. Introduction

Age-related loss of muscle mass and function, referred to as sarcopenia, is an inevitable process, affecting more than 40% of individuals above 80 years of age [1]. Sarcopenia and reduced aerobic capacity in elderly individuals are strong mediators of morbidity [2] and mortality [3,4]. The ability to perform activities of daily living in healthy individuals is progressively reduced with age, seemingly associated with a decrease in aerobic capacity [5]. Lower levels of aerobic capacity can contribute to a loss of independence, increased incidence of disability, frailty, and reduced quality of life in older people. Sarcopenia and age-related impaired aerobic capacity are related to a multitude of factors, including muscle mitochondrial degeneration [6,7].

It is well established that aerobic exercise training increases maximal aerobic exercise capacity (VO_{2peak}), accompanied by improvements in mitochondrial content, function, and enzyme expression in young, untrained individuals [8–11]. In elderly, findings have been equivocal. Some studies found that 6–16 weeks of intense aerobic exercise training improved aerobic capacity and mitochondrial enzyme activity [12–17], while others were not able to confirm significant effects of training in elderly [18–20]. Thus, it is unclear whether elderly have an attenuated response to training in aerobic capacity compared with young individuals [13,21,22]; in particular, it is not fully understood whether the plasticity for mitochondrial adaptations to aerobic training occurs to the same extent in young and elderly individuals.

A training-induced increase in muscle mitochondrial content and enzyme activity were shown to return to baseline with as little as 4–8 weeks of deconditioning in healthy, young individuals [23–27]. Thus, aerobic training and deconditioning are effective ways to provoke mitochondrial plasticity. In elderly, it could be hypothesized that the age-associated impairments in aerobic capacity and muscle mitochondrial function could relate to relatively faster loss of mitochondrial capacity with deconditiong, but the effect of deconditioning on mitochondrial content and enzyme activity has never been studied in elderly.

Mitochondria are important for many vital functions of the cell, including being a key initiator of programmed cell death (apoptosis). Studies in rats showed an increased apoptotic activity in the aging muscle, accompanied by a lowered expression of the mitochondrial outer membrane antiapoptotic B-cell lymphoma 2 (Bcl2) protein, which was reversed by 12 weeks of aerobic training [28–30]. Furthermore, cleavage of cysteine-dependent, aspartate-specific protease-3 (caspase-3), indicative of increased activation of caspase-3, is a key factor in induction of apoptosis, and it was found to be increased in skeletal muscle of 24-month-old compared to 12-month-old rats [31]. Collectively, these findings in rodents led to the idea that increased apoptotic activity driven by mitochondria could be a contributing mediator of age-related muscle loss in humans that can be reversed by exercise training [32]. These data imply that mitochondria-driven apoptosis could be a key factor behind age-related muscle function and mass loss. However, studies investigating mitochondrial and apoptotic biomarkers in skeletal muscle of elderly in response to aerobic training and deconditioning—and, thus, potential explanation for age-related muscle mass—are scarce.

The aim of this study was to investigate the effect of aerobic training and deconditioning on aerobic capacity and muscle mitochondrial function in elderly (>75 years old) and young healthy individuals (age < 30 years old). We hypothesized that elderly individuals would have indices of mitochondrial dysfunction, but that elderly would increase their aerobic and endurance capacity, as well as measures of mitochondrial content and function, to the same extent as the young individuals after aerobic training.

2. Materials and Methods

2.1. Individuals

The aim was to include a minimum of 10 elderly healthy individuals (age above 75 years old) and 10 healthy young individuals at the age of 20 to 30 years old. Exclusion criteria were nonsedentary, illness that required medication other than antihypertensive and antithrombotic treatment, severe musculoskeletal pain, neurological disorder, smoking, cardiovascular disease, attendance rate below 80% of total training sessions, additional training during the training phase, or failure to comply with instructions of inactivity during the deconditioning phase. Sedentary was defined as performing less than one hour of exercise a week at low to moderate intensity or a maximum of 5 km of cycling for transportation a day.

All participants completed a detailed medical history and electrocardiography, and all had a normal neurological examination before entering the study.

In total, 21 healthy individuals, 11 elderly (four women and seven men; 80 ± 4 years) and 10 young (five women and five men; 24 ± 3 years) individuals were included in the study. Every included participant completed the study in full.

All individuals gave oral and written consent to participate according to the Helsinki declaration. The study was approved by the Ethics Committee of the Capital Region (No. KF-293615). The individuals were all informed about the nature and risks of the study and gave written consent to participate before inclusion.

2.2. Study Design

The 11 elderly and 10 young participants completed a 6 week aerobic exercise training intervention on a bicycle ergometer followed by 8 weeks of deconditioning (Figure 1). Maximal aerobic exercise capacity (VO_{2peak}) and maximal workload were evaluated by an incremental test and aerobic endurance capacity evaluated by a time-to-exhaustion test at 80% of pretraining maximal workload before and after aerobic exercise training, and again after 4 and 8 weeks of deconditioning. Skeletal muscle biopsies were taken from vastus lateralis muscle before and after aerobic exercise training and after 8 weeks of deconditioning for measurement of mitochondrial and apoptotic markers. Dual-energy X-ray absorptiometry (DEXA) scanning of body composition was performed at baseline.

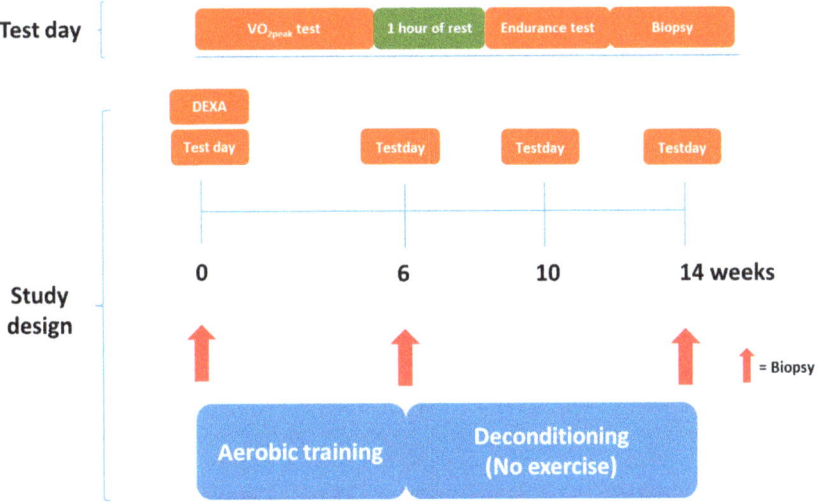

Figure 1. Study design overview. Twenty-one participants completed a 6 week aerobic exercise training intervention followed by 8 weeks of deconditioning (detraining—no exercise). Maximal aerobic exercise capacity and aerobic endurance capacity were evaluated using a maximal oxygen consumption rate test and an endurance time-to-exhaustion test, respectively, before and after aerobic exercise training and after subsequent 4 and 8 weeks of deconditioning. Skeletal muscle biopsies were taken from vastus lateralis muscle at baseline, after 6 weeks of aerobic training and after 8 weeks of deconditioning. DEXA: Dual-energy X-ray absorptiometry, VO_{2peak}: Peak oxygen consumption rate.

2.3. DEXA Scanning

A whole-body dual-energy X-ray absorptiometry (DEXA) scan (GE Medical Systems, Lunar, Prodigy, Chicago, IL) was performed prior to the intervention. Elderly and young individuals were instructed to drink 2.5 L of liquid and, hence, be well hydrated the day before the DEXA scan. They arrived overnight-fasted and were encouraged to empty their bladder prior to the scan.

They underwent the DEXA scan by lying straight and centered on the table with the hip region within two sets of hash marks on either side of the long edge of the table to ensure the entire body was within the scan area according to the manufacturer's instructions. The images were analyzed using enCORE™2004 Software (v.8.5) (GE Medical Systems, Lunar, Prodigy, Chicago, IL, USA). Reliability of this DEXA scanning procedure was recently described [33].

2.4. Maximal Oxygen Consumption Test

Before initial testing, individuals were familiarized with the equipment and test protocol on a separate day with a training session to reduce the impact that skill learning has on strength performance.

On each test day, individuals carried out an incremental cycling test to exhaustion on a stationary bicycle (Monark 939E, Sweden), and VO_2 was measured by pulmonary gas exchange with a breath-by-breath gas analyzer using an open-circuit online respirometer for indirect calorimetry measurements (Cosmed, Quark B2, Pavona, Italy). Load was set individually, increasing every other minute for the first 10 min, and thereafter every minute until exhaustion. Heart rate (HR) was measured during exercise, and the subject's self-assessed feeling of exertion, on a Borg scale, was assessed every minute. Maximal workload (Wmax) was the maximal power output (in Watt) achieved and sustained for at least 1 min during the incremental test.

2.5. Endurance Test

After the incremental test, individuals rested for 1 h before carrying out an endurance test on a stationary bicycle (Monark 939E, Sweden) evaluating time to exhaustion at 80% of pretraining Wmax, obtained under the test for maximal oxygen consumption. Exhaustion was achieved when individuals could not maintain a self-chosen pedal cadence rpm minus 10 rpm for 10 s (e.g., if a chosen rpm at 70 dropped to less than 60 rpm for more than 10 s, exhaustion was achieved). During this test, VO_2 was measured by pulmonary gas exchange as described above, and HR was also measured continuously throughout the test. Exercise economy during the endurance test was calculated as average VO_2 during the test divided by the workload (Watt).

2.6. Aerobic Exercise Training and Deconditioning Interventions

During the 6 week aerobic exercise training intervention, volunteers trained four times per week on a cycle ergometer. Each session lasted 35 min, and sessions alternated between continuous exercise bouts and intermittent exercise bouts. Continuous exercise sessions involved 35 min of continuous cycling at an intensity of 70% of the maximal heart rate (HRmax) reserve (the dynamic area between the resting HR (HRrest) and HRmax). Intermittent exercise consisted of 5 × 4 min intervals at an intensity of 95% of HRmax reserve, with 3 min of rest between intervals.

HRmax reserve has been shown to be well correlated to the intensity as percentage of VO_{2peak}. Heart rate intervals were estimated using the following formula, described by Swain et al. (2000) [34]:

$$HR\% \text{ intensity} = (HRmax - HRrest) \times \text{Intensity} (\%) + HRrest.$$

Heart rate intervals were set to the calculated HR ± 5 bpm. Training was carried out in a progressive manner, with an increasing workload during the training period to achieve the determined HR intervals. All training sessions were supervised to ensure correct exercise intensity and were carried out on stationary bikes (Monark 939E, Sweden or Tunturi T6, Finland). Heart rate was recorded during exercise by a heart-rate monitor. After 6 weeks of aerobic training, participants stopped the training program and returned to their habitual sedentary lifestyle and were instructed not to initiate any new form of training for the following eight weeks. Individuals wore a step counter during the entire study, i.e., the training and deconditioning period, to ensure that the level of daily activity during the training period corresponded to the activity level of the deconditioning period. Step counters were checked once per week throughout the period to ensure that the physical activity level did not vary more than 10% on a weekly basis.

2.7. Skeletal Muscle Biopsies

A skeletal muscle biopsy was performed after the endurance test in vastus lateralis right leg muscle pre- and post-training and after 8 weeks of deconditioning within 15 min of the endurance test. The biopsy was performed as previously described using a 5 mm percutaneous Bergström needle [35]. Needle entry was at least 3 cm away from the previous insertion to avoid scar tissue and interference with data due to post-biopsy edema. Muscle samples were immediately frozen in liquid isopentane cooled by liquid nitrogen before storage at −80 °C for later analysis.

2.8. Mitochondrial Enzyme Activities

Citrate synthase (CS) and mitochondrial complex I–IV enzyme activities were determined as previously described [23,36]. Muscle tissue was homogenized in 19 volumes of ice-cold medium containing protease and phosphatase inhibitor cocktail. Enzyme assays for CS and complex I–IV were performed at 25 °C in a Lambda 16 spectrophotometer (Perkin Elmer) [37]. Complex I specific activity was measured by following the decrease in absorbance due to the oxidation of nicotinamide adenine dinucleotide (NADH) at 340 nm with 425 nm as the reference wavelength. Sample was added to a buffer containing 25 mM potassium phosphate (pH 7.2), 5 mM MgCl2, 2 mM KCN, 2.5 mg/mL antimycin A, 0.13 mM NADH, 0.1 mg/mL sonicated phospholipids, and 75 µM decylubiquinone. Complex I activity was measured 3–5 min before addition of 2 µg/mL rotenone, after which the activity was measured for an additional 3 min. Complex I activity was the rotenone-sensitive activity [37,38]. Complex II specific activity was measured by following the reduction of 2,6-dichlorophenolindophenol (DCPIP) at 600 nm. Samples were preincubated in buffer containing 25 mM potassium phosphate (pH 7.2), 5 mM MgCl$_2$, and 20 mM succinate at 30 °C for 10 min. Antimycin A (2 µg/mL), 2 µg/mL rotenone, 2mM KCN, and 50 µM DCPIP were added, and a baseline rate was recorded for 3 min. The reaction was started with decylubiquinone (50 µM), and the enzyme-catalyzed reduction of DCPIP was measured for 3–5 min [37,38].

Complex III specific activity was determined in a reaction mixture containing the sample and 100 µM ethylenediaminetetraacetic acid (EDTA), 0.2% defatted bovine serum albumin (*w/v*), 3 mM/L sodium azide, and 60 µM/L ferricytochrome c in 50 mM/L potassium buffer (pH 8.0). The reaction was started by addition of 150 µM decylubiquinol in ethanol and monitored for 2 min at 550 nm [39]. Complex IV activity was measured by following the oxidation of cytochrome c (II) at 550 nm with 580 nm as the reference wavelength. The reaction buffer contained 20 mM potassium phosphate (pH 7.0) and 15 µM cytochrome c (II). Sample was added to the reaction buffer, and the initial activity was calculated from the apparent first-order rate constant after fully oxidizing cytochrome c [37,38].

CS activity was measured following the NADH changes at 340 nm at 25 °C by 50-fold dilution in a solution containing 100 µM acetoacetyl-CoA, 0.5 mM NAD (free acid), 1 mM sodium malate, 8 µg/mL malate dehydrogenase, 2.5 mM EDTA, and 10 mM Tris-HCl (pH 8.0). Samples were preincubated with 0.25% Triton X-100.

2.9. Western Blotting Analysis

Western blot analysis was performed as previously described [23,40]. For Western blotting, biopsies were sectioned on a cryostat (Microm HM550, Thermo Fisher Scientific, Waltham, MA, USA) at −20 °C and homogenized in ice-cold lysis buffer mixed with sample buffer. Proteins were separated on an SDS-PAGE gel, blotted to polyvinylidene difluoride (PVDF) membranes, and incubated in primary and secondary antibodies. Antibodies were directed toward Bcl2 (diluted 1:5000; Cell Signalling Technologies, Beverly, MA, USA) and alpha-tubulin (diluted 1:30.000; Abcam, UK, no 4074), with alpha-tubulin used as a loading control. Secondary goat anti-rabbit and goat anti-mouse antibodies coupled with horseradish peroxidase at a concentration of 1:10,000 were used to detect primary antibodies (DAKO, Glostrup, Denmark). Immunoreactive bands were detected by chemiluminescence using Clarity Max, (BioRad), quantified using a GBox XT16 darkroom, and GeneTools software was used to measure the intensities of immunoreactive bands (Syngene, Cambridge, UK). Immunoreactive band intensities were normalized to the intensity of the alpha-tubulin bands for each participant to correct for differences in total muscle protein loaded on the gel.

2.10. Bioplex Analysis

Muscle tissue was homogenized in the same way as described above (see Western blotting analysis). The prepared homogenates were diluted to a final protein concentration of 400 µg/mL. The Human Apoptosis 3-plex Panel (Invitrogen, CA, USA) was used for protein quantification of cleaved caspase-3 (cl. caspase-3) and a single-plex magnetic bead assay for beta-tubulin (loading control) (Millipore, Merck KGaA, Darmstadt, Germany). Then, 100 µL of prepared standards were added to separate wells and incubated at room temperature in the dark for 2 h. The plate was washed twice, before adding a 1× detection antibody to the wells, and then incubated for 1 h in darkness at room temperature. The plate was again washed twice, and 50 µL of streptavidin-R-Phycoerythrin (RPE) was added to the wells, followed by 30 min of incubation. The plate was washed three times, and 130 µL of wash solution was added to each well, upon reading the plate on a Luminex Bio-plex 200 system (Biorad, Hercules, CA, USA).

2.11. Statistical Analysis

All statistical analyses were carried out using SigmaPlot 11.0 and GraphPad PRISM 8 (GraphPad, La Jolla, CA, USA). All data are expressed as the mean ± standard error of mean (SE), except for baseline anthropometric characterization of participants shown as mean ± standard deviation (SD) (Table 1). A Shapiro–Wilk test was performed to test for normal distribution of data. The differences among groups were analyzed by a repeated-measures two-way analysis of variance (ANOVA) followed by Tukey's multiple comparison tests, when ANOVA revealed significant interactions. Baseline subject characteristics were evaluated with unpaired t-tests between young and elderly groups. Correlation analyses were performed with the Pearson's product-moment correlation coefficient. Differences were considered statistically significant when $p < 0.05$.

Table 1. General demographic data.

Demographic Parameter	Young Group	Elderly Group
Age, years	24 ± 3	80 ± 4 ***
Height, cm	175 ± 13	169 ± 9
Weight, kg	70 ± 14	76 ± 14
BMI, kg/m^2	22.5 ± 2.5	26.5 ± 3.5 *
FFM, kg	50.7 ± 14.3	48.4 ± 10.5
FM, kg	15.5 ± 6.0	26.0 ± 6.9 **
Body fat, %	24.2 ± 9.9	34.9 ± 7.7 *
VO$_{2\ peak}$, mL O$_2$/kg/min	37.5 ± 9.0	22.5 ± 6.1 ***

BMI, body mass index; FFM, fat-free mass; FM, fat mass, VO$_{2peak}$, maximal oxygen consumption rate. Data are shown as means ± SD. n = 10 in young and n = 11 in elderly. */**/*** Significantly different ($p < 0.05/0.01/0.001$) from young group.

3. Results

3.1. Anthropometry

Height, total body weight, and fat-free mass were similar among the young and the elderly individuals, whereas the elderly had a higher BMI (+15%), fat mass (+40%), and body fat% (+31%) and a lower VO$_{2peak}$ (−40%) compared with the young individuals ($p < 0.05$; Table 1).

3.2. Functional Parameters of Aerobic Capacity

The elderly individuals had lower absolute values of VO_{2peak} (~40%) and Wmax (~60%) compared with the young individuals ($p < 0.001$; Figure 2A,B). Six weeks of aerobic training improved VO_{2peak} and Wmax by 13% and 34%, respectively, in elderly individuals ($p < 0.05$) and to the same extent by 9% and 26%, respectively, in young individuals ($p < 0.05$) (Figure 2A,B). VO_{2peak} was lowered by 13% already after 4 weeks of deconditioning in the elderly only ($p < 0.05$), and VO_{2peak} returned to baseline in both the elderly and the young individuals after 8 weeks of deconditioning (Figure 2A). In the elderly individuals, Wmax also returned to pretraining level after 8 weeks of deconditioning, while Wmax was still increased by 11% in the young individuals compared with pretraining level ($p < 0.05$; Figure 2B). Endurance capacity, measured as time to exhaustion on 80% of pretraining Wmax, was improved to a similar extent by 2.4- and 1.5-fold in elderly and young individuals ($p < 0.05$), respectively (Figure 2C). Endurance capacity was impaired by 20% and 25% in the elderly by 4 and 8 weeks of deconditioning, but remained at post-training levels in the young individuals during deconditioning (Figure 2C).

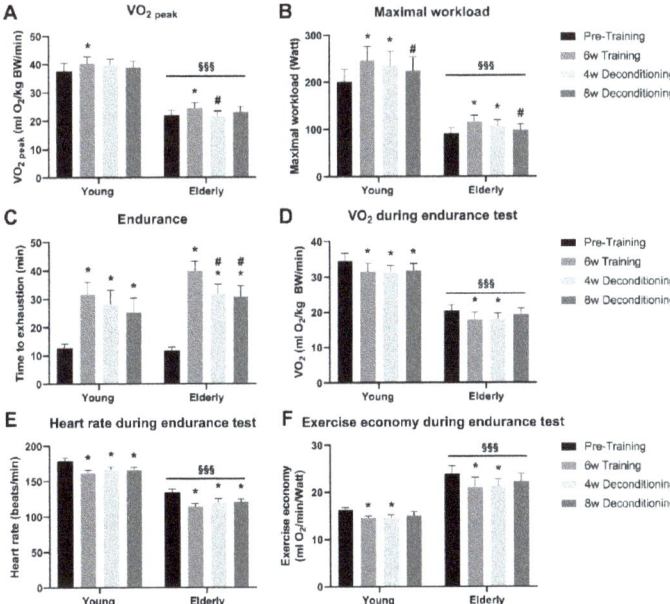

Figure 2. Functional parameters of aerobic capacity. (**A**) Maximal oxygen consumption rate (VO_{2peak}) and maximal workload (**B**) measured in an incremental bicycle test before and after 6 weeks of aerobic exercise training and after 4 and 8 weeks of subsequent deconditioning in elderly and young men and women. Time to exhaustion (**C**), average VO_2 (**D**), average heart rate (**E**), and exercise economy (**F**) during an endurance test on bicycle at 80% of maximal workload in elderly and young men and women. $n = 10$ in young and $n = 11$ elderly. * Significantly different ($p < 0.05$) from pretraining within age group. # Significantly different ($p < 0.05$) from 6 weeks of training within age group. §§§ Significantly different ($p < 0.001$) from young participants. All data are presented as means ± standard error (SE).

VO_2 (Figure 2D) and heart rate (Figure 2E) during the endurance test were overall ~30% lower in the elderly compared with the young individuals ($p < 0.001$). VO_2 (Figure 2D) and heart rate (Figure 2E) were ~15% decreased during the endurance test in both the elderly and the young subjects ($p < 0.05$) and remained so during 4 and 8 weeks of deconditioning. Exercise economy during the endurance test was improved by 12% and 10% in elderly and young individuals ($p < 0.05$), respectively, and remained improved after 4 weeks of deconditioning, but returned to pretraining levels after 8 weeks of deconditioning in both groups (Figure 2F). As a consequence of the relatively lower workload compared with oxygen use during the endurance test in the elderly, exercise economy during the endurance test was overall ~30% lower in the elderly compared with the young individuals ($p < 0.001$) (Figure 2F).

3.3. Mitochondrial Enzyme Activities

At baseline, maximal muscle CS and mitochondrial electron transport chain complex I–IV activities did not differ between elderly and young individuals (Figure 3A–E). Six weeks of aerobic training increased muscle CS activity by 31% in elderly individuals ($p < 0.05$), which was the same as that observed in the young individuals (45%) (Figure 3A). Eight weeks of deconditioning decreased CS activity in the elderly individuals by 18% ($p < 0.05$), while CS activity remained at post-training level in young individuals (Figure 3A). The training-induced increases in complex I (163% and 152%; Figure 3B), II (63% and 58%; Figure 3C), III (63% and 49%; Figure 3D), and IV (51% and 40%; Figure 3E) activities were similar in elderly and young individuals. In elderly individuals, 8 weeks of deconditioning decreased complex I (Figure 3B), II (Figure 3C), III (Figure 3D), and IV activities (Figure 3E) by 40%, 8%, 25%, and 26% ($p < 0.05$), respectively, whereas only complex I (26%; Figure 3B) and II (9%; Figure 3C) activities decreased in young individuals after 8 weeks of deconditioning ($p < 0.05$). Interestingly, the change in enzyme activity with deconditioning significantly correlated with change in endurance capacity for complex I ($r = 0.47$, $p < 0.05$) and tended to correlate for complex III ($r = 0.43$, $p = 0.05$) and CS ($r = 0.39$, $p = 0.09$), whereas the change in enzymatic activity for complex II and IV was not significantly correlated to the change in endurance capacity with deconditioning.

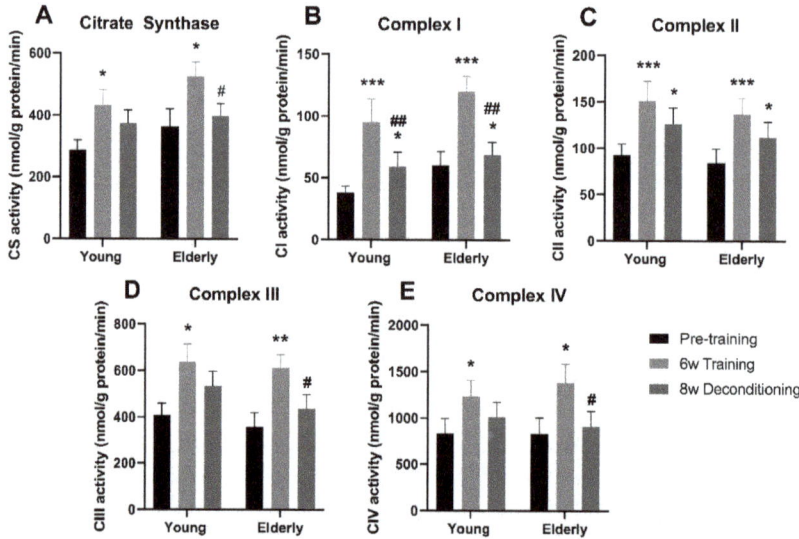

Figure 3. Mitochondrial enzyme activities. Maximal enzyme activity of citrate synthase (CS; **A**), and mitochondrial complex I (**B**), II (**C**), III (**D**), and IV (**E**) in skeletal muscle pre and post six weeks of aerobic exercise training and after subsequent 8 weeks of deconditioning in young and elderly individuals. $n = 10$ in young group and $n = 11$ in the elderly group. */**/*** $p < 0.05/0.01/0.001$, significantly different from pretraining within age group. #,## significantly different from 6 weeks of training within age group.

When correcting mitochondrial electron transport chain complex I–IV activities individually to CS activity, to take mitochondrial content into account, complex II (−26%) and III (−31%) activities were overall lower in the elderly compared with the young individuals pretraining and also after training and deconditioning ($p < 0.05$), whereas the CS-corrected complex I and IV activity was similar between young and elderly at all time points.

3.4. Apoptosis Markers: Cleaved Caspase 3 and Bcl2

There was no effect of aerobic training on cleaved caspase-3 protein content in either the elderly or the young individuals. Pretraining, elderly individuals had a 48% lower expression of cleaved caspase-3 protein content compared with young individuals ($p < 0.05$); however, after aerobic training and deconditioning, there was no longer any difference between the two groups (Figure 4A). Bcl2 protein expression decreased by 21% and 20% after aerobic training to a similar extent in the elderly and young individuals ($p < 0.05$), respectively; however, after 8 weeks of deconditioning, this was not different from pretraining levels in both groups (Figure 4B).

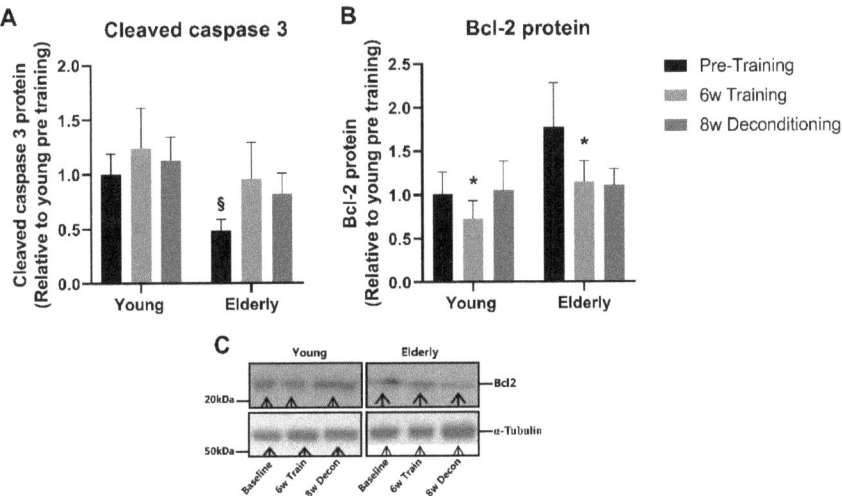

Figure 4. Apoptosis markers. Protein expression of cleaved caspase-3 (**A**) and B-cell lymphoma 2 (Bcl2) (**B**) in skeletal muscle pre and post 6 weeks of aerobic exercise training and after subsequent 8 weeks deconditioning period in young and elderly individuals. $n = 10$ in young group and $n = 11$ in the elderly group; however, due to lack of samples, only $n = 6$ in both groups in (**B**). (**C**) representative Western blots. Values are arbitrary units (means ± SE) and expressed relative to young group pretraining. § $p < 0.05$, young vs. elderly group within pretraining. * $p < 0.01$, main effect of training compared to pretraining independently of age.

4. Discussion

Age-related loss of muscle mass and function may be related to changes in mitochondrial function with age and an impaired response to adapt to the physical activity level. However, only a few studies investigated age-related changes in mitochondrial function in response to aerobic training and deconditioning. In the present study, we investigated age-related changes of aerobic capacity, mitochondrial function, and apoptotic signaling markers with aerobic training and deconditioning and found that (1) only 6 weeks of aerobic training efficiently improved maximal aerobic capacity and mitochondrial function in the elderly individuals, (2) the training effect on aerobic capacity, endurance, mitochondrial enzyme activities, and apoptosis signaling markers in the elderly individuals was similar to that found in the young individuals despite an age difference of more than 50 years, and (3) with deconditioning, the training-induced increases in endurance and mitochondrial enzyme activities decreased in a faster manner in elderly compared with young individuals.

It was suggested that differences in aerobic capacity in elderly versus young healthy humans, at least in part, may be a result of differences in the ability to gain and maintain VO_{2peak} with age [13,21,22]. However, in the present study, 6 weeks of intensive aerobic exercise training resulted in the same increase in VO_{2peak} in elderly individuals compared with that found in young, gender-matched, sedentary individuals, indicating a similar ability to increase oxidative capacity in elderly vs. young individuals. Although the training period was longer than in the present (8–16 weeks), the effect on aerobic capacity was overall the same as previously observed [12–17]. The increase in VO_{2peak} in the present study was found after only 6 weeks of aerobic training, suggesting that elderly individuals can increase oxidative capacity after a relatively short training period to the same extent as that seen in young healthy individuals.

Citrate synthase has been shown to be a strong marker of mitochondrial content. Thus, maximal CS activity strongly correlated with mitochondrial volume measured by electron microscopy in skeletal muscles of healthy, young men [41]. Moreover, maximal CS activity correlated with the improvement in mitochondrial volume after 6 weeks of aerobic training in skeletal muscle of young individuals [42]. In the literature, it has been debated whether there is an age-related decline in mitochondrial enzyme activities, since results from studies investigating this have been ambiguous. Several studies found decreased activity of CS and complex I–IV in muscle of elderly [15,43–47], indicating an age-related decline in mitochondrial content and function. Supporting this view, a study investigating the effect of age on mitochondrial content by transmission electron microscopy found a decrease in the content of mitochondria in elderly compared with young individuals [47]. In contrast, in the present study, CS and mitochondrial complex activities were similar at baseline between young and elderly, as we also recently showed between a similar cohort of young (~22 years) and elderly individuals (~82 years) [36] and in accordance with several other studies [13,48–50]. Interestingly, when mitochondrial complex activities were corrected relative to CS activity to take mitochondrial content into account, in the present study, complex II and III activities were lower in the elderly compared with the young individuals, implying a loss in the electron transport chain efficiency relative to mitochondrial content. It is possible that the mixed results from studies investigating the effect on age and mitochondrial function in part are related to differences in the pretraining level of physical activity in the investigated elderly individuals. Interestingly, in the present study, elderly individuals were able to increase CS activity (+31%) and mitochondrial complex activities (ranging between 61–163%) with training that matched that found in the healthy young individuals, which emphasizes that the ability to respond to an increase in demand in muscle enzymes in tricarboxylic acid (TCA) cycle and oxidative phosphorylation is preserved at least to the eighth decade of life. The few studies that investigated CS and/or mitochondrial complex activities in elderly of 60–80 years of age did not compare results to young but found a similar increase after 12–16 weeks of training [13,15,16,43], suggesting a similar ability of elderly of 60 and 80 years of age to respond to aerobic training. A recent study with only 6 weeks of high-intensity exercise training also showed improved CS activity and mitochondrial complex protein contents in "younger" elderly (63 years old) men and women [12], which, together with the intense protocol in the present study, underscores that mitochondria can adapt to even short-term training interventions in elderly of both 60 and 80 years of age, when the intensity and frequency of the training are high.

In addition to the exercise training intervention, we included a subsequent deconditioning period to evaluate mitochondrial dynamics in aged human skeletal muscle, which, to our knowledge, has not been studied previously in elderly healthy individuals. Deconditioning after exercise training was investigated in a few studies in healthy young individuals, and data implied that oxidative capacity, muscle mitochondrial protein content, and enzyme activities return to pretraining levels after 6–8 weeks in young individuals [23–27]. In the present study, mitochondrial content judged by CS and mitochondrial complex activities returned to pretraining levels after 8 weeks of deconditioning in the elderly, which was not seen in the young healthy individuals. Thus, enzyme activity of CS and complex I, III, and IV decreased in the elderly to a larger extent than in the young individuals. This indicates that the turnover rate of mitochondrial enzymes in the TCA cycle, as well as the oxidative phosphorylation, is fast and even more rapid in skeletal muscle of elderly. Thus, it seems as the ability to obtain oxidative capacity and increase mitochondrial volume with intensive aerobic training is preserved with age, but is lost faster in aged than in young muscle during subsequent deconditioning. A sedentary lifestyle in elderly individuals may, therefore, be even more deleterious to muscle health than in young individuals.

Endurance capacity is essential in order to maintain independence, reduce incidence of disability, and sustain a high quality of life in older people. In the present study, we found that 6 weeks of intensive aerobic exercise resulted in a remarkable increase in the time to exhaustion during an endurance test in the elderly individuals by 2.4-fold. Moreover, this training-induced increase in endurance was likely, at least in part, mediated by an improved exercise economy, reflecting the capacity to turn oxygen consumption into mechanical work and, hence, lower usage of VO_2 at the given power. This finding suggests a functional relevance of the training-induced increase in muscle mitochondrial respiratory enzyme activities, through an improved ability to sustain a high energy-production and also a more energy-efficient power production over a longer period of time. The present study is, to our knowledge, the first to demonstrate that the effect on aerobic capacity and muscle mitochondrial function and efficiency seemingly translates into functional improvement of endurance and exercise economy in elderly. In this line, it should be mechanistically studied in future investigations whether aerobic exercise training prevents sarcopenia by improving mitochondrial function and dynamics [51]. Interestingly, with deconditioning, a faster decrease in endurance capacity was observed among elderly compared with young individuals in accordance with similar decreases in CS and mitochondrial complex activities, indicating that, although elderly individuals improve endurance with training in the same manner as young individuals, aerobic endurance seems to be lost faster in elderly individuals, likely related to enhanced degradation of muscle mitochondrial enzymes. To support this notion, we found, despite the modest number of participants in the present study, that the loss of enzyme activity of CS and complex I and III in response to deconditioning tended to correlate to the reduction in endurance capacity. Of note, the faster decline in mitochondrial enzyme activity with deconditioning was in the present study observed in elderly of ~80 years of age, and it remains to be clarified whether 60–75-year-old individuals that are often investigated in the scientific literature would be more affected by deconditioning compared with young individuals. Importantly, a faster decline in endurance performance during deconditioning contrasts with the loss of strength performance after 6 weeks of resistance training, which we recently showed to be similar between young and elderly individuals (~82 years) after comparable 8 weeks of deconditioning [36].

Even though some studies in rodents indicated that apoptosis may play a role during muscle senescence [32], the involvement of age-related apoptosis of skeletal muscle and its regulation with training and deconditioning is poorly understood. Caspase-3 plays an important role in mediating cell death, and Bcl2 is thought to be an antiapoptotic driver. Interestingly, we found a lower muscle content of active caspase-3 (cleaved caspase-3) and a similar Bcl2 expression in the elderly compared with young individuals at baseline. This indicates, at least in healthy elderly individuals, that markers of the muscle intrinsic apoptotic pathway are not upregulated. These findings contrast with findings in rodents, in which increased apoptosis in old muscle of rodents was suggested on the basis of findings of an increased expression of proapoptotic marker cleaved caspase-3 protein [31] and a lower expression of the antiapoptotic Bcl2 protein [28–30]. Moreover, in the present study, caspase-3 activity remained similar in elderly and young skeletal muscle after 6 weeks of aerobic training, indicating that exercise training does not induce a higher apoptosis activity. In contrast, Bcl2 protein content decreased slightly in response to training to the same extent in young and elderly, implying either less antiapoptotic signaling after training independently of age or that Blc2 content is not directly coupled to apoptosis rate. To our knowledge, this study is the first to investigate apoptotic markers with training and deconditioning in human muscle of elderly compared with young individuals. Although we only investigated a few markers of a complex signaling, the present results do not substantiate the hypothesis that increased apoptosis with time is the mediator of age-related muscle mass. The faster decline with deconditioning in endurance capacity and mitochondrial enzyme activity could relate to an age-related decline in mitochondrial fusion/fission regulation or an impaired matching of lysosomal mitophagy flux to the demand in aged muscle during deconditioning [51]. In support of the latter, we previously showed in young individuals that 3 weeks of one-legged aerobic training improved the capacity for autophagosomal formation [40], which is also found to occur in elderly [52], emphasizing the importance of physical activity to improve or maintain lysosomal mitophagic capacity. From studies in rodents [53–55] and humans [52], it is known that both muscle disuse and aging are associated with impaired mitophagy regulation, and it is, hence, likely that impaired mitophagy and mitochondrial function with deconditioning contribute to accelerated impairment in elderly, which should be addressed in future studies. Overall, accelerated decline in mitochondrial function and sarcopenia seems not to be driven by increased muscle apoptosis in human muscle, and further investigations are needed to elucidate the responsible molecular mechanisms driving sarcopenia and age-related inactivity-induced mitochondrial impairments.

The present study had some limitations that must be acknowledged. It was suggested that potential sex-specific adaptations to aerobic training exist [12]. We recognize that the present study included both men and women but that the number of participants was not optimal to detect an intervention × sex interaction; however, the present study was primarily designed to investigate the effects of training and deconditioning in elderly vs. young individuals. Studies with more subjects are warranted to evaluate potential sex-specific age-related adaptations to training and deconditioning.

5. Conclusions

In the present study, we found that 6 weeks of aerobic training efficiently improved maximal aerobic capacity and mitochondrial function in elderly individuals to the seemingly same extent as in young individuals despite an age difference of more than 50 years. This implies that aerobic exercise training is a potent tool to combat age-related loss of aerobic capacity and mitochondrial function. However, with deconditioning, we present the novel finding that the training-induced increases in performance and mitochondrial enzyme activities seemingly decreased in a faster manner in elderly compared with young individuals. This accelerated loss of mitochondrial function in the elderly with deconditioning could play a role in the development of mitochondrial dysfunction and sarcopenia during aging, and responsible mechanisms need to be investigated further in future studies.

Author Contributions: Conceptualization, S.P.A. and T.D.J.; methodology, S.P.A., F.D.T., T.K., and T.D.J.; investigation, A.M.F., S.P.A., K.A.N.Q., F.D.T., T.K., M.C.Ø., and T.D.J.; resources, T.K., J.V. and T.D.J.; data curation, A.M.F., S.P.A., K.A.N.Q., T.D.K.; writing—original draft preparation, A.M.F., K.A.N.Q., T.D.J.; writing—review and editing, A.M.F., S.P.A., K.A.N.Q., F.D.T., T.K., M.C.Ø., J.V. and T.D.J.; visualization, A.M.F.; supervision, T.K., J.V. and T.D.J.; project administration, S.P.A. and T.D.J.; funding acquisition, J.V. All authors have read and agreed to the published version of the manuscript.

Funding: A.M.F. was supported by a research grant from the Danish Diabetes Academy (grant number NNF17SA0031406), which was funded by the Novo Nordisk Foundation. A.M.F. was further supported by the Alfred Benzon Foundation.

Acknowledgments: We thank Tessa Munkeboe Hornsyld and Danuta Goralska-Olsen at the Copenhagen Neuromuscular Center, University of Copenhagen, Denmark for excellent technical assistance. Lastly, we would like to gratefully recognize the volunteers for participating in this invasive and demanding study.

Conflicts of Interest: The authors declare no conflict of interest.

References

1. Fuggle, N.; Shaw, S.; Dennison, E.; Cooper, C. Sarcopenia. *Best Pr. Res. Clin. Rheumatol.* **2017**, *31*, 218–242. [CrossRef] [PubMed]
2. Proctor, D.N.; Joyner, M.J. Skeletal muscle mass and the reduction of VO2 max in trained older subjects. *J. Appl. Physiol.* **1997**, *82*, 1411–1415. [CrossRef] [PubMed]
3. Myers, J.; Prakash, M.; Froelicher, V.; Do, D.; Partington, S.; Atwood, J.E. Dat Exercise Capacity and Mortality among Men Referred for Exercise Testing. *N. Engl. J. Med.* **2002**, *346*, 793–801. [CrossRef] [PubMed]

4. Blair, S.N.; Kohl, H.W., III; Paffenbarger, R.S., Jr.; Clark, D.G.; Cooper, K.H.; Gibbons, L.W. Physical fitness and all-cause mortality. A prospective study of healthy men and women. *JAMA* **1989**, *262*, 2395–2401. [CrossRef]
5. Posner, J.D.; McCully, K.K.; Landsberg, L.A.; Sands, L.; Tycenski, P.; Hofmann, M.T.; Wetterholt, K.L.; Shaw, C.E. Physical determinants of independence in mature women. *Arch. Phys. Med. Rehabil.* **1995**, *76*, 373–380. [CrossRef]
6. Peterson, C.M.; Johannsen, D.L.; Ravussin, E. Skeletal Muscle Mitochondria and Aging: A Review. *J. Aging Res.* **2012**, *2012*, 1–20. [CrossRef]
7. Johnson, M.L.; Robinson, M.M.; Nair, K.S. Skeletal muscle aging and the mitochondrion. *Trends Endocrinol. Metab.* **2013**, *24*, 247–256. [CrossRef]
8. Turner, D.L.; Hoppeler, H.; Claassen, H.; Vock, P.; Kayser, B.; Schena, F.; Ferretti, G. Effects of endurance training on oxidative capacity and structural composition of human arm and leg muscles. *Acta Physiol. Scand.* **1997**, *161*, 459–464. [CrossRef]
9. Hoppeler, H.; Howald, H.; Conley, K.; Lindstedt, S.L.; Claassen, H.; Vock, P.; Weibel, E.R. Endurance training in humans: Aerobic capacity and structure of skeletal muscle. *J. Appl. Physiol.* **1985**, *59*, 320–327. [CrossRef]
10. Holloszy, J.O. Biochemical adaptations in muscle. Effects of exercise on mitochondrial oxygen uptake and respiratory enzyme activity in skeletal muscle. *J. Boil. Chem.* **1967**, *242*, 2278–2282.
11. Tarnopolsky, M.A.; Rennie, C.D.; Robertshaw, H.A.; Fedak-Tarnopolsky, S.N.; Devries, M.C.; Hamadeh, M.J. Influence of endurance exercise training and sex on intramyocellular lipid and mitochondrial ultrastructure, substrate use, and mitochondrial enzyme activity. *Am. J. Physiol. Integr. Comp. Physiol.* **2007**, *292*, R1271–R1278. [CrossRef] [PubMed]
12. Chrøis, K.M.; Dohlmann, T.L.; Søgaard, D.; Hansen, C.V.; Dela, F.; Helge, J.W.; Larsen, S. Mitochondrial adaptations to high intensity interval training in older females and males. *Eur. J. Sport Sci.* **2019**, *20*, 135–145. [CrossRef] [PubMed]
13. Konopka, A.R.; Suer, M.K.; Wolff, C.A.; Harber, M.P. Markers of Human Skeletal Muscle Mitochondrial Biogenesis and Quality Control: Effects of Age and Aerobic Exercise Training. *J. Gerontol. Ser. A Boil. Sci. Med. Sci.* **2013**, *69*, 371–378. [CrossRef]
14. Menshikova, E.V.; Ritov, V.B.; Fairfull, L.; Ferrell, R.E.; Kelley, D.E.; Goodpaster, B.H. Effects of Exercise on Mitochondrial Content and Function in Aging Human Skeletal Muscle. *J. Gerontol. Ser. A Boil. Sci. Med. Sci.* **2006**, *61*, 534–540. [CrossRef]
15. Short, K.R.; Vittone, J.L.; Bigelow, M.L.; Proctor, D.N.; Rizza, R.A.; Coenen-Schimke, J.M.; Nair, K.S. Impact of aerobic exercise training on age-related changes in insulin sensitivity and muscle oxidative capacity. *Diabetes* **2003**, *52*, 1888–1896. [CrossRef] [PubMed]
16. Konopka, A.R.; Douglass, M.D.; Kaminsky, L.A.; Jemiolo, B.; Trappe, T.A.; Trappe, S.; Harber, M.P. Molecular Adaptations to Aerobic Exercise Training in Skeletal Muscle of Older Women. *J. Gerontol. Ser. A Boil. Sci. Med. Sci.* **2010**, *65*, 1201–1207. [CrossRef]
17. Broskey, N.T.; Greggio, C.; Boss, A.; Boutant, M.; Dwyer, A.; Schlueter, L.; Hans, D.; Gremion, G.; Kreis, R.; Boesch, C.; et al. Skeletal Muscle Mitochondria in the Elderly: Effects of Physical Fitness and Exercise Training. *J. Clin. Endocrinol. Metab.* **2014**, *99*, 1852–1861. [CrossRef]
18. Seals, D.R.; Hagberg, J.M.; Hurley, B.F.; Ehsani, A.A.; Holloszy, J.O. Endurance training in older men and women. I. Cardiovascular responses to exercise. *J. Appl. Physiol. Respir. Environ. Exerc. Physiol.* **1984**, *57*, 1024–1029. [CrossRef]
19. Seals, D.R.; Reiling, M.J. Effect of regular exercise on 24-hour arterial pressure in older hypertensive humans. *Hypertension* **1991**, *18*, 583–592. [CrossRef]
20. De Vito, G.; Bernardi, M.; Forte, R.; Pulejo, C.; Figura, F. Effects of a low-intensity conditioning programme on V˙O2max and maximal instantaneous peak power in elderly women. *Graefes Arch. Clin. Exp. Ophthalmol.* **1999**, *80*, 227–232. [CrossRef]
21. Wang, E.; Næss, M.S.; Hoff, J.; Albert, T.L.; Pham, Q.; Richardson, R.S.; Helgerud, J. Exercise-training-induced changes in metabolic capacity with age: The role of central cardiovascular plasticity. *AGE* **2013**, *36*, 665–676. [CrossRef] [PubMed]
22. Örlander, J.; Aniansson, A. Effects of physical training on skeletal muscle metabolism and ultrastructure in 70 to 75-year-old men. *Acta Physiol. Scand.* **1980**, *109*, 149–154. [CrossRef]

23. Fritzen, A.M.; Thøgersen, F.D.; Thybo, K.; Vissing, J.; Krag, T.O.B.; Ruiz-Ruiz, C.; Risom, L.; Wibrand, F.; Høeg, L.D.; Kiens, B.; et al. Adaptations in Mitochondrial Enzymatic Activity Occurs Independent of Genomic Dosage in Response to Aerobic Exercise Training and Deconditioning in Human Skeletal Muscle. *Cells* **2019**, *8*, 237. [CrossRef] [PubMed]
24. Coyle, E.F.; Martin, W.H.; Sinacore, D.R.; Joyner, M.J.; Hagberg, J.M.; Holloszy, J.O. Time course of loss of adaptations after stopping prolonged intense endurance training. *J. Appl. Physiol.* **1984**, *57*, 1857–1864. [CrossRef] [PubMed]
25. Coyle, E.F.; Martin, W.H.; Bloomfield, S.A.; Lowry, O.H.; Holloszy, J.O. Effects of detraining on responses to submaximal exercise. *J. Appl. Physiol.* **1985**, *59*, 853–859. [CrossRef]
26. Klausen, K.; Andersen, L.B.; Pelle, I. Adaptive changes in work capacity, skeletal muscle capillarization and enzyme levels during training and detraining. *Acta Physiol. Scand.* **1981**, *113*, 9–16. [CrossRef]
27. Jeppesen, T.D.; Schwartz, M.; Olsen, D.B.; Wibrand, F.; Krag, T.O.B.; Duno, M.; Hauerslev, S.; Vissing, J. Aerobic training is safe and improves exercise capacity in patients with mitochondrial myopathy. *Brain* **2006**, *129*, 3402–3412. [CrossRef]
28. Song, W.; Kwak, H.-B.; Lawler, J.M. Exercise Training Attenuates Age-Induced Changes in Apoptotic Signaling in Rat Skeletal Muscle. *Antioxid. Redox Signal.* **2006**, *8*, 517–528. [CrossRef]
29. Kwak, H.-B.; Song, W.; Lawler, J.M. Exercise training attenuates age-induced elevation in Bax/Bcl-2 ratio, apoptosis, and remodeling in the rat heart. *FASEB J.* **2006**, *20*, 791–793. [CrossRef]
30. Chung, L.; Ng, Y.-C. Age-related alterations in expression of apoptosis regulatory proteins and heat shock proteins in rat skeletal muscle. *Biochim. Biophys. Acta* **2006**, *1762*, 103–109. [CrossRef]
31. Dirks-Naylor, A.J.; Leeuwenburgh, C. Aging and lifelong calorie restriction result in adaptations of skeletal muscle apoptosis repressor, apoptosis-inducing factor, X-linked inhibitor of apoptosis, caspase-3, and caspase-12. *Free Radic. Boil. Med.* **2004**, *36*, 27–39. [CrossRef] [PubMed]
32. Leeuwenburgh, C. Role of Apoptosis in Sarcopenia. *J. Gerontol. Ser. A Boil. Sci. Med. Sci.* **2003**, *58*, M999–M1001. [CrossRef] [PubMed]
33. Dordevic, A.L.; Bonham, M.P.; Ghasem-Zadeh, A.; Evans, A.; Barber, E.M.; Day, K.; Kwok, A.; Truby, H. Reliability of Compartmental Body Composition Measures in Weight-Stable Adults Using GE iDXA: Implications for Research and Practice. *Nutrients* **2018**, *10*, 1484. [CrossRef] [PubMed]
34. Swain, D.P. Energy cost calculations for exercise prescription: An update. *Sports Med.* **2000**, *30*, 17–22. [CrossRef]
35. Bergstrom, J. Percutaneous needle biopsy of skeletal muscle in physiological and clinical research. *Scand. J. Clin. Lab. Invest.* **1975**, *35*, 609–616. [CrossRef] [PubMed]
36. Fritzen, A.M.; Thøgersen, F.D.; Qadri, K.A.N.; Krag, T.; Sveen, M.-L.; Vissing, J.; Jeppesen, T.D. Preserved Capacity for Adaptations in Strength and Muscle Regulatory Factors in Elderly in Response to Resistance Exercise Training and Deconditioning. *J. Clin. Med.* **2020**, *9*, 2188. [CrossRef]
37. Wibrand, F.; Jeppesen, T.D.; Frederiksen, A.L.; Olsen, D.B.; Duno, M.; Schwartz, M.; Vissing, J. Limited diagnostic value of enzyme analysis in patients with mitochondrial tRNA mutations. *Muscle Nerve* **2009**, *41*, 607–613. [CrossRef]
38. Birchmachin, M.; Briggs, H.; Saborido, A.; Bindoff, L.A.; Turnbull, D. An Evaluation of the Measurement of the Activities of Complexes I-IV in the Respiratory Chain of Human Skeletal Muscle Mitochondria. *Biochem. Med. Metab. Boil.* **1994**, *51*, 35–42. [CrossRef]
39. Krähenbühl, S.; Talos, C.; Wiesmann, U.; Hoppel, C.L. Development and evaluation of a spectrophotometric assay for complex III in isolated mitochondria, tissues and fibroblasts from rats and humans. *Clin. Chim. Acta* **1994**, *230*, 177–187. [CrossRef]
40. Fritzen, A.M.; Madsen, A.B.; Kleinert, M.; Treebak, J.T.; Lundsgaard, A.-M.; Jensen, T.E.; Richter, E.A.; Wojtaszewski, J.F.; Kiens, B.; Frøsig, C. Regulation of autophagy in human skeletal muscle: Effects of exercise, exercise training and insulin stimulation. *J. Physiol.* **2016**, *594*, 745–761. [CrossRef]
41. Larsen, S.; Nielsen, J.; Hansen, C.N.; Nielsen, L.B.; Wibrand, F.; Stride, N.; Schrøder, H.D.; Boushel, R.; Helge, J.W.; Dela, F.; et al. Biomarkers of mitochondrial content in skeletal muscle of healthy young human subjects. *J. Physiol.* **2012**, *590*, 3349–3360. [CrossRef] [PubMed]
42. Lundby, A.-K.M.; Jacobs, R.A.; Gehrig, S.; De Leur, J.; Hauser, M.; Bonne, T.C.; Flück, D.; Dandanell, S.; Kirk, N.; Kaech, A.; et al. Exercise training increases skeletal muscle mitochondrial volume density by enlargement of existing mitochondria and not de novo biogenesis. *Acta Physiol.* **2017**, *222*, e12905. [CrossRef]

43. Ghosh, S.; Lertwattanarak, R.; Lefort, N.; Molina-Carrion, M.; Joya-Galeana, J.; Bowen, B.P.; Garduño-García, J.J.; Abdul-Ghani, M.; Richardson, A.; DeFronzo, R.A.; et al. Reduction in Reactive Oxygen Species Production by Mitochondria From Elderly Subjects With Normal and Impaired Glucose Tolerance. *Diabetes* **2011**, *60*, 2051–2060. [CrossRef]
44. Boffoli, D.; Scacco, S.; Vergari, R.; Solarino, G.; Santacroce, G.; Papa, S. Decline with age of the respiratory chain activity in human skeletal muscle. *Biochim. Biophys. Acta* **1994**, *1226*, 73–82. [CrossRef]
45. Rooyackers, O.E.; Adey, D.B.; Ades, P.A.; Nair, K.S. Effect of age on in vivo rates of mitochondrial protein synthesis in human skeletal muscle. *Proc. Natl. Acad. Sci. USA* **1996**, *93*, 15364–15369. [CrossRef] [PubMed]
46. Tonkonogi, M.; Fernström, M.; Walsh, B.; Ji, L.L.; Rooyackers, O.; Hammarqvist, F.; Wernerman, J.; Sahlin, K. Reduced oxidative power but unchanged antioxidative capacity in skeletal muscle from aged humans. *Pflügers Arch.* **2003**, *446*, 261–269. [CrossRef]
47. Crane, J.D.; Devries, M.C.; Safdar, A.; Hamadeh, M.J.; Tarnopolsky, M.A. The Effect of Aging on Human Skeletal Muscle Mitochondrial and Intramyocellular Lipid Ultrastructure. *J. Gerontol. Ser. A Boil. Sci. Med. Sci.* **2009**, *65*, 119–128. [CrossRef]
48. Brierley, E.; Johnson, M.; James, O.; Turnbull, D. Effects of physical activity and age on mitochondrial function. *QJM Int. J. Med.* **1996**, *89*, 251–258. [CrossRef]
49. Barrientos, A.; Casademont, J.; Rötig, A.; Miro, O.; Urbano-Márquez, Á.; Rustin, P.; Cardellach, F. Absence of Relationship between the Level of Electron Transport Chain Activities and Aging in Human Skeletal Muscle. *Biochem. Biophys. Res. Commun.* **1996**, *229*, 536–539. [CrossRef]
50. Gouspillou, G.; Sgarioto, N.; Kapchinsky, S.; Purves-Smith, F.; Norris, B.; Pion, C.H.; Barbat-Artigas, S.; Lemieux, F.; Taivassalo, T.; Morais, J.A.; et al. Increased sensitivity to mitochondrial permeability transition and myonuclear translocation of endonuclease G in atrophied muscle of physically active older humans. *FASEB J.* **2013**, *28*, 1621–1633. [CrossRef]
51. Casuso, R.A.; Huertas, J.R. The emerging role of skeletal muscle mitochondrial dynamics in exercise and ageing. *Ageing Res. Rev.* **2020**, *58*, 101025. [CrossRef] [PubMed]
52. Arribat, Y.; Broskey, N.T.; Greggio, C.; Boutant, M.; Alonso, S.C.; Kulkarni, S.S.; Lagarrigue, S.; Carnero, E.A.; Besson, C.; Canto, C.; et al. Distinct patterns of skeletal muscle mitochondria fusion, fission and mitophagy upon duration of exercise training. *Acta Physiol.* **2018**, *225*, e13179. [CrossRef] [PubMed]
53. Kang, C.; Yeo, D.-W.; Ji, L.L. Muscle immobilization activates mitophagy and disrupts mitochondrial dynamics in mice. *Acta Physiol.* **2016**, *218*, 188–197. [CrossRef] [PubMed]
54. Vainshtein, A.; Tryon, L.D.; Pauly, M.; Hood, D.A. Role of PGC-1α during acute exercise-induced autophagy and mitophagy in skeletal muscle. *Am. J. Physiol. Physiol.* **2015**, *308*, C710–C719. [CrossRef]
55. Carter, H.N.; Kim, Y.; Erlich, A.T.; Zarrin-Khat, D.; Hood, D.A.; Erlich, A.T. Autophagy and mitophagy flux in young and aged skeletal muscle following chronic contractile activity. *J. Physiol.* **2018**, *596*, 3567–3584. [CrossRef]

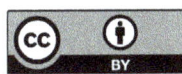

© 2020 by the authors. Licensee MDPI, Basel, Switzerland. This article is an open access article distributed under the terms and conditions of the Creative Commons Attribution (CC BY) license (http://creativecommons.org/licenses/by/4.0/).

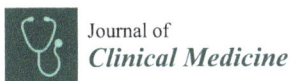

Article

Low Physical Activity in Patients with Complicated Type 2 Diabetes Mellitus Is Associated with Low Muscle Mass and Low Protein Intake

Ilse J. M. Hagedoorn [1,*], Niala den Braber [1,2], Milou M. Oosterwijk [1], Christina M. Gant [3,4], Gerjan Navis [3], Miriam M. R. Vollenbroek-Hutten [1,2], Bert-Jan F. van Beijnum [2], Stephan J. L. Bakker [3] and Gozewijn D. Laverman [1]

1. Division of Nephrology, Department of Internal Medicine, Ziekenhuisgroep Twente, 7609 PP Almelo, The Netherlands; n.braber@zgt.nl (N.d.B); Mi.oosterwijk@zgt.nl (M.M.O.); m.vollenbroek@zgt.nl (M.M.R.V.-H.); g.laverman@zgt.nl (G.D.L.)
2. Faculty of Electrical Engineering, Mathematics and Computer Science, University of Twente, 7522 NB Enschede, The Netherlands; b.j.f.vanbeijnum@utwente.nl
3. Division of Nephrology, Department of Internal Medicine, University of Groningen, University Medical Center Groningen, 9713 GZ Groningen, The Netherlands; cm.gant@meandermc.nl (C.M.G.); g.j.navis@umcg.nl (G.N); s.j.l.bakker@umcg.nl (S.J.L.B.)
4. Department of Internal Medicine, Meander Medisch Centrum, 3813 TZ Amersfoort, The Netherlands
* Correspondence: ilse_hagedoorn10@hotmail.com; Tel.: +31-6-44-019-033

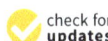

Received: 21 August 2020; Accepted: 23 September 2020; Published: 25 September 2020

Abstract: Objective: In order to promote physical activity (PA) in patients with complicated type 2 diabetes, a better understanding of daily movement is required. We (1) objectively assessed PA in patients with type 2 diabetes, and (2) studied the association between muscle mass, dietary protein intake, and PA. Methods: We performed cross-sectional analyses in all patients included in the Diabetes and Lifestyle Cohort Twente (DIALECT) between November 2016 and November 2018. Patients were divided into four groups: <5000, 5000–6999, 7000–9999, ≥ 10,000 steps/day. We studied the association between muscle mass (24 h urinary creatinine excretion rate, CER) and protein intake (by Maroni formula), and the main outcome variable PA (steps/day, Fitbit Flex device) using multivariate linear regression analyses. Results: In the 217 included patients, the median steps/day were 6118 (4115–8638). Of these patients, 48 patients (22%) took 7000–9999 steps/day, 37 patients (17%) took ≥ 10,000 steps/day, and 78 patients (36%) took <5000 steps/day. Patients with <5000 steps/day had, in comparison to patients who took ≥10,000 steps/day, a higher body mass index (BMI) (33 ± 6 vs. 30 ± 5 kg/m^2, p = 0.009), lower CER (11.7 ± 4.8 vs. 14.8 ± 3.8 mmol/24 h, p = 0.001), and lower protein intake (0.84 ± 0.29 vs. 1.08 ± 0.22 g/kg/day, p < 0.001). Both creatinine excretion (β = 0.26, p < 0.001) and dietary protein intake (β = 0.31, p < 0.001) were strongly associated with PA, which remained unchanged after adjustment for potential confounders. Conclusions: Prevalent insufficient protein intake and low muscle mass co-exist in obese patients with low physical activity. Dedicated intervention studies are needed to study the role of sufficient protein intake and physical activity in increasing or maintaining muscle mass in patients with type 2 diabetes.

Keywords: type 2 diabetes; physical activity; muscle mass; protein intake; accelerometer

1. Introduction

Type 2 diabetes is a predominately lifestyle-related disease and has become one of the major global public health concerns, with highest prevalence in older adults [1]. Sufficient physical activity (PA) is a main focus of treatment, in addition to improving diet quality. There are two different aspects of PA: aerobic training and resistance exercise. While guidelines first mainly recommended moderate to vigorous PA, contemporary public health guidelines state that 'some physical activity is better than none' by suggest reducing the time spent in sedentary behaviour [2]. Total steps per day is a good indicator of the overall volume of physical activity [3].

However, the vast majority of patients with type 2 diabetes do not adhere to the American Diabetes Association (ADA) guidelines of >150 min per week of moderate to vigorous PA, which is comparable with 7000 steps per day [3–5]. Traditionally, a goal of 10,000 steps per day has been advocated by popular media, although this goal is under debate in scientific literature [6,7]. In order to promote PA and reduce sedentary behaviour, a better understanding of total daily movement is required, especially in patients with complicated type 2 diabetes.

In regard to PA, sufficient muscle mass is mandatory to perform PA, and conversely, PA promotes an increase in muscle mass. Compared with non-diabetic subjects, patients with type 2 diabetes show decreased muscle strength and mass [8,9]. In type 2 diabetes, reduced muscle mass and muscle function, defined as sarcopenia, have been implicated both as a cause and as a consequence of increased insulin resistance [8–10]. Furthermore, it is known that low muscle mass in obese individuals is associated with frailty, disability, and increased morbidity and mortality [11].

However, dietary counselling (such as is performed in the geriatric population) consists mainly of caloric restriction, and not the preservation of muscle mass. Adequate protein intake is an important requirement for sustaining, and especially increasing, muscle mass, which has been confirmed by several observational and intervention studies [12–17]. Moreover, combining physical exercise with protein intake has a positive synergistic effect on muscle protein synthesis [16,17]. Therefore, adequate protein intake might be a current blind spot in the treatment of type 2 diabetes.

We hypothesize that in patients with complicated type 2 diabetes, low protein intake and low muscle mass are associated with low PA, and the former could be an important actionable item to improve PA. Therefore, here we (1) objectively measure PA (in steps/day) in patients with complicated type 2 diabetes, and (2) investigate the association between protein intake and muscle mass and PA.

2. Materials and Methods

2.1. Patient Inclusion

This study was performed in the DIAbetes and LifEstyle Cohort Twente (DIALECT), an observational cohort study in patients with complicated type 2 diabetes mellitus, treated in the secondary healthcare level in the outpatient clinic of the Ziekenhuisgroep Twente (ZGT), Almelo and Hengelo, the Netherlands. The study consists of two sub-cohorts: DIALECT-1 and DIALECT-2. The general procedures have been described extensively previously [18]. In DIALECT-2, the data collection at baseline is more extensive, including a one-week PA registration.

The study was performed in accordance with the Helsinki agreement and the guidelines of good clinical practice, has been approved by the local institutional review boards (METC-registration numbers NL57219.044.16 and 1009.68020) and is registered in the Netherlands Trial Register (NTR trial code 5855). Prior to participation, all patients signed an informed consent form. All adult patients with type 2 diabetes treated in the secondary healthcare level in the outpatient clinic of internal medicine in ZGT Hospital were eligible for participation. The patients were treated in the secondary healthcare level because the diabetes care became complex for primary healthcare services (for example, in the presence of complications such as nephropathy or because of a complex insulin schedule). Exclusion criteria were renal replacement therapy, inability to understand the informed consent procedure, and inability to walk. We report here on all patients included in DIALECT-2 between November 2016 and November 2018.

2.2. Data Collection

Participation in DIALECT-2 consisted of at least two hospital visits with one week in between. Information on medical condition and medication was obtained from electronic patient files and verified with the patient during the baseline visit. Smoking habits were collected through questionnaires. Anthropometric measurements, leg length, and presence of diabetic polyneuropathy were obtained from physical examination at baseline. Leg length was measured using a tape measure from the anterior superior iliac spine to the ground. Polyneuropathy was assessed by touch test (Semmes Weinstein monofilament) and vibration (Vibratip) by the on–off method; both tests have been validated as screening methods for polyneuropathy [19]. Polyneuropathy was present if at least one of the two tests was positive. Body composition parameters were determined by Bio impedance using a TANITA device (type BC-418MA, Tokyo, Japan), which calculates segmental body composition, including fat percentage and predicted muscle mass. Blood samples were taken from a single non-fasting venapunction, and patients collected 24 h urine to provide objective data on nutritional intake, including protein intake. We used the 24 h urinary creatinine excretion rate (CER) as a measure of muscle mass [11,20,21]. The estimated daily protein intake (g/kg/day) was calculated using the universally adopted formula of Maroni, ((24 h urea excretion × 0.18) + 15 + 24 h protein excretion)/weight (kg) [22]. Blood pressure was measured in supine position by an automated device for 15 min with one-minute intervals (Dinamap®; GE Medical systems, Milwaukee, WI, USA). The mean systolic and diastolic pressure of the last three measurements was used for further analysis.

2.3. Main Outcome: Physical Activity

During 8 consecutive days, daily movement was measured by a triaxial Fitbit accelerometer worn around the wrist on the non-dominant side. The devices used were either a Fitbit Flex (Fitbit Inc., Boston, MA, USA), a Fitbit charge HR (Fitbit, San Francisco, CA, USA), or Fitbit Charge 2 (Fitbit Inc., San Francisco, CA, USA). These Fitbit devices share the same recording mechanisms and record the number of steps taken on a minute-to-minute basis. Patients were asked to adhere to their daily activities as normal and were blinded from the online activity data. Also, the Fitbit screens showed no results. Only during swimming or showering was the Fitbit removed. At visit 2 (day 8), the patients returned the Fitbit and data were transferred to a hospital server for further analysis. Patients were asked to write down information regarding non-wearing time in a lifestyle diary. Valid days were defined as days without significant non-wearing time (i.e., >2 h non-wearing time during waking hours). Patients with more than two days of significant non-wearing time were excluded. To indicate the total daily movement, we used the average of the total steps per day, excluding day 1 and 8 from the average because of non-wearing time.

2.4. Statistical Analysis

Statistical procedures were performed by using SPSS statistics (IBM Statistics for Windows, Version 23.0, Armonk, NY, USA). Normality of data was determined by visual inspection of histograms. Data were presented as mean ± standard deviation (normal distribution), as median and interquartile range (IQR 25th–75th percentiles, skewed data), or as number and percentage (dichotomous and categorical data). To compare the characteristics of total steps per day, the population was divided into four different groups based on reference values from current literature (i.e., <5000, 5000–6999, 7000–9999, ≥10,000 steps per day) [3]. Differences between the groups were analysed using One-Way ANOVA, Kruskal–Wallis, or Chi-square test when appropriate. A two-sided $p < 0.05$ was considered statistically significant. The estimated daily protein intake was divided into three groups (i.e., <0.8 g/kg/day, 0.8–1.2 g/kg/day, and >1.2 g/kg/day). The recommended dietary protein intake is ≥0.8 g/kg/day [12,23].

To investigate whether 24 h CER and protein intake were associated with total steps/day, we performed multivariate linear regression analyses. First, we identified possible confounders using univariate analyses. Model 2, adjusted for age and gender, was the main basis for confounder selection. Parameters with a $p < 0.15$ were considered contenders for the multivariate model. For each group of closely associated variables (for example, body mass index (BMI), waist circumference, and hip circumference as measures of body size), we included the variable with the highest β for the multivariate model. Potential interaction of protein intake and CER with total steps/day was evaluated by inclusion of the product term in the linear regression analysis. We considered a $p < 0.10$ to be statistically significant for the product term. To graphically represent the interaction between protein intake, CER, and total steps per day, we created nine groups based on the tertiles of protein intake and tertiles of muscle mass. Low, medium, and high represent respectively the lowest, middle, and highest tertiles of protein intake and muscle mass.

3. Results

3.1. Baseline Characteristics and Total Steps per Day

Of 231 eligible participants, 217 patients were included in the study. The reasons for exclusion were: hardware malfunction ($n = 6$), non-fitting wristband ($n = 4$), patient dropped out during participation ($n = 2$), and patient not able to walk ($n = 2$) (Figure S1). Patient characteristics stratified by total steps per day are shown in Table 1.

Median total steps per day was 6118 (4115–8638, data not shown). Of the total study population, 85 patients (39%) took ≥7000 steps/day, of whom 37 patients (17%) reached ≥10,000 steps/day (Table 1).

The mean age of the total study population was 65 ± 12 years, two-thirds were men, and the mean BMI was 32 ± 6 kg/m². Of all patients, 64% used insulin, and the mean HbA1c was 60 ± 13 mmol/mol (7.6% ± 3.3%). The prevalence of micro- (74%) and macrovascular (35%) complications was high. Compliance with wearing of the Fitbit sensor was good; 22 patients reported significant non-wearing time (>2 h/day) at any day during day 2 until day 7, however, no patient had more than two days of non-wearing time (compliance data not shown).

The mean age was highest (69 ± 11 years) in the group of patients with <5000 steps per day ($p < 0.001$). There were no differences in gender between the groups ($p = 0.99$). Patients with <5000 steps/day had the highest BMI (33 ± 6 kg/m², $p = 0.009$) and the highest waist- and hip circumference (waist: 116 ± 14 cm, $p = 0.001$; hip: 115 ± 14 cm, $p = 0.009$). Both measurements of muscle mass (i.e., 24 h CER and percentage of predicted muscle mass (PMM) using bio-impedance) were lowest in patients with 5000 steps/day ($p = 0.001$ and $p = 0.06$, respectively).

No significant differences were observed in HbA1c, insulin use, and years of diabetes between the groups. Patients with <5000 steps per day had the most pack-years of smoking ($p = 0.005$), the lowest diastolic blood pressure (0.02), and the lowest HDL-cholesterol ($p = 0.03$). The prevalence of micro- and macrovascular complications was consistently and progressively lower in each group of increasing number of steps/day, especially for diabetic kidney disease ($p = 0.004$), polyneuropathy ($p = 0.008$), and cerebrovascular disease ($p = 0.008$). Protein intake was also lowest in patients with <5000 steps/day (0.84 g/kg/day, $p < 0.001$, Figure 1). Almost half of all patients with <5000 steps per day had a protein intake <0.8 g/kg/day.

Table 1. Patient characteristics stratified by total steps per day.

Characteristics	n	Total Population (n = 217)	<5000 steps/day (n = 78)	5000–6999 steps/day (n = 54)	7000–9999 steps/day (n = 48)	≥10,000 steps/day (n = 37)	p-Value
Age, years	217	65 ± 12	69 ± 11	64 ± 10	62 ± 13 [a]	60 ± 10 [a]	<0.001
Gender, men n (%)	217	144 (66)	51 (65)	36 (67)	32 (67)	25 (68)	0.99
BMI, kg/m²	217	32 ± 6	33 ± 6	31 ± 5	31 ± 5	30 ± 5 [a]	0.009
Education level, n (%) [b]	185						0.10
Low		65 (35)	31 (44)	16 (36)	11 (28)	7 (23)	
Medium		81 (44)	29 (41)	17 (38)	16 (41)	19 (63)	
High		39 (21)	11 (16)	12 (27)	12 (31)	4 (13)	
Waist circumference, cm	216	112 ± 13	116 ± 14	109 ± 12 [a]	111 ± 13	107 ± 10 [a]	0.001
Hip circumference, cm	216	111 ± 13	115 ± 14	109 ± 12	110 ± 11	108 ± 9 [a]	0.009
Leg length, cm	120	98 ± 7	96 ± 8	97 ± 6	100 ± 8	99 ± 7	0.11
Fat percentage, %	206	33 ± 9	34 ± 8	33 ± 9	32 ± 10	30 ± 8	0.10
Predicted muscle mass, % [c]	206	64 ± 8	62 ± 8	63 ± 8	65 ± 8	67 ± 8	0.06
Creatinine excretion, mmol/24 h	215	13.2 ± 5	11.7 ± 4.8	13.6 ± 4.3	14.3 ± 5.1 [a]	14.8 ± 3.8 [a]	0.001
Systolic blood pressure, mmHg	211	130 ± 15	132 ± 16	127 ± 14	131 ± 16	133 ± 13	0.26
Diastolic blood pressure, mmHg	211	74 ± 9	72 ± 9	76 ± 9	73 ± 8	77 ± 12 [a]	0.02
Pulse rate, bpm	211	71 ± 12	71 ± 13	73 ± 11	69 ± 10	70 ± 13	0.44
Diabetes duration, years	217	13 (8–19)	14 (8–20)	14 (8–19)	13 (5–20)	11 (7–18)	0.65
Insulin use, yes n (%)	215	138 (64)	56 (73)	32 (59)	25 (52)	25 (70)	0.09
Units of insulin	135	62 (34–101)	66 (40–118)	78 (38–114)	53 (26–105)	50 (35–77)	0.53
Alcohol intake units/month	213	3 (0–25)	0 (0–24)	5 (0–26)	2 (0–11)	8 (0–30)	0.27
Smoking, pack-years	199	8 (0–24)	14 (1–32)	7 (0–28)	1 (0–19) [a]	1 (0–21) [a]	0.005
HbA1c, mmol/mol (%)	215	60 ± 13 (7.6 ± 3.3)	60 ± 13 (7.6 ± 3.3)	60 ± 11 (7.6 ± 3.1)	62 ± 14 (7.8 ± 3.4)	59 ± 11 (7.5 ± 3.1)	0.69
Total cholesterol, mmol/L	215	4.2 ± 1.0	4.2 ± 1.1	4.2 ± 1.0	4.4 ± 0.9	4.2 ± 0.8	0.85
HDL-cholesterol, mmol/L	214	1.13 ± 0.3	1.10 ± 0.3	1.16 ± 0.3	1.15 ± 0.4	1.24 ± 0.3 [a]	0.03
LDL-cholesterol, mmol/L	200	2.04 ± 0.8	2.0 ± 0.9	2.03 ± 0.9	2.16 ± 0.8	1.97 ± 0.6	0.67
Microvascular complications, n (%)	217	160 (74)	66 (85)	37 (69)	27 (56)	16 (43)	<0.001
Diabetic kidney disease, n (%)	211	106 (50)	48 (66)	27 (50)	19 (40)	12 (33)	0.004
eGFR < 60 mL/min/1.73 m², n (%)	217	70 (32)	38 (59)	17 (32)	10 (21)	5 (14)	<0.001
Micro-albuminuria, n (%)	211	83 (39)	40 (55)	20 (37)	14 (29)	9 (25)	0.006
Polyneuropathy, n (%)	217	97 (45)	46 (59)	24 (44)	17 (36)	10 (28)	0.008
Retinopathy, n (%)	210	41 (20)	18 (24)	10 (19)	6 (13)	7 (19)	0.532
Macrovascular complications, n (%)	217	75 (35)	33 (42)	22 (41)	12 (25)	8 (22)	0.05
Peripheral arterial diseases, n (%)	217	8 (4)	4 (5)	1 (2)	2 (4)	1 (3)	0.78
Coronary artery diseases, n (%)	216	54 (25)	23 (30)	18 (34)	8 (17)	5 (14)	0.06
Cerebrovascular accident or TIA, n (%)	217	27 (12)	17 (22)	6 (11)	1 (2)	3 (8)	0.008
Amputation, n (%)	217	3 (2)	3 (4)	0 (0)	0 (0)	0 (0)	0.14
Urea excretion, mmol/24 h	206	387 (291–510)	342 (242–448)	402 (274–505)	432 (327–508) [a]	465 (331–528) [a]	0.02
Protein intake, g/day	202	88 ± 28	79 ± 27	90 ± 31	93 ± 24 [a]	96 ± 24 [a]	0.004
Protein intake, g/kg/day	202	0.95 ± 0.30	0.84 ± 0.29	0.99 ± 0.33 [a]	0.99 ± 0.27 [a]	1.08 ± 0.22 [a]	<0.001
<0.8 g/kg/day, n (%)		64 (31)	35 (46)	15 (28)	10 (24)	4 (11)	
0.8–1.2 g/kg/day, n (%)		102 (50)	32 (42)	28 (53)	22 (54)	20 (56)	0.006
>1.2 g/kg/day, n (%)		40 (19)	9 (12)	10 (19)	9 (22)	12 (33)	

[a] Significant difference from <5000 steps/day. [b] Education level according to the International Standard Classification of Education (ISCED), as follows: Low: ISCED 1–2; Medium: ISCED 3; High ISCED 4–8; [c] Predicted Muscle Mass %: TANITA predicted muscle mass (kg) divided by total body weight (kg). Data presented as mean ± standard deviation, as median and interquartile range (IQR 25th–75th), or in number and (percentage). eGFR: estimated glomerular filtration rate. TIA: transient ischemic attack.

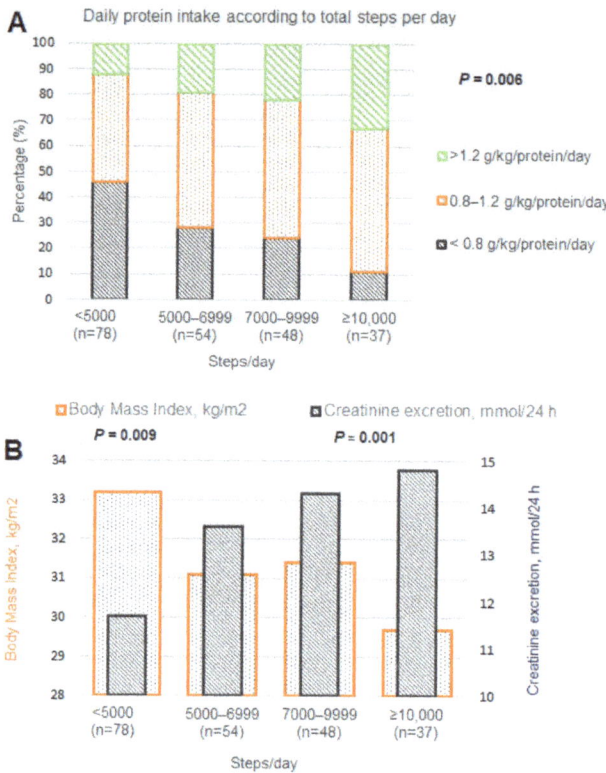

Figure 1. Protein intake, body mass index (BMI), and 24 h urinary creatinine excretion according to total steps per day. Distribution of total protein intake (**A**) and urinary creatinine excretion and body mass index (**B**) in four groups of total steps per day. (**A**) demonstrates that insufficient protein intake is significantly more prevalent in patients with <5000 steps/day. (**B**) shows higher body mass index and lower creatinine excretion in patients with <5000 steps/day, demonstrating a more unfavourable body composition.

3.2. Association between Urinary Creatinine Excretion, Total Protein Intake, and Total Steps per Day

To analyse the association between total steps per day, muscle mass (24 h CER), and daily dietary protein intake, we performed linear regression analyses. Unadjusted, both CER ($\beta = 0.28$, $p = 0.03$) and dietary protein intake ($\beta = 0.29$, $p = 0.004$) (Model 1) were positively associated with steps/day. When adjusting for possible confounders (Table S1), both for CER and protein intake, the association with total steps/day did not markedly change (Table 2). It should be noted that the predicted variance of both models remained low (0.23 and 0.24, respectively). There was a significant interaction between CER and protein intake on total steps per day, where higher CER combined with higher protein was associated with more steps/day ($p = 0.096$, Figure 2). As there was a very strong correlation between CER and dietary protein intake ($R = 0.57$), both variables could not be inserted simultaneously in the analysis.

Table 2. Multivariate linear regression analyses on the associations between CER, protein intake and total steps/day (dependent variable)

Independent Variables		Total Steps per day (Dependent)			Independent Variables	Total Steps per day (Dependent)		
		Standardized Beta	p-Value	R^2		Standardized Beta	p-Value	R^2
Model 1	CER	0.28	0.003	0.08	Protein intake	0.29	0.004	0.08
Model 2	CER	0.23	0.03	0.10	Protein intake	0.28	0.004	0.13
Model 3	CER	0.23	0.04	0.19	Protein intake	0.18	0.10	0.19
Model 4	CER	0.26	0.04	0.21	Protein intake	0.23	0.04	0.22
Model 5	CER	0.26	0.02	0.23	Protein intake	0.23	0.04	0.24

CER: creatinine excretion rate. Model 1 is unadjusted; Model 2 is adjusted for model 1 and age and gender; Model 3 is adjusted for model 2 and BMI and leg length; Model 4 is adjusted for model 3 and pack-years; Model 5 is adjusted for model 4 and eGFR < 60 mL/min/1.73 m^2, polyneuropathy, and presence of macrovascular disease.

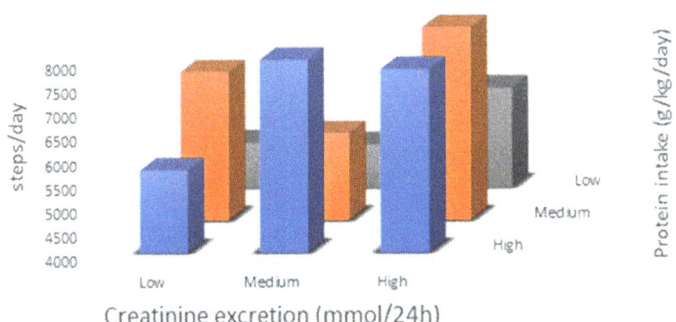

Figure 2. Low, medium, and high represent the lowest, middle, and highest tertiles of protein intake and creatinine excretion. The figure shows the interaction between urinary creatinine excretion (CER) and protein intake on total steps per day. Both high CER and high protein intake were associated with more steps/day, and total steps per day was highest in those with both high CER and high protein intake.

4. Discussion

We investigated the total daily physical activity (PA) of patients with complicated type 2 diabetes. We found that more than one-third of the study participants had limited activity (less than 5000 steps per day). On the other hand, 39% of participants took ≥7000 steps per day, which has been advocated as the movement target for adults ≥ 65 years and/or patients with chronic diseases [3], demonstrating that sufficient PA in a complicated type 2 diabetes population is indeed a reachable goal.

Our main finding was that low muscle mass was an important determinant of low PA. Additionally, protein intake was significantly and relevantly lower in patients with both low PA and low muscle mass. It is tempting to speculate on a downward spiral of reduced protein intake, lower muscle mass, and reduced PA, against the background of a sedentary lifestyle. The insight that insufficient protein intake is associated with low muscle mass and physical inactivity may provide an important actionable item to improve physical fitness in patients with type 2 diabetes: namely, increase protein intake.

Low muscle mass is increasingly recognized as an important health concern in patients with chronic disease, diminishing physical fitness and PA. In contrast to previous beliefs, declining muscle mass is not only due to ageing and physical inactivity, but has many other contributing causes, such as mitochondrial dysfunction [11,24,25]. This is especially important in patients with type 2 diabetes, as data suggest skeletal muscle lipid content is associated with systemic insulin resistance [11]. Damage to the skeletal muscles, with pronounced and accelerated decline in muscle quality, has been described as a new complication of diabetic patients attributed to their longer survival [8]. Insulin resistance and oxidative stress are components of the pathophysiological basis of sarcopenia, which would be related to characteristic components of diabetes, such as vascular alterations, chronic inflammation, and lipid infiltration in muscles [8,11]. In regard to our population, 24 h CER in the group with ≤5000 steps per day (11.7 ± 4.8 mmol/24 h) was significantly lower compared to the total study population (13.2 ± 5 mmol/24 h), and also lower when compared to the general Dutch population (13.3 ± 4.1 mmol/24 h, based on data from the Lifelines cohort study) [12]. However, it should be noted that no diagnostic methods or definitive cut-off points exist to identify patients who might benefit from muscle-boosting therapy.

Adequate protein intake is an important requirement for sustaining, and especially increasing, muscle mass, which has been confirmed by several observational and intervention studies [12–17]. Moreover, combining physical exercise with protein intake has a positive synergistic effect on muscle protein synthesis [16,17].

The recommended dietary allowance (RDA) and the Netherlands Nutrition Centre [12,23] recommend a dietary protein intake of ≥0.8 g/kg/day. However, for elderly adults, the Dutch guideline suggests a higher protein intake (1.2–2.0 g/kg/day) to maintain optimal muscle health [26,27]. We found that almost half of all patients (46%) in the group of <5000 steps per day had a daily protein intake < 0.8 g/kg/day, and only 12% had an intake of >1.2 g/kg/day. To our knowledge, this is the first study in patients with type 2 diabetes that has highlighted the insufficient protein intake of inactive patients with type 2 diabetes. However, BMI and waist circumference were higher in patients with low PA, consistent with altered body composition in inactive patients. This is in line with previous studies in patients with type 2 diabetes [4,28,29]. Low muscle mass and function have strong negative prognostic impacts in obese individuals, which may lead to frailty disability and increased morbidity and mortality [11]. However, awareness of the importance of muscle maintenance in obesity is low among clinicians and scientists [11]. The European Society for Clinical Nutrition and Metabolism (ESPEN) and the European Association for the study of Obesity (EASO) recognize and identify obesity with altered body composition due to low skeletal muscle function and mass as a scientific and clinical priority for researchers and clinicians. ESPEN and EASO therefore call for action in particular regard to optimal nutritional therapy. Generally, the first step in treating obese patients with type 2 diabetes is weight loss interventions by following a caloric restricted diet, which, however, might increase the risk for undesirable decreases in muscle mass.

To our knowledge, this is the first study to objectively measure daily PA by using steps/day in complicated type 2 diabetes. Most of the previous studies in type 2 diabetes used metabolic equivalent (MET) or counts per minute (CPM) to measure daily movement, which makes it somewhat difficult to compare previous results with our findings [4,24,25,28–34]. However, in a study population with older patients (≥55 years) with type 2 diabetes, the average total steps per day was similar to our results [34]. In contrast to this previous study, which showed that older women had fewer steps per day, we found no difference in steps/day between genders.

Additionally, we found that the presence of micro- and macrovascular complications was higher in patients with physical inactivity. This is in line with a recent review on diabetic polyneuropathy and nephropathy [35]. Interestingly, diabetic polyneuropathy is associated with lower muscle strength measured by knee extension force [25,32,35], providing an alternative cause of muscle mass decline in addition to reduced dietary protein intake. Additionally, in patients with chronic kidney disease, uremic muscle mass decline has been suggested by a significant inverse association between uremic toxin indoxyl sulphate and skeletal muscle mass [33,35]. Of note, in our study, a third of the patients with ≥10,000 steps per day had polyneuropathy and nephropathy (28% and 33%, respectively), suggesting that sufficient PA is indeed possible in spite of the presence of these complications. However, in contrast to other studies in patients with type 2 diabetes, we found associations between HDL-cholesterol, diastolic blood pressure, macrovascular complications, and physical activity [4,28,29].

Strengths of our study included the objective measurements of daily movement by the Fitbit Flex, a light and simple wristband, well applicable in daily life clinical practice that hardly interferes with daily activities. We chose to present steps/day, which is easily interpretable by clinicians and patients. Another strength of our study was muscle mass estimation by 24 h CER, which is well accepted for estimation of total body skeletal muscle mass, even in patients with advanced renal failure [12,21]. Additionally, we objectively determined protein intake by 24 h urinary urea excretion. In the future, we plan to extend our analysis to also include muscle quality using gait speed, as well as quality of life questionnaires. An important limitation of our study is the cross-sectional design, which allows only research of associations and not causality. Additional prospective studies are warranted to confirm our findings. Another limitation is that one-week record of the Fitbit may not be sufficiently representative of PA, as certain activities, such as swimming, and seasonal variations were not taken into account. However, only 8 patients of the total 217 patients (4%) recorded swimming in their lifestyle diary. Secondly, we had the sampling periods of our population distributed over the seasons. Making these effect negligible.

Our study has important clinical implications. We found clear associations between low protein intake, loss of muscle mass, and low PA in patients with complicated type 2 diabetes. Our study suggests that optimizing protein intake might be a first step to improving physical fitness in patients with type 2 diabetes. As current dietary guidelines focus on reducing overall caloric intake, and carbohydrate intake in particular, adequate protein intake might be an important blind spot in current nutritional management. This has also been advocated in previous studies, which suggest that dietary protein should be prescribed together with physical exercise in order to optimize muscle health [12,16,17,36]. The review by Scot and colleagues also emphasizes that lifestyle modification programs for older adults with type 2 diabetes, particularly for those with sarcopenia, should incorporate progressive resistance training, along with adequate intakes of protein and vitamin D, which may improve both functional and metabolic health and prevent undesirable decreases in muscle mass associated with weight loss intervention [9]. In the future, we want to include data from the Food Frequency Questionnaire (FFQ) in the analyses in order to investigate how intakes of total energy, carbohydrate, fat, and vitamin D may contribute to muscle mass and physical activity. It is important to note that the source of dietary protein (animal or vegetable) should also be taken into account, as we have previously shown that higher vegetable protein intake is associated with lower prevalence of renal function impairment [37].

5. Conclusions

In conclusion, our study shows that prevalent low protein intake and low muscle mass co-exist in patients with complicated type 2 diabetes with low physical activity. Dedicated intervention studies are needed to study the role of sufficient protein intake and PA in increasing or maintaining muscle mass in patients with type 2 diabetes.

Supplementary Materials: The following are available online at http://www.mdpi.com/2077-0383/9/10/3104/s1, Figure S1: flow chart of patient inclusion, Table S1: linear regression analyses for total steps per day.

Author Contributions: I.J.M.H. researched data and wrote the manuscript. N.d.B. analyzed the Fitbit data and reviewed/edited the manuscript. C.M.G., G.D.L., G.N., S.J.L.B. and M.M.R.V.-H. researched data and reviewed/edited the manuscript. M.M.O. and B.-J.F.v.B. reviewed/edited the manuscript. G.D.L. is the principal investigator of DIALECT and the guarantor. All authors have read and agreed to the published version of the manuscript.

Funding: Funding was provided from the ZGT hospital research fund.

Acknowledgments: The authors would like to thank Nicole Oosterom, Annis Jalving, Roos Nijboer, and all of the students who have participated in DIALECT 1 and 2, Ziekenhuisgroep Twente, for their general contributions to DIALECT, including patient inclusion.

Conflicts of Interest: The authors report no potential conflicts of interest relevant to this article.

References

1. Wild, S.; Roglic, G.; Green, A.; Sicree, R.; King, H. Global prevalence of diabetes: Estimates for the year 2000 and projections for 2030. *Diabetes Care* **2004**, *27*, 1047–1053. [CrossRef] [PubMed]
2. Weggemans, R.M.; Backx, F.J.G.; Borghouts, L.; Chinapaw, M.; Hopman, M.T.E.; Koster, A.; Kremers, S.; van Loon, L.J.C.; May, A.; Mosterd, A.; et al. The 2017 Dutch Physical Activity Guidelines. *Int. J. Behav. Nutr. Phys. Act.* **2018**, *15*, 58. [CrossRef] [PubMed]

3. Tudor-Locke, C.; Craig, C.L.; Aoyagi, Y.; Bell, R.C.; Croteau, K.A.; De Bourdeaudhuij, I.; Ewald, B.; Gardner, A.W.; Hatano, Y.; Lutes, L.D.; et al. How many steps/day are enough? For older adults and special populations. *Int. J. Behav. Nutr. Phys. Act.* **2011**, *8*, 1–19.
4. Jakicic, J.M.; Greg, E.; Knowler, W.; Kelley, D.E.; Lang, W.; Miller, G.D.; Pi-Sunyer, F.X.; Regensteiner, J.G.; Rejeski, W.J.; Ribisl, P.; et al. Activity patterns of obese adults with Type 2 Diabetes in the look AHEAD study. *Med. Sci. Sports. Exerc.* **2010**, *42*, 1995–2005. [CrossRef] [PubMed]
5. Oosterom, N.; Gant, C.M.; Ruiterkamp, N.; van Beijnum, B.J.F.; Hermens, H.; Bakker, S.J.L.; Navis, G.; Vollenbroek-Hutten, M.M.R.; Laverman, G.D. Physical activity in patients with type 2 diabetes: The case for objective measurement in routine clinical care. *Diabetes Care* **2018**, *41*, e50–e51. [CrossRef]
6. Min Lee, I.; Shiroma, E.J.; Kamada, M.; Basset, D.R.; Matthews, C.E.; Buring, J. E Association of Step Volume and Intensity with All-Cause Mortality in Older Women. *JAMA Intern. Med.* **2019**, *179*, 1105–1112.
7. Saint-Maurice, P.F.; Troiano, R.P.; Bassett, D.R.; Graubard, B.I.; Carlson, S.A.; Shirom, E.J.; Fulton, J.E.; Matthews, C.E. Association of Daily Step Count and Step Intensity with Mortality Among US Adults. *J. Am. Med. Assoc.* **2020**, *323*, 1151–1160. [CrossRef]
8. Trierweiler, H.; Kisielewicz, G.; Hoffmann Jonasson, T.; Rasmussen Petterle, R.; Aguiar Moreira, C.; Cochenski Borba, V.Z. Sarcopenia: A chronic complication of type 2 diabetes mellitus. *Diabetol. Metab. Syndr.* **2018**, *10*, 1–9. [CrossRef]
9. Scot, D.; Courten de, B.; Ebeling, P.R. Sarcopenia: A potential cause and consequence of type 2 diabetes in Australia's ageing population? *Med. J. Aust.* **2016**, *205*, 329–333. [CrossRef]
10. Mesinovic, J.; Zengin, A.; Courten, B.; Ebeling, P.R.; Scott, D. Sarcopenia and type 2 diabetes mellitus: A bidirectional relationship. *Diabetes Metab. Syndr. Obes. Targets Ther.* **2019**, *2*, 1057–1072. [CrossRef]
11. Barazzoni, R.; Bischoff, S.C.; Boiirie, Y.; Busetto, L.; Cederholm, T.; Dicker, D.; Toplak, H.; Van Gossum, A.; Yumuk, V.; Vettor, R. Sarcopenic obesity: Time to meet the challenge. *Clin. Nutr.* **2018**, *37*, 1787–1793. [CrossRef] [PubMed]
12. Alexandrov, N.V.; Eelderink, C.; Singh-Povel, C.M.; Navis, G.J.; Bakker, S.J.L.; Corpeleijn, E. Dietary protein sources and muscle mass over the life course: The Lifelines Cohort study. *Nutrients* **2018**, *10*, 1471. [CrossRef] [PubMed]
13. Housten, D.K.; Nicklas, B.J.; Ding, J.; Harris, T.B.; Tylavsky, F.A.; Newman, A.B.; Lee, J.S.; Sahyoun, N.R.; Visser, M.; Kritchevsky, S.B.; et al. Dietary protein intake is Associated with Lean Mass Change in Older, Community-Dwelling Adults: The Health, Aging, and Body Composition (Health ABC) study. *Am. J. Clin. Nutr.* **2008**, *87*, 150–155. [CrossRef]
14. Huang, R.Y.; Yang, K.C.; Chang, H.H.; Lee, L.T.; Lu, C.W.; Huang, K.C. The association between total protein and vegetable protein intake and low muscle mass among the community-dwelling elderly population in Northern Taiwan. *Nutrients* **2016**, *8*, 373. [CrossRef] [PubMed]
15. Sahni, S.; Mangano, K.M.; Hannan, M.T.; Kiel, D.P.; McLean, R.R. Higher Protein Intake is Associated with Higher Lean Mass and Quadriceps Muscle Strength in Adults Men and Women. *J. Nutr.* **2015**, *145*, 1569–1575. [CrossRef]
16. Tieland, M.; Borgonjen-Van den Berg, K.J.; van Loon, L.J.; de Groot, L.C. Dietary Protein Intake in Community-Dwelling, Frail, and Institutionalized Elderly People: Scope for Improvement. *Eur. J. Nutr.* **2012**, *51*, 173–179. [CrossRef]
17. Liao, C.D.; Tsauo, J.Y.; Wu, Y.T.; Cheng, C.-P.; Chen, H.-C.; Huang, Y.C.; Liou, T.-H. Effects of protein supplementation combined with resistance exercise on body composition and physical function in older adults: A systematic review and meta-analysis. *Am. J. Clin. Nutr.* **2017**, *106*, 1078–1091. [CrossRef]
18. Gant, C.M.; Binnenmars, S.H.; Berg, E.V.D.; Bakker, S.J.L.; Navis, G.; Laverman, G.D. Integrated assessment of pharmacological and nutritional cardiovascular risk management: Blood pressure control in the DIAbetes and LifEstyle Cohort Twente (DIALECT). *Nutrients* **2017**, *9*, 709. [CrossRef]
19. Olaleye, D.; Perkins, B.A.; Bril, V. Evaluation of three screening tests and a risk assessment model for diagnosing peripheral neuropathy in the diabetes clinic. *Diabetes Res. Clin. Pract.* **2015**, *4*, 115–128.
20. Proctor, D.N.; O'Brien, P.C.; Atkinson, E.J.; Nair, K.S. Comparison of techniques to estimate total body skeletal muscle mass in people of different age groups. *Am. J. Physiol.* **1999**, *277*, 489. [CrossRef]
21. Heymsfield, S.B.; Arteaga, C.; McManus, C.; Smith, J.; Moffitt, S. Measurement of muscle mass in humans: Validity of the 24-hour urinary creatinine method. *Am. J. Clin. Nutr.* **1983**, *37*, 478–494. [CrossRef] [PubMed]

22. Maroni, B.J.; Steinman, T.I.; Mitch, W.E. A method for estimating nitrogen intake of patients with chronic renal failure. *Kidney Int.* **1985**, *27*, 58–65. [CrossRef] [PubMed]
23. Trumbo, P.; Schlicker, S.; Yates, A.A.; Poos, M.; Food and nutrition board of the institute of medicine; The National Academies. Dietary references intakes for Energy, Carbohydrate, Fiber, fat, fatty acids, cholesterol, protein and amino acids. *J. Am. Diet. Assoc.* **2002**, *102*, 1621–1630. [CrossRef]
24. Cruz-Jentoft, A.J.; Bahat, G.; Bauer, J.; Boirie, Y.; Bruyère, O.; Cederholm, T.; Cooper, C.; Landi, F.; Rolland, Y.; Sayer, A.A.; et al. Guidelines. Sarcopenia: Revised European consensus on definition and diagnosis. *Age Aging* **2019**, *48*, 16–31. [CrossRef]
25. Nomura, T.; Ishiguro, T.; Ohira, M.; Ikeda, Y. Diabetic polyneuropathy is a risk factor for decline of lower extremity strength in patients with type 2 diabetes. *J. Diabetes Investig.* **2018**, *91*, 86–192. [CrossRef]
26. Baum, J.I.; Kim, I.Y.; Wolfe, R.R. Protein consumption and the Elderly: What is the optimal level of intake? *Nutrients* **2016**, *8*, 359. [CrossRef]
27. Nowson, C.; Connell, S. Protein requirements and recommendations for older people: A review. *Nutrients* **2015**, *7*, 6574–6599. [CrossRef]
28. Healy, G.N.; Winkler, E.A.H.; Brakenridge, C.L.; Reeves, M.M.; Eakin, E.G. Accelerometer-Derived sedentary and physical activitiy time in overweight/obese adults with type 2 diabetes; Cross-sectional associations with cardiometabolic biomarkers. *PLoS ONE* **2015**, *10*, e0119140. [CrossRef]
29. Balducci, S.; D'Errico, V.; Haxhi, J.; Sacchetti, M.; Orlando, G.; Cardelli, P.; Di Biase, N.; Bollanti, L.; Conti, F.; Zanuso, S. Level and correlates of physical activity and sedentary behavior in patients with type 2 diabetes: A cross-sectional analysis of the Italian Diabetes and Exercise Study_2. *PLoS ONE* **2017**, *12*, e0173337. [CrossRef]
30. Cooper, A.R.; Sebire, S. Sedentary time, breaks in sedentary time and metabolic variables in people with newly diagnosed type 2 diabetes. *Diabetologia* **2012**, *55*, 589–599. [CrossRef]
31. Cichosz, S.L.; Fleischer, J.; Hoeyem, P.; Laugesen, E.; Poulsen, P.L.; Christinansen, J.S.; Ejskjær, N.; Hansen, T.K. Objective measurements of activity patterns in people with newly diagnosed Type 2 diabetes demonstrate a sedentary lifestyle. *Diabet. Med.* **2013**, *30*, 1063–1066. [CrossRef] [PubMed]
32. Andersen, H.; Nielsen, S.; Mogensen, C.E.; Jakobsen, J. Muscle strenght in type 2 diabetes. *Diabetes* **2004**, *53*, 1543–1548. [PubMed]
33. Sato, E.; Mori, T.; Mishima, E.; Suzuki, A.; Sugawara, S.; Saigusa, D.; Miura, D.; Morikawa-Ichinose, T.; Saito, R.; Saito, R.; et al. Metabolic alterations by indoxyl sulfate in skeletal muscle induce uremic sarcopenia in chronic kidney disease. *Sci. Rep.* **2016**, *6*, 36618. [PubMed]
34. Joan, J.K.; Edney, K.; Moran, C.; Strikanth, V.; Calisaya, M. Gender differences in physical activity levels of older people with type 2 diabetes mellitus. *J. Phys. Act. Health* **2016**, *13*, 409–415.
35. Nomura, T.; Kawae, T.; Kataoka, H.; Ikeda, Y. Aging, physical activity and diabetic complications related to loss of muscle strength in patients with type 2 diabetes. *Phys. Ther. Res.* **2018**, *21*, 33–38. [PubMed]
36. Landi, F.; Calvani, R.; Tosato, M.; Martone, A.M.; Ortolani, E.; Savera, G.; D'Angelo, E.; Sisto, A.; Marzetti, E. Protein intake and muscle health in old age: From biological plausibility to clinical evidence. *Nutrients* **2016**, *8*, 295.
37. Oosterwijk, M.M.; Soedamah-Muthu, S.; Geleijnse, J.M.; Bakker, S.J.L.; Navis, G.; Binnenmars, S.H.; Gant, C.M.; Laverman, G.D. High Dietary intake of vegetable protein is associated with lower prevalence of renal function impairment: Results of the Dutch DIALECT-1 Cohort. *Kidney Int. Rep.* **2019**, *4*, 710–719.

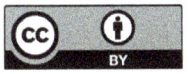 © 2020 by the authors. Licensee MDPI, Basel, Switzerland. This article is an open access article distributed under the terms and conditions of the Creative Commons Attribution (CC BY) license (http://creativecommons.org/licenses/by/4.0/).

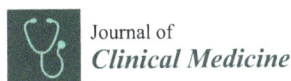

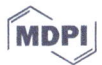

Article

Respiratory Muscle Strengths and Their Association with Lean Mass and Handgrip Strengths in Older Institutionalized Individuals

Francisco Miguel Martínez-Arnau [1,2], Cristina Buigues [2,3], Rosa Fonfría-Vivas [2,3] and Omar Cauli [2,3,*]

1. Department of Physiotherapy, University of Valencia, 46010 Valencia, Spain; Francisco.m.martinez@uv.es
2. Frailty and Cognitive Impairment Research Group (FROG), University of Valencia, 46010 Valencia, Spain; cristina.buigues@uv.es (C.B.); rosa.fonfria@uv.es (R.F.-V.)
3. Department of Nursing, University of Valencia, 46010 Valencia, Spain
* Correspondence: Omar.Cauli@uv.es

Received: 15 July 2020; Accepted: 19 August 2020; Published: 24 August 2020

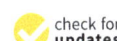

Abstract: The study of reduced respiratory muscle strengths in relation to the loss of muscular function associated with ageing is of great interest in the study of sarcopenia in older institutionalized individuals. The present study assesses the association between respiratory muscle parameters and skeletal mass content and strength, and analyzes associations with blood cell counts and biochemical parameters related to protein, lipid, glucose and ion profiles. A multicenter cross-sectional study was performed among patients institutionalized in nursing homes. The respiratory muscle function was evaluated by peak expiratory flow, maximal respiratory pressures and spirometry parameters, and skeletal mass function and lean mass content with handgrip strength, walking speed and bioimpedance, respectively. The prevalence of reduced respiratory muscle strength in the sample ranged from 37.9% to 80.7%. Peak expiratory flow significantly ($p < 0.05$) correlated to handgrip strength and gait speed, as well as maximal inspiratory pressure ($p < 0.01$). Maximal expiratory pressure significantly ($p < 0.01$) correlated to handgrip strength. No correlation was obtained with muscle mass in any of parameters related to reduced respiratory muscle strength. The most significant associations within the blood biochemical parameters were observed for some protein and lipid biomarkers e.g., glutamate-oxaloacetate transaminase (GOT), urea, triglycerides and cholesterol. Respiratory function muscle parameters, peak expiratory flow and maximal respiratory pressures were correlated with reduced strength and functional impairment but not with lean mass content. We identified for the first time a relationship between peak expiratory flow (PEF) values and GOT and urea concentrations in blood which deserves future investigations in order to manage these parameters as a possible biomarkers of reduced respiratory muscle strength.

Keywords: spirometry; urea; fatigue; respiratory system; skeletal muscles; lipids; transaminases

1. Introduction

Sarcopenia is a geriatric syndrome that according to the European Working Group on Sarcopenia in Older People (EWGSOP) guidelines, is defined as a progressive and generalized loss of skeletal muscle mass and strength, with a risk of adverse outcomes, such as functional capacity impairment, dependence, falls and fractures, negative impact on quality of life, hospitalization and death [1]. In older individuals, sarcopenia has a widespread effect on all skeletal muscles throughout the body, but the features of sarcopenia in the respiratory muscles and its relationship with established sarcopenia parameters such as reduced lean mass, poor muscular strength and functional impairment [1,2] have been less widely investigated in older individuals [3,4], and no studies have been performed in nursing home residents, a significant population in western societies with a huge burden of comorbidities, including sarcopenia [5–8]. Besides the loss of muscular mass and strength, aging leads to proteolysis of elastic fiber and an increase in collagen in the pulmonary parenchyma, which coupled with an increase in the rigidity of the chest wall generates a mechanical disadvantage, and weakness of the respiratory muscles over time [9,10]. These changes results in a diminished respiratory muscle strength (RMS), referred to as sarcopenia of the respiratory muscle or reduced respiratory muscle strength as just it is analysed by quantifying the decline in respiratory function [3]. Respiratory muscles are also responsible of producing a proper pressure difference between inspiration and expiration to generate a correct airway flow rate, which guarantees a good respiratory function [11]. Other respiratory parameters, such as vital capacity (VC), forced vital capacity (FVC), forced expiratory volume in 1 s (FEV1), and peak expiratory flow rate (PEF) are also affected as a result of changes in elastic recoil and thorax compliance associated with aging [3,11,12]. RMS is therefore related to FEV1, FVC, and PEF. Even in patients without airway obstruction, these functions may decline due to age-induced weakness of the respiratory muscles. PEF measurements were recommended over RMS measurements for the assessment of respiratory function in the EWGSOP consensus report published in 2010 [2]. However, the EWGSOP report also indicated that PEF measurements should be used in association with other assessments, because there is a limited evidence about the relationship between PEF and skeletal muscle mass/sarcopenia in older adults. A previous study revealed that PEF is a significant predictor of mortality in older adults [13,14]. Further studies have demonstrated that sarcopenia is related to an increased incidence of pulmonary complications after surgery [15–17] and aspiration pneumonia mortality [18]. Izawa et al. [19] evaluated the relationship between maximal inspiratory pressure (MIP) and physical function as a measure of sarcopenia in older patients with heart disease, and found that sarcopenic patients presented lower values of MIP which also correlated with reduced skeletal muscle mass index, gait speed and hand grip strength. There is a lack of studies demonstrating the association between respiratory muscle weakness and sarcopenia parameters (reduced lean mass and muscular strength and low physical performance) in older institutionalized individuals. Moreover, no studies about the relationship of respiratory muscle function and blood analytical parameters in sarcopenic individuals have been performed. The objectives in this study were therefore to compare respiratory muscle function with lean mass content, handgrip strength and functional impairment (walking speed) in order to assess whether there is an association between respiratory muscle parameters such as the maximum respiratory pressures and peak expiratory flow and parameters of skeletal muscular function. Since skeletal sarcopenia have been associated to malnutrition and undernutrition, which in turn is accompanied by several alterations detectable in blood regarding both blood cell counts and biochemical metabolic markers [20–23] we also evaluated the associations between the parameters related to respiratory muscle strength and skeletal sarcopenia with blood cell counts and biochemical parameters related to protein, lipid, glucose and indirectly with energy production (glucose, creatinine, transaminases, and ions concentrations).

2. Materials and Methods

2.1. Design and Study Population

A cross-sectional study was conducted in individuals institutionalized in nursing homes and long-stay centers for the older individuals in the province of Valencia, Spain (GeroResidencias La Saleta, Valencia). We selected nursing home residents of both genders. Participants were excluded if they were unable to understand the content of questionnaires (moderate-severe cognitive impairment), had a poorly controlled major psychiatric disease (schizophrenia, bipolar disorders, etc.), acute infections, or a known cancer condition. According to the requirements of the Declaration of Helsinki, written consent was obtained from all of the selected subjects before beginning the study, after informing them about the procedures involved and the purpose of the research. The entire study protocol was approved by the local ethical committee at the University of Valencia (H1524420647893, approved 5 July 2018).

2.2. Sociodemographic and Clinical Variables

Socio-demographic variables and medical conditions were recorded, including the number of medications taken, the type and number of any comorbidities using the Charlson index, and several hematological and biochemical parameters. The Charlson index was used to assess comorbidity (with a Cronbach's Alpha of 0.78) [24]. This index assesses 16 diseases that are explicitly defined and scored by a continuous variable from 0 to 31. With this index, the 10-year survival prediction is estimated for patients with comorbidity [25].

2.3. Measurement of Respiratory Muscle Function

The assessment of respiratory function was carried out through two different tests, the assessment of lung volumes and flows by performing a forced spirometry, and the assessment of the maximum respiratory pressures that the respiratory muscles are capable of generating at mouth level as a result of maximum effort.

The spirometric assessment followed the standardized recommendations of the European Respiratory Society [26]. The patient was placed in a seated position, with his back supported by the backrest and with nasal clamps to avoid air leakage. The maneuver was explained in detail to the patient to minimize errors, requesting an initial maximum inspiration to reach total lung capacity, which allows the subsequent performance of a forced maximum expiration for at least 6 s, until the limit of expiration is reached. At least three manoeuvres are performed, with a rest of 1 min between each one, and the highest value of the three repetitions is recorded.

By carrying out this test, the following volumes and forced pulmonary capacities in absolute and relative values were obtained: forced vital capacity (FVC), forced expiratory volume in the first second (FEV1), FEV1/FVC, forced expiratory volume in smaller than 1mm diameter tracks (FEV2575) and peak expiratory flow (PEF). At least three repetitions of the maneuver were performed (with a maximum of 8 repetitions) to achieve the correct execution of the test, discarding those spirometric maneuvers with artifacts in their performance or variations of more than 0.150 L between the highest FEV1 and/or FVC values, as recommended by the ATS/ERS [26].

For the assessment of respiratory muscle strength, maximum static respiratory pressures in the mouth, inspiratory (MIP) and expiratory (MEP) were measured. These parameters allow us to know in a simple way the global force that the respiratory muscles are capable of exerting. The tests require the collaboration of the patient to perform a maximum isometric effort. The standardized regulations for this test were followed [27,28]. To evaluate the MIP, the patient was instructed to start from the residual volume and for the MEP to start from the total lung capacity, so that the maximum value of the three maneuvers could be collected, with a variation of less than 10% between them and a 1-min pause between each of the repetitions. This excluded those attempts where there was more than 10% variation between them, as recommended by Laveneziana, et al. [28].The proposed cut-off points for PEF and maximum respiratory pressures (MIP and MEP) were used to establish the existence of respiratory sarcopenia. The cut-off point for PEF was set at 4.40 L/s for men and 3.21 L/s for women [22]. The cut-off point for MIP was set at less than or equal to 55 H_2O cm for men and less than or equal to 45 H_2O cm for women, while for MEP it was set at less than or equal to 60 H_2O cm for men and less than or equal to 50 H_2O cm for women [4]. Before the test was conducted, the steps for correctly performing the test were carefully explained to the participants. Once explained, a test of all the steps to be followed was carried out, without demanding maximum effort from the participants to avoid accumulated fatigue. Afterwards, the tests were carried out in accordance with international standards [28].

The older institutionalized population has a high prevalence of cognitive impairment, which could make this type of testing difficult. However, we excluded patients with moderate and severe cognitive impairment, so that the collaboration of patients included was adequate to perform these tests. In addition, an adaptation procedure was carried out on the study subjects before the definitive test, excluding from the sample those subjects who presented poor coordination and, therefore, difficulty in carrying out the test at the discretion of the evaluator. In all the centres, assessments were made in the morning between 8 and 11 am and in the same period of time. To avoid inter-observer errors, all measurements were taken by the same trained investigator.

In addition, to analyze reliability, we assessed the stability of the measure obtaining values of intraclass correlation coefficient (ICC; one-way, mixed-effects model) between PEF values in the three centers of 0.71, what was indicative of moderate to good reliability.

2.4. Measurement of Sarcopenia

Muscle skeletal sarcopenia was assessed by indirect measures of muscle function and muscle mass, such as handgrip strength assessed by hand-dynamometry, walking speed and bioimpedance respectively. Hand-dynamometer was assessed in the dominant hand by means of a JAMAR dynamometer (Lafayette Instrument Company, Lafayette, IN, USA) as previously described [29]. The subject was placed in a standard position: in a sitting position, with the shoulder at 0° of flexion, the elbow attached to the body at 90° of flexion and the forearm in a neutral position. After the subject is positioned appropriately, the examiner asks the patient to squeeze as hard as possible for 3 s and then relax. Three attempts were made, with 1 min rest in between. The mean value obtained was recorded. The cut-offs for handgrip strength were ≤ 30 kg/m^2 for men and ≤ 20 kg/m^2 for women [2]. The walking speed was assessed using the 4-m walking test [30]. The patient was asked to walk at usual pace and from a standing start and using their usual walking aid. The time required to cover this distance was recorded and, based on this, the walking speed in m/s was calculated. The cut-off for low walking speed was ≤ 0.8 m/s walking through 4 m [2]. The body composition was assessed by bioelectrical impedance analysis (BIA) with a BF-300 device (Tanita, Tokyo, Japan) as previously described [31,32]. The BIA measure was performed with a standard technique using a single frequency of 50 KHz and 550 mA, and the placement of four electrodes in a distal position (four electrodes at feet) while participant was in a standing position. BIA measurements were carried out in the early morning following the next considerations: (1) No physical exercise in the previous hours; (2) 2–3 h of fasting, including drinking plenty of water or alcohol; (3) urination 30 min before the test; (4) no metal parts at the time of the test. The values of reactance and resistance were then recorded once the patient was stabilized. The repeatability and accuracy of the resistance and reactance measurements enabled the smallest changes to be recorded to a resolution of 0.1 Ω. Muscle mass was calculated using the formula of Janssen et al. [31]: muscle mass (kg) = [(height^2/R × 0.401) + (3.825 × sex) + (−0.701 × age) + 5.102] where height is expressed in cm, R in Ω, age in years and female sex has a value of zero and males a value of one. The muscle mass index (MMI) is defined as the muscle mass a person has, corrected by body surface area (muscle mass/height^2). The bioimpedance test was performed early in the morning while the patient is at rest, after overnight fasting (food and drink) and removing all metal elements. The cut-off for the loss of muscle mass assessed by bioimpedance of the whole body were ≤ 5.5 kg/m^2 for women and ≤ 7.25 kg/m^2 for men [2]. These muscle mass values are adjusted with the cut-off values for the Spanish population being 8.31 kg/m^2 for men and 6.68 kg/m^2 for women [33]. In order to minimize the influence of physical performance across the time of the day, all measurements were always conducted between 8–11 a.m.

2.5. Haemogram and Analytical Parameters

To obtain the analytical determinations, the usual blood controls carried out in residential centers were used. Thus, blood samples were collected from each subject at approximately 8 am (after 8–10 h fasting). 10 mL of blood plasma was collected into Vacutainer tubes (BD, Franklin Lakes, NJ, USA) containing EDTA.

Clinical laboratories belonging to local public health centers were used to analyze the different hematological parameters (white blood cells, hemoglobin, erythrocytes, and platelets) and biochemical parameters (glucose, urea, urate, cholesterol, triglycerides, creatinine, glutamic oxaloacetic transaminase [GOT], and serum glutamic pyruvic transaminase [GPT], sodium ions [Na^+], potassium ions [K^+], and Calcium [Ca^{++}]). Within public health centers, the variation range of metabolites in plasma sample varies between 0.4–1.1% dependent on the metabolite.

2.6. Statistical Analysis

Quantitative variables were analysed using descriptive statistics, specifically central tendency measures (means), standard error of the mean (SEM), 95% confidence interval and ranges. Frequencies and percentages were used to describe the qualitative variables. The normal distribution of the variables, in order to determine whether to carry out parametric or non-parametric tests, was analysed using the Shapiro-Wilk test. Outliers were identified on the boxplot drawn in SPSS program which uses a step of 1.5 × IQR (Interquartile range). No outliers were identified and all data were included in the statistical analysis. Differences in quantitative variables between the two groups were analyzed with the two-tailed tests e.g., parametric Student t-test or the nonparametric Mann-Whitney U-test. To analyze the correlation between quantitative variables, the parametric Pearson test or the non-parametric Spearman's test was used depending on their distribution. Statistical significance was considered at $p < 0.05$. SPSS version 25.0 statistical package (SPSS Inc., Chicago, IL, USA) was used to perform the statistical analyses.

3. Results

3.1. Sociodemographic and Clinical Parameters of the Study Sample

A total of 58 subjects (67.2% female) living in three nursing care centers located in the province of Valencia (Spain) were enrolled in the study (Table 1). All the participants were Caucasian. Their age ranged from 55 to 93 years, and the mean age was 78.6 ± 8.9 years. 63.8% of the subjects were independent in their walking ability (they did not require external aids such as a cane or walker). Smokers were 15.5% ($n = 9$) of the sample. A percentage of 21.1% ($n = 12$) in the study sample used bronchodilators as a usual treatment. Among individuals using bronchodilators, $n = 6$ used bronchodilator therapy containing glucocorticoids. Regarding the use of common medications affecting the muscular system, none of the individuals received oral glucocorticoid treatment, 37.9% ($n = 22$) used statins to lower cholesterol levels and 5.2% ($n = 3$) used muscle relaxant drugs. Mean body mass index was 28.8 ± 5.8 (Range 18.7–50.2). The Charlson comorbidity index score adjusted for age was 5.4 ± 1.9 (Range 1.0–11.0). The occurrence of the most common comorbidities are indicated in Table 1.

Respiratory function assessment showed an absence of respiratory failure related to oxyhemoglobin saturation, with 95.9 ± 1.9% (range 91.0–99.0). Respiratory functional exploration showed spirometric values within normal ranges for a population of these characteristics (FVC at 84.0 ± 23.6% (Range 23.0–149.0) and FEV1 at 83.3 ± 28.3% (Range 20.0–160.0)), except for a small reduction in the permeability of the smaller diameter airway, with an FEV2575 at 54.5 ± 25.7% (Range 12.0–149.0). Respiratory muscle strength was diminished, at both inspiratory (36.5 ± 17.4 H_2O cm) and expiratory (58.9 ± 23.7 H_2O cm) levels. The maximal respiratory pressures (MIP and MEP) and spirometric parameter values (FVC, FEV1, FEV1/FVC, FEV2575 and PEF) are shown in Table 2.

A positive correlation was found between oxyhemoglobin saturation and FVC ($r = 0.287$ $p = 0.034$, Pearson test) and oxyhemoglobin saturation and FEV1 ($r = 0.269$ $p = 0.047$, Pearson test). No correlations were found between heart rate and any other respiratory parameters.

Table 1. Characteristics of the study sample.

Clinical and Demographic Characteristics of Participants	Mean Value ± SD (Range) or Percentage
Age (years)	78.6 ± 8.9 (55–93)
Sex	Male 32.8% Female 67.2%
IBM (kg/m^2)	28.9 ± 6.1 (18.7–50.2)
Smokers	15.5%
Use of bronchodilators as a usual treatment	21.1%
Walking ability	Independent 63.8% Can 3.4% Walker 32.8%
Comorbidities (Charlson index)	5.4 ± 1.9 (1–11)
Diabetes	31.0%
Chronic obstructive pulmonary disease	17.2%
Hypertension	32.8%
Hypercholesterolemia	37.9%
Congestive heart failure	10.3%
Renal failure	12.1%
Osteoporosis	20.7%
Depression	19.0%

Table 2. Respiratory function parameters.

Respiratory Parameters	Mean Value (± SD)	Range
SatO$_2$ (%)	95.9 ± 1.9	91.0–99.0
Heart rate (bpm)	77.1 ± 14.2	49.0–114.0
FVC (L/s)	1.8 ± 0.7	0.3–4.4
FEV1 (L/s)	1.3 ± 0.5	0.3–2.9
FEV1/FVC (%)	76.5 ± 12.1	45.9–100.0
FEV25-75 (L/s)	1.2 ± 0.5	0.3–3.1
PEF (L/s)	2.8 ± 1.2	0.7–5.7
MIP (H$_2$O cm)	36.5 ± 17.4	7.0–77.0
MEP (H$_2$O cm)	58.9 ± 23.7	10.0–99.0

A positive correlation can be found between the various parameters that describe the spirometric function by analyzing the correlation between the different parameters of respiratory function. There was a significant correlation between FVC percentage values and FEV1 percentage values (r = 0.894, $p < 0.001$, Pearson test), FEV2575 percentage values (r = 0.473, $p < 0.001$, Pearson test) and PEF (r = 0.281 $p = 0.033$, Pearson test). Significant correlations were also found between FEV1 percentage values and FEV2575 percentage values (r = 0.689, $p < 0.001$, Pearson test). There was a correlation between PEF and maximum respiratory pressures, with both MIP (r = 0.419, $p < 0.001$, Pearson test) and with MEP (r = 0.575, $p < 0.001$, Pearson test), and the maximum respiratory pressures between them (r = 0.559, $p < 0.001$, Pearson test).

Based on the PEF cut-off points established by Kera et al., (22), the prevalence of respiratory sarcopenia in the sample studied was 70.7%. On the other hand, if the values of MIP and MEP established by Ohara et al., (4) are taken as the benchmark, the prevalence of respiratory sarcopenia was 80.7% and 37.9%, respectively.

3.2. Evaluation of Skeletal Muscle Mass and Function

According to the EWGSOP guidelines, 17.6% of the subjects were classified as sarcopenic, with 17.6% meeting the criteria of reduced lean mass, 65.4% meeting the criteria of low physical performance and 84.5% meeting the criteria of reduced muscle strength. The mean values of each criterion were skeletal muscle-mass index of 9.21 ± 2.793 kg/m^2, walking speed of 0.66 ± 0.331 m/s and handgrip strength of 17.90 ± 8.506 kg. The data from the anthropometric characteristics of all the participants in this study are summarized in Table 3.

Table 3. Anthropometric analysis and sarcopenia parameters.

Anthropometric Analysis	Mean Value (± SD)	Range	% of Individuals Fulfilling the EWGSOP Criterion for Sarcopenia
Muscle mass (Janssen)	22.8 ± 8.2	13.2–49.5	Reduced lean mass: 17.6%
Skeletal muscle mass index (Janssen)	9.2 ± 2.8	5.5–20.1	Reduced lean mass: 17.6%
Hand grip in dominant hand (Kg)	17.9 ± 8.5	6.5–42.0	Muscle strength (dominant hand): 84.5%
Hand grip in non-dominant hand (Kg)	16.5 ± 7.6	3.3–36.7	Muscle strength (non-dominant hand): 84.5%
Walking speed (m/s)	0.6 ± 0.3	0.1–1.5	Physical performance: 65.4%

3.3. Evaluation of the Relationship between Muscle Skeleñata Parameters (Mass and Function) and Muscle Respiratory Function

There was a significant and positive correlation between physical performance and PEF absolute values (r = 0.563, $p < 0.001$, Spearman's test), PEF percentage values (r = 0.440, $p = 0.001$, Pearson test) and MIP values (r = 0.354, $p = 0.011$, Spearman's test). No correlation between physical performance and MEP was found (r = 0.268, $p = 0.268$, Spearman's test). No significant correlation was found between the other parameters of respiratory function and physical performance ($p > 0.05$ in all cases).

There was a significant and positive correlation between handgrip strength and MIP values (r = 0.599, $p < 0.001$, Spearman's test), MEP values (r = 0.465, $p < 0.001$, Spearman's test) and PEF absolute values (r = 0.375, $p = 0.004$, Spearman's test). There was also a significant but negative correlation between handgrip strength and FEV1 percentage values (r = −0.307, $p = 0.019$, Spearman's test). No significant correlation was found between other parameters of respiratory function and handgrip strength ($p > 0.05$ in all cases) (Figure 1).

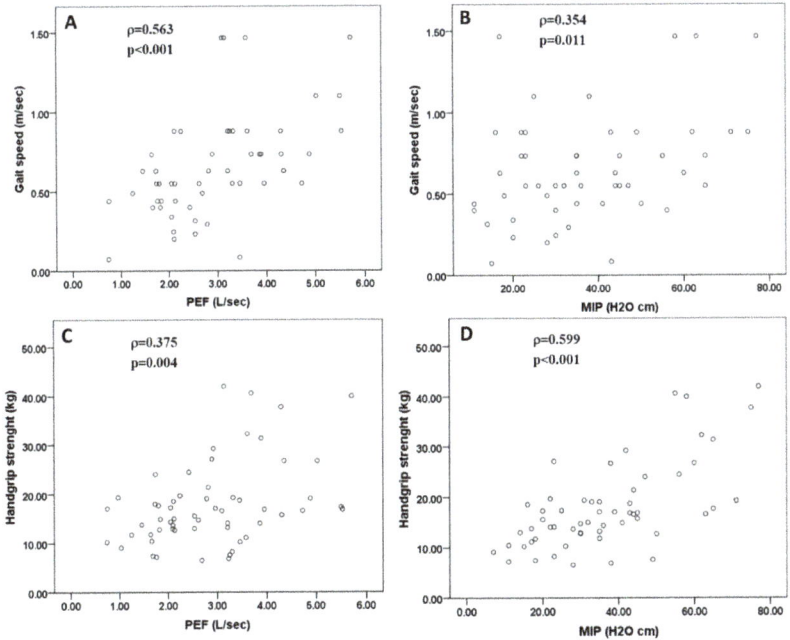

Figure 1. Representation of the significant correlations between skeletal and respiratory muscle sarcopenia parameters. Significant correlations between gait speed and PEF (**A**) or MIP (**B**) and between handgrip strength and PEF (**C**) or MIP (**D**).

No significant correlations were found between skeletal muscle mass index and respiratory function parameters, in relation to either PEF absolute values (r = 0.252, p = 0.074, Spearman's test), or MIP (r = 0.143, p = 0.322, Spearman's test), or MEP (r = 0.225, p = 0.112, Spearman's test).

We categorized patients based on cut-off scores for skeletal sarcopenia (see Methods section) and we evaluated whether there were any differences in the respiratory parameters and respiratory muscle parameters (Figure 2).

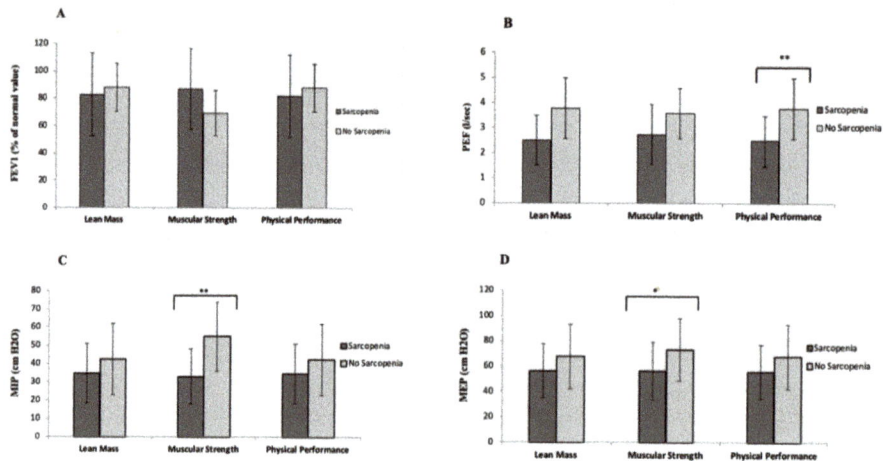

Figure 2. Mean difference of respiratory parameters ((**A**): FEV1; (**B**): PEF; (**C**): MIP; (**D**): MEP) according to the presence or not of the three cut-off values for sarcopenia parameters * $p < 0.05$; ** $p < 0.001$.

As for physical performance, differences were observed in both PEF (NS = 3.78 vs. S = 2.49, MeanDiff = 1.29 [95%CI: 0.67–1.91], $p < 0.001$) and PEF% (NS = 64.11 vs. S = 47.21, MeanDiff = 16.90 [95%CI: 6.59–27.22], $p = 0.002$).

For the handgrip strength, different maximal respiratory pressures were observed in both groups, MIP (NS = 54.89 vs. S = 33.06, MeanDiff = 21.83 [95%CI: 10.48–33.18], $p < 0.001$) and MEP (NS = 73.22 vs. S = 56.69, MeanDiff = 16.92 [95%CI: 0.13–37.70], $p = 0.048$). When analyzing the PEF we observed no statistically significant differences, although a trend was observed in them (NS = 3.57 vs. S = 2.74, MeanDiff = 0.86 [95%CI: −0.006–1.72], $p = 0.052$).

No significant differences for lean mass content were observed for any of the comparisons ($p > 0.05$) (Figure 2).

We also categorized patients based on respiratory muscle sarcopenia according to Kera et al. (22) and Ohara et al. (4) (see methods), and we evaluated whether there were any differences in the somatic sarcopenia parameters, such as skeletal muscle mass index, handgrip strength and gait speed (Figure 3).

For MIP, differences were observed in both gait speed (NS = 0.89 vs. S = 0.59, MeanDiff = 0.30 [95%CI: 0.51–0.85], $p = 0.007$) and handgrip strength (NS = 27.35 vs. S = 15.64, MeanDiff = 11.71 [95%CI: 4.75–18.66], $p = 0.003$). No differences were found for skeletal muscle mass index ($p = 0.844$).

As regards MEP, a different maximal handgrip strength were observed in both groups, (NS = 20.31 vs. S = 13.96, MeanDiff = 6.35 [95%CI: 2.59–10.11], $p = 0.001$). No statistically significant differences were found in gait speed or skeletal muscle mass index ($p = 0.156$ and $p = 0.214$, respectively).

For PEF, differences were observed in gait speed (NS = 0.82 vs. S = 0.58, MeanDiff = 0.24 [95%CI: 0.32–0.45], $p = 0.025$), but not in handgrip strength (NS = 17.90 vs. S = 17.90, MeanDiff = 0.01 [95%CI: −4.99–4.98], $p = 0.997$) (Figure 3).

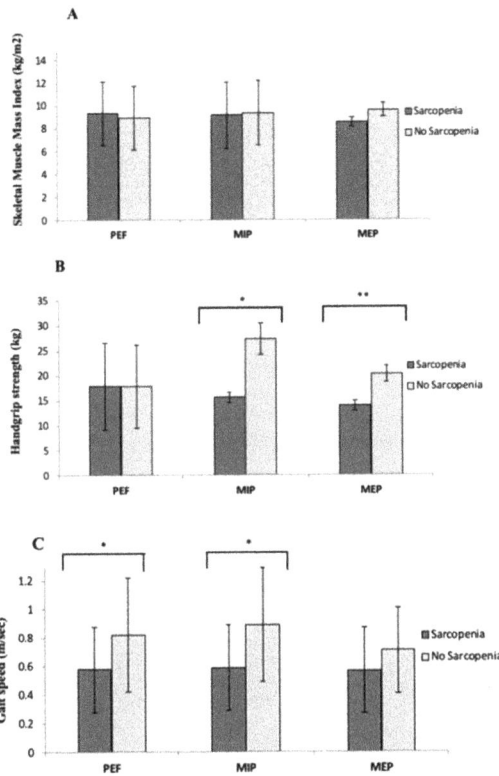

Figure 3. Mean difference of muscle mass (**A**), Handgrip strength (**B**) and gait speed (**C**) according to the presence of each respiratory muscle sarcopenia criteria. * $p < 0.05$; ** $p < 0.001$.

3.4. Evaluation of the Relationship between Sarcopenia Parameters and Blood Analytical Markers

No significant associations were found when analyzing the possible correlations between the parameters of the hemogram (white blood cells, hemoglobin, erythrocytes, and platelets) and the parameters of respiratory sarcopenia and somatic sarcopenia ($p > 0.05$ in all cases).

The relationship between respiratory sarcopenia parameters and biochemical parameters (glucose, urea, urate, cholesterol, triglycerides, creatinine, glutamic oxaloacetic transaminase [GOT], and serum glutamic pyruvic transaminase [GPT], sodium ions [Na^+], potassium ions [K^+], Calcium [Ca^{++}]) was subsequently studied. There was a significant and positive correlation between PEF values and GOT ($r = 0.387$, $p = 0.004$, Spearman's test) and a significant and negative correlation between PEF values and urea ($r = -0.366$, $p = 0.007$, Pearson test) (Figure 4). No significant correlation was found between other parameters of biochemical markers and respiratory sarcopenia parameters values ($p > 0.05$ in all cases, Pearson's and Spearman's correlation test).

We also categorized patients based on criteria of respiratory sarcopenia according to Kera et al. (22) and Ohara et al. (4) (see methods) and we evaluated whether there were any differences on blood analytical markers.

Significant differences were found in urea values for the presence of sarcopenia estimated by PEF (NS = 32.58 vs. S = 46.70, MeanDiff = 14.12 [95%CI: −23.59–4.64], $p = 0.005$) but not in GOT values (NS = 18.50 vs. S = 14.97, MeanDiff = 3.53 [95%CI: −1.18–8.23], $p = 0.132$).

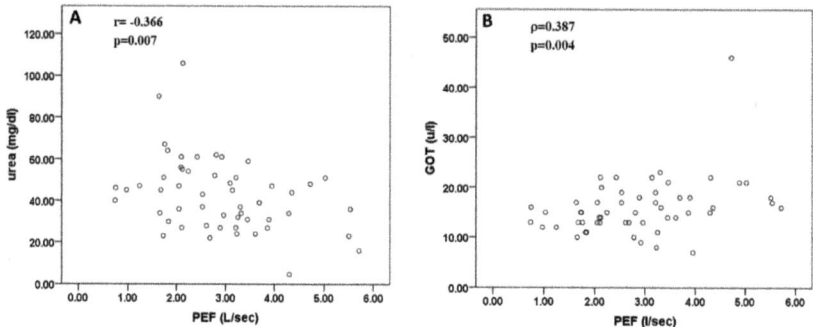

Figure 4. Correlation between PEF and urea (**A**) and GOT (**B**) concentration.

Studying the possible correlations between somatic sarcopenia values and biochemical parameters showed a significant and positive correlation between handgrip strength and urate concentration (r = 0.279, p = 0.041, Spearman's test) and between gait speed and GOT (r = 0.390, p = 0.006, Spearman's test). There was also a significant and negative correlation between skeletal muscle mass index and total cholesterol (r = −0.405, p = 0.004, Spearman's test) and triglycerides (r = −0.357, p = 0.017, Spearman's test), and between urea and gait speed (r = −0.36, p = 0.012, Spearman's test). No significant correlation was found between other parameters of biochemical markers and muscle mass and function values (p > 0.05 in all cases, Spearman's correlation test) (Figure 5).

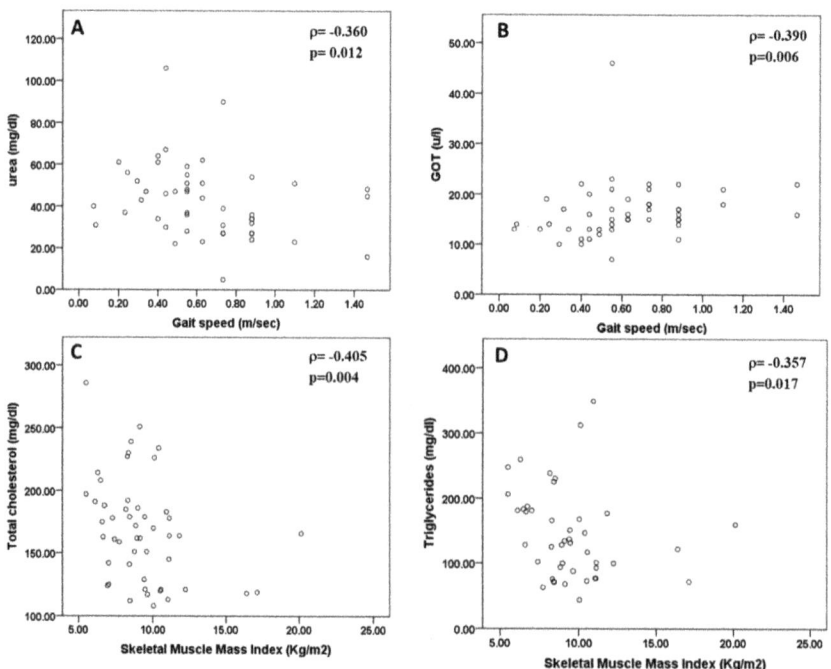

Figure 5. Correlation between skeletal muscle sarcopenia parameters and urea (**A**), GOT (**B**) and lipids ((**C**): total cholesterol; (**D**): triglycerides) concentration in blood.

We also categorized the patients based on the cut-off scores of the three parameters studied for the evaluation of sarcopenia (see Methods section) and evaluated if there were any differences in blood analytical markers.

For the gait speed, there were statistically significant differences in urea values (NS = 34.72 vs. S = 45.82, MeanDiff = 11.10 [95%CI: −20.44–1.76], p = 0.042) but not in GOT values (NS = 17.0 vs. S = 16.42, MeanDiff = 0.58 [95%CI: −2.31–3.48], p = 0.685).

For the presence of sarcopenia according to lean mass content, there were statistically significant differences in total cholesterol values (NS = 162.29 vs. S = 199.13, MeanDiff = 36.83 [95%CI:−71.58—2.08], p = 0.04) but not in tryglicerides (NS = 135.92 vs. S = 180.75, MeanDiff = 44.83 [95%CI: −99.94–10.27], p = 0.101)

As for handgrip strength, no differences were observed in urate values between groups (NS = 4.74 vs. S = 4.79, MeanDiff = 0.05 [95%CI: −0.94–0.85], p = 0.807).

4. Discussion

This study, which analyzes sarcopenia parameters in older people living in nursing homes, shows the direct relationship between respiratory muscle function and skeletal muscle function, especially with regard to the muscular strength and walking speed, and we report on the correlation between sarcopenia parameters and several biochemical markers obtained in routine blood analysis. This is the first study, to our knowledge, that considers the relationship between respiratory muscle strength and blood biochemical markers, finding a relationship between peak expiratory flow (PEF) values and glutamate-oxaloacetate transaminase (GOT) and urea concentration. We also observed associations between musculoskeletal parameters of sarcopenia with some blood markers, e.g., muscle mass and total cholesterol and triglyceride values, walking speed and urea and GOT values and handgrip strength and urate values. We discuss these new findings below.

The prevalence of sarcopenia in the sample of nursing home residents, following the EWGSOP criteria [2] and adjusting the skeletal muscle mass index to the Spanish population according to the cut-off points proposed by Masanés and coworkers [33], was 17.6%. These data are lower than those previously proposed for the Spanish institutionalized population [8], 41.4% applying the same assessment criteria, but are consistent with those described in a literature review that includes studies in several countries of patients residing in long-term care homes [6], like the population of our study. It is possible that the exclusion of patients who were not able to understand the content of the questionnaires influences the prevalence of the sample in the present study, since the presence of cognitive impairment increases the rates of sarcopenia [34].

The relationship between respiratory function parameters and somatic sarcopenia in community-dwelling older people has been studied in recent years, given the objectivity of these parameters and the ease and speed of assessment, but no studies in nursing home residents displaying higher levels of functional impairment and comorbidity burdens have been reported. Three parameters of respiratory function that have been established in the literature as determinants of respiratory sarcopenia, PEF [35] and maximum inspiratory (MIP) and expiratory (MEP) respiratory pressures [4].

Prevalence scores of respiratory sarcopenia according to PEF values were 70.7%, while maximum respiratory pressures were 80.7% according for MIP and 37.9% for MEP. The highest prevalence values of respiratory sarcopenia were obtained for both MIP and PEF, as in the study by Bahat et al. [36]. This may be due to the fact that loss of respiratory muscle strength occurs first in the inspiratory muscles, and is related to deterioration of type IIx and/or IIb muscle fibers of the diaphragm [3]. Loss of inspiratory muscle strength (MIP) leads to a reduced volume of inspired air prior to glottal closure and contraction of the expiratory muscle, preventing effective maximal expiration (PEF) [37,38]. In addition, it implies an inability to fully inflate the lungs, which is necessary to achieve the optimization of the length-tension relationship of the expiratory muscles, stimulate lung surfactant production and distribution, and open the collapsed peripheral airways that often accompany the hypoventilation processes associated with age and the aging process [39–41].

Furthermore, the greater relevance of the inspiratory muscles in the deterioration of the peripheral muscles was also justified by the decline in handgrip strength (84.5% of the sample studied) and the decline in walking speed (65.4% of the sample studied), as established in previous studies [4,19].

PEF was considered the most relevant parameter for establishing respiratory sarcopenia by Kera et al. [35,42] due to the involvement of the respiratory muscles in its execution and the minimal impact of the deterioration of the airway on its values, since it is measured at the beginning of forced expiration, and is not affected by the modifications in elastic recoil and thorax compliance associated with age [43]. The authors highlighted their preference for this test over respiratory muscle strength because of the lesser effort required and to avoid maneuvers that involve an increase in intracranial pressure, with the risks that this entails [35].

The results of this study confirm the results obtained by Kera et al. [42] in community-dwelling older people, but obtain higher values of correlation than Kera in the criterion of strength (handgrip strength) ($r = 0.375$ vs. $r = 0.283$) and in the criterion of functional performance (gait speed) ($r = 0.563$ vs. $r = 0.167$). No correlation was obtained in this study with the index of musculoskeletal mass, with muscle function more relevant than the amount of existing lean muscle mass in sarcopenic older individuals. In turn, Kera et al. [35] obtained differences between patients categorized as respiratory sarcopenic for the three determining variables of somatic sarcopenia, which were always higher in non-sarcopenic patients, while these differences were only obtained for gait speed in this study, possibly due to the high rates of sedentarism among nursing home residents and their more limited independence in their basic activities of daily life. In our study, no associations were found between respiratory muscle function and lean mass content and it could be explained in part by the obesity paradox [44]. The body mass index in the study sample widely varies among the participants enrolled in the study (range 18.7–50.2) and one third of patients have overweight and obesity grade I. This paradoxical benefit of a medically unfavorable phenotype is particularly strong in the overweight and class I obesity, and less pronounced in the more severe or morbidly obese populations (class II–III and greater). Rather than an obesity paradox, it is possible that this phenomenon may represent a "lean paradox", in which individuals classified as normal weight or underweight may have a reduced lean mass, as a result of a progressive catabolic state and lean mass loss [45–47] whereas overweight and obese patients maintain an adequate lean mass content compared to under and normo-weight individuals [44,48]. Likely, the reduced respiratory muscle strength in overweight and obese individuals could be explained by other pathophysiological factors related to excessive fat accumulation in the thoracic-abdominal region which limits the chest wall expansion and diaphragm contraction, lengthens abdominal muscles, reduces the upper airway calibre, modifies airway configuration, and increases in intra-abdominal pressure and these effects may reduce respiratory muscle function independently on lean mass content [49–51]. Alternatively the reduced muscular function in obese individuals may be also related to chronic low-grade inflammation characterized by the predominance of interleukin-1β, interleukin-6, and tumor necrosis factor-α (TNF-α) observed in obese patients [52]. Further studies with larger sample should evaluate in details the comparison the effects of underweight, obesity with or without sarcopenia on respiratory muscle strengths in order to shed new lights on these apparent discrepancies between muscular strength and lean mass content.

Other reports suggested that valuable markers of reduced respiratory muscle strength are the values related to the maximum respiratory pressures (MIP and MEP), because these parameters are a more direct measurement of the maximum strength of respiratory muscles [4,19,36,53]. In our study, MIP correlated with both walking speed and handgrip strength ($r = 0.599$ and $r = 0.354$, respectively), while MEP correlated with handgrip strength ($r = 0.465$). This parameter, which is slightly more difficult to evaluate than the PEF due to its assessment procedure, is directly related to the loss of strength in the peripheral muscles, as seen in previous studies not only of older people living in the community [19,53] and in nursing homes [4], but also in healthy [54] and hospitalized young adults [55]. On the other hand, no relationship could be found between skeletal muscle mass index and maximum respiratory pressures, like those reported in previous studies of healthy older patients [53] and older patients with cardiovascular diseases [19].

These parameters of maximum respiratory strength appear to be good indicators of reduced respiratory muscle strength in older institutionalized individuals, since patients who presented sarcopenia according to these cut-off values presented significantly lower values of gait speed and handgrip strength that were as good as those recently shown by community dwelling older adults [4].

We demonstrated that parameters related to reduced respiratory muscle strength, e.g., PEF values, are significantly associated with urea and GOT concentrations in blood, which have not been previously reported for the respiratory muscle function. GOT, also known as aspartate aminotransferase, is a mitochondrial and cytoplasmic enzyme, with an important role in cell energy production [56]. Alterations in GOT levels in blood are considered well-known markers of hepatic, myocardial and skeletal muscle cytolysis, while GPT also known as alanine aminotransferase, is mainly a hepatic cytoplasmic enzyme [57–59]. In our study, the lack of a significant association between PEF and GPT levels in blood suggests that the association between PEF and GOT levels is related to myocardial or skeletal muscle metabolism. High serum GOT with normal serum GPT is highly prevalent among community dwelling older individuals who are underweight, and might reflect skeletal muscle pathology [60]. Furthermore, high levels of GOT in serum are present in obese subjects, regardless of age, which may be associated with sarcopenic obesity, reduced muscle mass and overweight, in some of the subjects studied [61,62]. However, the processes involved in regulating blood GOT levels in both underweight and obese subjects remain unknown, but they seem to be related to low muscle mass and function, and in this respect we found a new association with PEF values. The role of cardiac diseases cannot be ruled out, since 30% of the sample presents a comorbidity of this type. However, due to the limited size of the sample of nursing home residents with preserved cognitive function necessary to perform spirometry analysis, it was impossible to study selective pathologies.

However, confirming the association between GOT levels and muscular metabolism and function, GOT levels were also found to be significantly associated with gait speed and almost significantly with grip strength ($p = 0.05$). PEF values were also inversely and significantly associated with urea concentration in blood. Elevated serum urea, a breakdown product of protein, is generally considered a marker of muscle wasting in several conditions [63,64]. Another possible explanation for increased urea levels could be an alteration in kidney function, but the creatinine levels in our study were not significantly associated with any of the sarcopenia parameters and the correlation between urea levels and PEF therefore suggested effects based on muscle metabolism. A recent study with a machine learning approach found that urea concentration is one of risk factors for the development of predictive models for patients with sarcopenia [65], and we also reported an association between urea levels and gait speed. In relation to the positive correlation between uric acid levels and muscle strength reported in our study, this finding replicates the association reported in community dwelling-older individuals in the "InCHIANTI" study [66], which observed that higher urate levels were significantly associated with higher measures of muscle strength, and concluded that high urate levels could create a protective reaction that would counteract the excessive production of free radicals that damage muscle proteins and reduce muscle strength. Likewise, Can et al. [67], focusing on markers of inflammation and oxidative stress, analyzed a sample of 72 geriatric patients confirmed that patients with sarcopenia had significantly lower levels of uric acid than non-sarcopenic patients. Moreover, high serum urate levels are a good positive predictor of grip strength in nonagenarian older individuals, and may delay the progression of sarcopenia [68]. The skeletal muscle criterion of lean mass content was the only criterion that was significantly (and inversely) correlated with blood lipid (cholesterol and triglycerides) concentration. The aging process stimulates the appearance of fat infiltration in muscle tissue, and obesity enhances fat deposits at visceral level, in the liver, heart, pancreas and skeletal muscle, which generates a negative effect on sarcopenia. These lipids cause a pro-inflammatory effect that secretes paracrine and cytokine hormones, promoting a feedforward cycle by producing intramyocellular lipids. This toxicity generated by fats hinders the contraction of muscle fibers and the synthesis of muscle proteins, favoring the development of sarcopenia [69,70].

A study by the South Korean KNHANES conducted an evaluation of sarcopenic obesity subjects and showed a link to an increased risk of dyslipemia in these patients [71]. Mesinovic et al. [72] recently determined the associations between metabolic syndrome and components of sarcopenia, including muscle mass and quality, absolute and relative strength, and physical performance, in 84 overweight and obese older adults, and demonstrated that triglyceride levels had a negative association with leg extension strength and lower-limb relative strength. Lu et al. [73] reported that serum triglycerides and high-density lipoprotein cholesterol were independently associated with sarcopenic obesity. All the biomarkers found to be significantly associated with sarcopenia indexes can be obtained in a routine blood analysis, as they can be rapidly, inexpensively, and reproducibly assayed. Future longitudinal investigations should test these biomarkers as a part of a valuable panel of metabolites to diagnose sarcopenia and monitor the efficacy of clinical interventions in sarcopenic individuals. This is the first study to demonstrate an independent relationship between respiratory muscle strength and some aspects of body sarcopenia in institutionalized elderly people with high rates of comorbidities and polypharmacy. The fact that respiratory sarcopenia is associated with muscle strength and gait speed supports the beneficial effect of various exercises and rehabilitation interventions on breathing muscles [74–76]. New randomized clinical trial should evaluate the effects of such interventions not only for skeletal sarcopenia but also to improve respiratory muscle strength thus allowing a better respiratory function which can influence many respiratory tract diseases since the impairment of (inspiratory and expiratory) respiratory muscles is a common clinical finding, not only in patients with neuromuscular disease but also in those with respiratory diseases affecting the lung parenchyma or airways [77–79]. We provided further evidence for the use of suitable cut-off points for respiratory muscle strength which can be tested in future researches prior its proposal as indicator of muscle respiratory function in clinical settings. Loss of mass and function of the respiratory muscles could be prevented by properly applying these exercises. More studies on sarcopenia and its effects on respiratory muscle strength are needed to improve life expectancy and quality of life in the older institutionalized individuals.

Author Contributions: Conceptualization, F.M.M.-A., C.B., R.F.-V., O.C.; Methodology, F.M.M.-A., C.B., R.F.-V., O.C.; formal analysis, F.M.M.-A., O.C.; investigation, F.M.M.-A., C.B., R.F.-V., O.C.; data curation, F.M.M.-A., C.B., R.F.-V., O.C.; writing—Original draft preparation, F.M.M.-A., O.C.; writing—Review and editing, F.M.M.-A., C.B., R.F.-V., O.C. All authors have read and agreed to the published version of the manuscript.

Funding: This research received no external funding.

Conflicts of Interest: The authors declare no conflict of interest.

Abbreviations

95% CI	95% Confidence interval
EDTA	Ethylenediaminetetraacetic acid
EWGSOP	European Working Group for Sarcopenia in Older People
FEV1	Forced Expiratory Volume in first second
FEV2575	Mesoexpiratory volume
FVC	Forced vital capacity
GOT	Glutamic oxaloacetic transaminase
GPT	Glutamic pyruvic transaminase
MEP	Maximal expiratory pressure
MIP	Maximal inspiratory pressure
NS	Non-sarcopenic individuals
PEF	Peak expiratory flow
RMS	Respiratory muscle strength
S	Sarcopenic individuals
Sat O_2	Oxyhemoglobinic saturation
SD	Standard deviation
VC	Vital capacity

References

1. Cruz-Jentoft, A.J.; Bahat, G.; Bauer, J.; Boirie, Y.; Bruyère, O.; Cederholm, T.; Cooper, C.; Landi, F.; Rolland, Y.; Sayer, A.A.; et al. Sarcopenia: Revised {European} consensus on definition and diagnosis. *Age Ageing* **2019**, *48*, 16–31. [CrossRef] [PubMed]
2. Cruz-Jentoft, A.J.; Baeyens, J.P.; Bauer, J.M.; Boirie, Y.; Cederholm, T.; Landi, F.; Martin, F.C.; Michel, J.P.; Rolland, Y.; Schneider, S.M.; et al. Sarcopenia: European consensus on definition and diagnosis. *Age Ageing* **2010**, *39*, 412–423. [CrossRef] [PubMed]
3. Elliott, J.E.; Greising, S.M.; Mantilla, C.B.; Sieck, G.C. Functional impact of sarcopenia in respiratory muscles. *Respir. Physiol. Neurobiol.* **2016**, *226*, 137–146. [CrossRef] [PubMed]
4. Ohara, D.G.; Pegorari, M.S.; Oliveira dos Santos, N.L.; de Fátima Ribeiro Silva, C.; Monteiro, R.L.; Matos, A.P.; Jamami, M. Respiratory Muscle Strength as a Discriminator of Sarcopenia in Community-Dwelling Elderly: A Cross-Sectional Study. *J. Nutr. Health Aging* **2018**, *22*, 952–958. [CrossRef] [PubMed]
5. Papadopoulou, S.K.; Tsintavis, P.; Potsaki, G.; Papandreou, D. Differences in the Prevalence of Sarcopenia in Community-Dwelling, Nursing Home and Hospitalized Individuals. A Systematic Review and Meta-Analysis. *J. Nutr. Heal. Aging* **2020**, *24*, 83–90. [CrossRef]
6. Rodríguez-Rejón, A.I.; Ruiz-López, M.D.; Wanden-Berghe, C.; Artacho, R. Prevalence and Diagnosis of Sarcopenia in Residential Facilities: A Systematic Review. *Adv. Nutr.* **2019**, *10*, 51–58. [CrossRef]
7. Shen, Y.; Chen, J.; Chen, X.; Hou, L.S.; Lin, X.; Yang, M. Prevalence and Associated Factors of Sarcopenia in Nursing Home Residents: A Systematic Review and Meta-analysis. *J. Am. Med. Dir. Assoc.* **2019**, *20*, 5–13. [CrossRef]
8. Bravo-José, P.; Moreno, E.; Espert, M.; Romeu, M.; Martínez, P.; Navarro, C. Prevalence of sarcopenia and associated factors in institutionalised older adult patients. *Clin. Nutr. ESPEN* **2018**, *27*, 113–119. [CrossRef]
9. Kovacs, E.; Lowery, E.; Kuhlmann, E.; Brubaker, A. The aging lung. *Clin. Interv. Aging* **2013**, *8*, 1489. [CrossRef]
10. Skloot, G.S. The Effects of Aging on Lung Structure and Function. *Clin. Geriatr. Med.* **2017**, *33*, 447–457. [CrossRef]
11. Conn, P.M. *Handbook of Models for Human Aging*; Elsevier Academic Press: Cambridge, MA, USA, 2006; ISBN 9780080460062.
12. Sharma, G.; Goodwin, J. Effect of aging on respiratory system physiology and immunology. *Clin. Interv. Aging* **2006**, *1*, 253–260. [CrossRef]
13. Vaz Fragoso, C.A.; Gahbauer, E.A.; Van Ness, P.H.; Concato, J.; Gill, T.M. Peak Expiratory Flow as a Predictor of Subsequent Disability and Death in Community-Living Older Persons. *J. Am. Geriatr. Soc.* **2008**, *56*, 1014–1020. [CrossRef]
14. Roberts, M.H.; Mapel, D.W. Limited Lung Function: Impact of Reduced Peak Expiratory Flow on Health Status, Health-Care Utilization, and Expected Survival in Older Adults. *Am. J. Epidemiol.* **2012**, *176*, 127–134. [CrossRef] [PubMed]
15. Ida, S.; Watanabe, M.; Yoshida, N.; Baba, Y.; Umezaki, N.; Harada, K.; Karashima, R.; Imamura, Y.; Iwagami, S.; Baba, H. Sarcopenia is a Predictor of Postoperative Respiratory Complications in Patients with Esophageal Cancer. *Ann. Surg. Oncol.* **2015**, *22*, 4432–4437. [CrossRef] [PubMed]
16. Zhang, S.; Tan, S.; Jiang, Y.; Xi, Q.; Meng, Q.; Zhuang, Q.; Han, Y.; Sui, X.; Wu, G. Sarcopenia as a predictor of poor surgical and oncologic outcomes after abdominal surgery for digestive tract cancer: A prospective cohort study. *Clin. Nutr.* **2018**. [CrossRef] [PubMed]
17. Nishigori, T.; Okabe, H.; Tanaka, E.; Tsunoda, S.; Hisamori, S.; Sakai, Y. Sarcopenia as a predictor of pulmonary complications after esophagectomy for thoracic esophageal cancer. *J. Surg. Oncol.* **2016**, *113*, 678–684. [CrossRef]
18. Maeda, K.; Akagi, J. Muscle Mass Loss Is a Potential Predictor of 90-Day Mortality in Older Adults with Aspiration Pneumonia. *J. Am. Geriatr. Soc.* **2017**, *65*, e18–e22. [CrossRef]
19. Izawa, K.P.; Watanabe, S.; Oka, K.; Kasahara, Y.; Morio, Y.; Hiraki, K.; Hirano, Y.; Omori, Y.; Suzuki, N.; Kida, K.; et al. Respiratory muscle strength in relation to sarcopenia in elderly cardiac patients. *Aging Clin. Exp. Res.* **2016**, *28*, 1143–1148. [CrossRef]
20. Omran, M.L.; Morley, J.E. Assessment of protein energy malnutrition in older persons, part II: Laboratory evaluation. *Nutrition* **2000**, *16*, 131–140. [CrossRef]

21. Zhang, Z.; Pereira, S.L.; Luo, M.; Matheson, E.M. Evaluation of blood biomarkers associated with risk of malnutrition in older adults: A systematic review and meta-analysis. *Nutrients* **2017**, *9*, 829. [CrossRef]
22. Li, S.; Zhang, J.; Zheng, H.; Wang, X.; Liu, Z.; Sun, T. Prognostic Role of Serum Albumin, Total Lymphocyte Count, and Mini Nutritional Assessment on Outcomes After Geriatric Hip Fracture Surgery: A Meta-Analysis and Systematic Review. *J. Arthroplast.* **2019**, *34*, 1287–1296. [CrossRef] [PubMed]
23. Shakersain, B.; Santoni, G.; Faxén-Irving, G.; Rizzuto, D.; Fratiglioni, L.; Xu, W. Nutritional status and survival among old adults: An 11-year population-based longitudinal study. *Eur. J. Clin. Nutr.* **2016**, *70*, 320–325. [CrossRef] [PubMed]
24. Zelada Rodríguez, M.A.; Gómez-Pavón, J.; Sorando Fernández, P.; Franco Salinas, A.; Mercedes Guzmán, L.; Baztán, J.J. Fiabilidad interobservador de los 4 índices de comorbilidad más utilizados en pacientes ancianos. *Rev. Esp. Geriatr. Gerontol.* **2012**, *47*, 67–70. [CrossRef]
25. Charlson, M.E.; Pompei, P.; Ales, K.L.; MacKenzie, C.R. A new method of classifying prognostic comorbidity in longitudinal studies: Development and validation. *J. Chronic Dis.* **1987**, *40*, 373–383. [CrossRef]
26. Miller, M.R.; Hankinson, J.; Brusasco, V.; Burgos, F.; Casaburi, R.; Coates, A.; Crapo, R.; Enright, P.; van der Grinten, C.P.M.; Gustafsson, P.; et al. Standardisation of spirometry. *Eur. Respir. J.* **2005**, *26*, 319–338. [CrossRef] [PubMed]
27. American Thoracic Society. ATS/ERS Statement on respiratory muscle testing. *Am. J. Respir. Crit. Care Med.* **2002**, *166*, 518–624. [CrossRef]
28. Laveneziana, P.; Albuquerque, A.; Aliverti, A.; Babb, T.; Barreiro, E.; Dres, M.; Dubé, B.P.; Fauroux, B.; Gea, J.; Guenette, J.A.; et al. ERS statement on respiratory muscle testing at rest and during exercise. *Eur. Respir. J.* **2019**, *53*. [CrossRef]
29. Roberts, H.C.; Denison, H.J.; Martin, H.J.; Patel, H.P.; Syddall, H.; Cooper, C.; Sayer, A.A. A review of the measurement of grip strength in clinical and epidemiological studies: Towards a standardised approach. *Age Ageing* **2011**, *40*, 423–429. [CrossRef]
30. Studenski, S.; Perera, S.; Patel, K.; Rosano, C.; Faulkner, K.; Inzitari, M.; Brach, J.; Chandler, J.; Cawthon, P.; Connor, E.B.; et al. Gait speed and survival in older adults. *JAMA J. Am. Med. Assoc.* **2011**, *305*, 50–58. [CrossRef]
31. Janssen, I.; Heymsfield, S.B.; Baumgartner, R.N.; Ross, R. Estimation of skeletal muscle mass by bioelectrical impedance analysis. *J. Appl. Physiol.* **2000**, *89*, 465–471. [CrossRef]
32. Martínez-Arnau, F.M.; Fonfría-Vivas, R.; Buigues, C.; Castillo, Y.; Molina, P.; Hoogland, A.J.; van Doesburg, F.; Pruimboom, L.; Fernández-Garrido, J.; Cauli, O. Effects of leucine administration in sarcopenia: A randomized and placebo-controlled clinical trial. *Nutrients* **2020**, *12*, 932. [CrossRef] [PubMed]
33. Masanés, F.; Rojano i Luque, X.; Salvà, A.; Serra-Rexach, J.A.; Artaza, I.; Formiga, F.; Cuesta, F.; López Soto, A.; Ruiz, D.; Cruz-Jentoft, A.J. Cut-off points for muscle mass—not grip strength or gait speed—determine variations in sarcopenia prevalence. *J. Nutr. Heal. Aging* **2017**, *21*, 825–829. [CrossRef]
34. Liu, X.; Hou, L.; Xia, X.; Liu, Y.; Zuo, Z.; Zhang, Y.; Zhao, W.; Hao, Q.; Yue, J.; Dong, B. Prevalence of sarcopenia in multi ethnics adults and the association with cognitive impairment: Findings from West-China health and aging trend study. *BMC Geriatr.* **2020**, *20*. [CrossRef] [PubMed]
35. Kera, T.; Kawai, H.; Hirano, H.; Kojima, M.; Watanabe, Y.; Motokawa, K.; Fujiwara, Y.; Ihara, K.; Kim, H.; Obuchi, S. Definition of Respiratory Sarcopenia With Peak Expiratory Flow Rate. *J. Am. Med. Dir. Assoc.* **2019**, *20*, 1021–1025. [CrossRef] [PubMed]
36. Bahat, G.; Tufan, A.; Ozkaya, H.; Tufan, F.; Akpinar, T.S.; Akin, S.; Bahat, Z.; Kaya, Z.; Kiyan, E.; Erten, N.; et al. Relation between hand grip strength, respiratory muscle strength and spirometric measures in male nursing home residents. *Aging Male* **2014**, *17*, 136–140. [CrossRef]
37. Schramm, C.M. Current concepts of respiratory complications of neuromuscular disease in children. *Curr. Opin. Pediatr.* **2000**, *12*, 203–207. [CrossRef] [PubMed]
38. Kang, S.W.; Bach, J.R. Maximum insufflation capacity: Vital capacity and cough flows in neuromuscular disease. *Am. J. Phys. Med. Rehabil.* **2000**, *79*, 222–227. [CrossRef] [PubMed]
39. Lowery, E.M.; Brubaker, A.L.; Kuhlmann, E.; Kovacs, E.J. The aging lung. *Clin. Interv. Aging* **2013**, *8*, 1489–1496. [PubMed]
40. Lalley, P.M. The aging respiratory system-Pulmonary structure, function and neural control. *Respir. Physiol. Neurobiol.* **2013**, *187*, 199–210. [CrossRef]

41. Schmidt-Nowara, W.W.; Altman, A.R. Atelectasis and neuromuscular respiratory failure. *Chest* **1984**, *85*, 792–795. [CrossRef]
42. Kera, T.; Kawai, H.; Hirano, H.; Kojima, M.; Fujiwara, Y.; Ihara, K.; Obuchi, S. Relationships among peak expiratory flow rate, body composition, physical function, and sarcopenia in community-dwelling older adults. *Aging Clin. Exp. Res.* **2018**, *30*, 331–340. [CrossRef] [PubMed]
43. Janssens, J.P.; Pache, J.C.; Nicod, L.P. Physiological changes in respiratory function associated with ageing. *Eur. Respir. J.* **1999**, *13*, 197–205. [CrossRef] [PubMed]
44. Elagizi, A.; Kachur, S.; Lavie, C.J.; Carbone, S.; Pandey, A.; Ortega, F.B.; Milani, R.V. An Overview and Update on Obesity and the Obesity Paradox in Cardiovascular Diseases. *Prog. Cardiovasc. Dis.* **2018**, *61*, 142–150. [CrossRef] [PubMed]
45. Do, J.G.; Park, C.H.; Lee, Y.T.; Yoon, K.J. Association between underweight and pulmonary function in 282,135 healthy adults: A cross-sectional study in Korean population. *Sci. Rep.* **2019**, *9*, 14308. [CrossRef] [PubMed]
46. Jeon, Y.K.; Shin, M.J.; Kim, M.H.; Mok, J.H.; Kim, S.S.; Kim, B.H.; Kim, S.J.; Kim, Y.K.; Chang, J.H.; Shin, Y.B.; et al. Low pulmonary function is related with a high risk of sarcopenia in community-dwelling older adults: The Korea National Health and Nutrition Examination Survey (KNHANES) 2008–2011. *Osteoporos. Int.* **2015**, *26*, 2423–2429. [CrossRef] [PubMed]
47. Park, C.H.; Yi, Y.; Do, J.G.; Lee, Y.T.; Yoon, K.J. Relationship between skeletal muscle mass and lung function in Korean adults without clinically apparent lung disease. *Medicine* **2018**, *97*. [CrossRef]
48. Yanek, L.R.; Vaidya, D.; Kral, B.G.; Dobrosielski, D.A.; Moy, T.F.; Stewart, K.J.; Becker, D.M. Lean Mass and Fat Mass as Contributors to Physical Fitness in an Overweight and Obese African American Population. *Ethn Dis.* **2015**, *25*, 214–219.
49. Carbone, S.; Billingsley, H.E.; Rodriguez-Miguelez, P.; Kirkman, D.L.; Garten, R.; Franco, R.L.; Lee, D.-C.; Lavie, C.J. Lean Mass Abnormalities in Heart Failure: The Role of Sarcopenia, Sarcopenic Obesity, and Cachexia. *Curr. Probl. Cardiol.* **2019**, 100417. [CrossRef]
50. Magnani, K.L.; Cataneo, A.J.M. Respiratory muscle strength in obese individuals and influence of upper-body fat distribution. *Sao Paulo Med. J.* **2007**, *125*, 215–219. [CrossRef]
51. Lin, C.K.; Lin, C.C. Work of breathing and respiratory drive in obesity. *Respirology* **2012**, *17*, 402–411. [CrossRef]
52. Lima, T.R.L.; Almeida, V.P.; Ferreira, A.S.; Guimarães, F.S.; Lopes, A.J. Handgrip strength and pulmonary disease in the elderly: What is the link? *Aging Dis.* **2019**, *10*, 1109–1129. [CrossRef] [PubMed]
53. iee Shin, H.; Kim, D.K.; Seo, K.M.; Kang, S.H.; Lee, S.Y.; Son, S. Relation between respiratory muscle strength and skeletal muscle mass and hand grip strength in the healthy elderly. *Ann. Rehabil. Med.* **2017**, *41*, 686–692. [CrossRef] [PubMed]
54. Sawaya, Y.; Ishizaka, M.; Kubo, A.; Sadakiyo, K.; Yakabi, A.; Sato, T.; Shiba, T.; Onoda, K.; Maruyama, H. Correlation between skeletal muscle mass index and parameters of respiratory function and muscle strength in young healthy adults according to gender. *J. Phys. Ther. Sci.* **2018**, *30*, 1424–1427. [CrossRef]
55. Peterson, S.J.; Park, J.; Zellner, H.K.; Moss, O.A.; Welch, A.; Sclamberg, J.; Moran, E.; Hicks-McGarry, S.; Becker, E.A.; Foley, S. Relationship Between Respiratory Muscle Strength, Handgrip Strength, and Muscle Mass in Hospitalized Patients. *J. Parenter. Enter. Nutr.* **2019**. [CrossRef] [PubMed]
56. Chowdhury, M.S.I.; Rahman, A.Z.; Haque, M.; Nahar, N.; Taher, A. Serum Aspartate Aminotransferase (AST) and Alanine Aminotransferase (ALT) Levels in Different Grades of Protein Energy Malnutrition. *J. Bangladesh Soc. Physiol.* **1970**, *2*, 17–19. [CrossRef]
57. Karaphillis, E.; Goldstein, R.; Murphy, S.; Qayyum, R. Serum alanine aminotransferase levels and all-cause mortality. *Eur. J. Gastroenterol. Hepatol.* **2017**, *29*, 284–288. [CrossRef]
58. Nathwani, R.A.; Pais, S.; Reynolds, T.B.; Kaplowitz, N. Serum alanine aminotransferase in skeletal muscle diseases. *Hepatology* **2005**, *41*, 380–382. [CrossRef]
59. Malakouti, M.; Kataria, A.; Ali, S.K.; Schenker, S. Elevated Liver Enzymes in Asymptomatic Patients—What Should I Do? *J. Clin. Transl. Hepatol.* **2017**, *5*, 1–10. [CrossRef]
60. Shibata, M.; Nakajima, K.; Higuchi, R.; Iwane, T.; Sugiyama, M.; Nakamura, T. Nakamura High Concentration of Serum Aspartate Aminotransferase in Older Underweight People: Results of the Kanagawa Investigation of the Total Check-Up Data from the National Database-2 (KITCHEN-2). *J. Clin. Med.* **2019**, *8*, 1282. [CrossRef]

61. Zamboni, M.; Mazzali, G.; Fantin, F.; Rossi, A.; Di Francesco, V. Sarcopenic obesity: A new category of obesity in the elderly. *Nutr. Metab. Cardiovasc. Dis.* **2008**, *18*, 388–395. [CrossRef]
62. Stenholm, S.; Harris, T.B.; Rantanen, T.; Visser, M.; Kritchevsky, S.B.; Ferrucci, L. Sarcopenic obesity: Definition, cause and consequences. *Curr. Opin. Clin. Nutr. Metab. Care* **2008**, *11*, 693–700. [CrossRef] [PubMed]
63. Haines, R.W.; Zolfaghari, P.; Wan, Y.; Pearse, R.M.; Puthucheary, Z.; Prowle, J.R. Elevated urea-to-creatinine ratio provides a biochemical signature of muscle catabolism and persistent critical illness after major trauma. *Intensive Care Med.* **2019**, *45*, 1718–1731. [CrossRef] [PubMed]
64. Lattanzi, B.; D'Ambrosio, D.; Merli, M. Hepatic Encephalopathy and Sarcopenia: Two Faces of the Same Metabolic Alteration. *J. Clin. Exp. Hepatol.* **2019**, *9*, 125–130. [CrossRef] [PubMed]
65. Kang, Y.J.; Yoo, J.I.; Ha, Y.C. Sarcopenia feature selection and risk prediction using machine learning: A cross-sectional study. *Medicine* **2019**, *98*, e17699. [CrossRef]
66. Macchi, C.; Molino-Lova, R.; Polcaro, P.; Guarducci, L.; Lauretani, F.; Cecchi, F.; Bandinelli, S.; Guralnik, J.M.; Ferrucci, L. Higher circulating levels of uric acid are prospectively associated with better muscle function in older persons. *Mech. Ageing Dev.* **2008**, *129*, 522–527. [CrossRef]
67. Can, B.; Kara, O.; Kizilarslanoglu, M.C.; Arik, G.; Aycicek, G.S.; Sumer, F.; Civelek, R.; Demirtas, C.; Ulger, Z. Serum markers of inflammation and oxidative stress in sarcopenia. *Aging Clin. Exp. Res.* **2017**, *29*, 745–752. [CrossRef]
68. Molino-Lova, R.; Sofi, F.; Pasquini, G.; Vannetti, F.; Del Ry, S.; Vassalle, C.; Clerici, M.; Sorbi, S.; Macchi, C. Higher uric acid serum levels are associated with better muscle function in the oldest old: Results from the Mugello Study. *Eur. J. Intern. Med.* **2017**, *41*, 39–43. [CrossRef]
69. Batsis, J.A.; Villareal, D.T. Sarcopenic obesity in older adults: Aetiology, epidemiology and treatment strategies. *Nat. Rev. Endocrinol.* **2018**, *14*, 513–537. [CrossRef]
70. Carnio, S.; LoVerso, F.; Baraibar, M.A.; Longa, E.; Khan, M.M.; Maffei, M.; Reischl, M.; Canepari, M.; Loefler, S.; Kern, H.; et al. Autophagy Impairment in Muscle Induces Neuromuscular Junction Degeneration and Precocious Aging. *Cell Rep.* **2014**, *8*, 1509–1521. [CrossRef]
71. Baek, S.J.; Nam, G.E.; Han, K.D.; Choi, S.W.; Jung, S.W.; Bok, A.R.; Kim, Y.H.; Lee, K.S.; Han, B.D.; Kim, D.H. Sarcopenia and sarcopenic obesity and their association with dyslipidemia in Korean elderly men: The 2008-2010 Korea National Health and Nutrition Examination Survey. *J. Endocrinol. Investig.* **2014**, *37*, 247–260. [CrossRef]
72. Mesinovic, J.; McMillan, L.; Shore-Lorenti, C.; De Courten, B.; Ebeling, P.; Scott, D. Metabolic Syndrome and Its Associations with Components of Sarcopenia in Overweight and Obese Older Adults. *J. Clin. Med.* **2019**, *8*, 145. [CrossRef] [PubMed]
73. Lu, C.W.; Yang, K.C.; Chang, H.H.; Lee, L.T.; Chen, C.Y.; Huang, K.C. Sarcopenic obesity is closely associated with metabolic syndrome. *Obes. Res. Clin. Pract.* **2013**, *7*. [CrossRef] [PubMed]
74. Buchman, A.S.; Boyle, P.A.; Wilson, R.S.; Leurgans, S.; Shah, R.C.; Bennett, D.A. Respiratory muscle strength predicts decline in mobility in older persons. *Neuroepidemiology* **2008**, *31*, 174–180. [CrossRef] [PubMed]
75. Kim, J.; Davenport, P.; Sapienza, C. Effect of expiratory muscle strength training on elderly cough function. *Arch. Gerontol. Geriatr.* **2009**, *48*, 361–366. [CrossRef]
76. Kim, J.; Sapienza, C.M. Implications of expiratory muscle strength training for rehabilitation of the elderly: Tutorial. *J. Rehabil. Res. Dev.* **2005**, *42*, 211–223. [CrossRef]
77. Laghi, F.; Tobin, M.J. Disorders of the respiratory muscles. *Am. J. Respir. Crit. Care Med.* **2003**, *168*, 10–48. [CrossRef]
78. Meek, P.M.; Schwartzstein, R.M.; Adams, L.; Altose, M.D.; Breslin, E.H.; Carrieri-Kohlman, V.; Gift, A.; Hanley, M.V.; Harver, A.; Jones, P.W.; et al. Dyspnea: Mechanisms, assessment, and management: A consensus statement. *Am. J. Respir. Crit. Care Med.* **1999**, *159*, 321–340.
79. Caruso, P.; De Albuquerque, A.L.P.; Santana, P.V.; Cardenas, L.Z.; Ferreira, J.G.; Prina, E.; Trevizan, P.F.; Pereira, M.C.; Iamonti, V.; Pletsch, R.; et al. Métodos diagnósticos para avaliação da força muscular inspiratória e expiratória. *J. Bras. Pneumol.* **2015**, *41*, 110–123. [CrossRef]

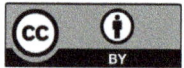

© 2020 by the authors. Licensee MDPI, Basel, Switzerland. This article is an open access article distributed under the terms and conditions of the Creative Commons Attribution (CC BY) license (http://creativecommons.org/licenses/by/4.0/).

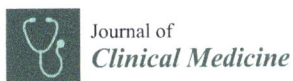

Article

Preserved Capacity for Adaptations in Strength and Muscle Regulatory Factors in Elderly in Response to Resistance Exercise Training and Deconditioning

Andreas Mæchel Fritzen [1,2,*], Frank D. Thøgersen [1], Khaled Abdul Nasser Qadri [1], Thomas Krag [1], Marie-Louise Sveen [1,3], John Vissing [1] and Tina D. Jeppesen [1]

1. Department of Neurology, Copenhagen Neuromuscular Center, Rigshospitalet, DK-2100 Copenhagen, Denmark; frank.thogersen@gmail.com (F.D.T.); khaled_qadri@hotmail.com (K.A.N.Q.); thomas.krag@regionh.dk (T.K.); mqsv@novonordisk.com (M.-L.S.); john.vissing@regionh.dk (J.V.); tina@dysgaard.dk (T.D.J.)
2. Molecular Physiology Group, Department of Nutrition, Exercise, and Sports, Faculty of Science, University of Copenhagen, DK-2100 Copenhagen, Denmark
3. Novo Nordisk A/S, DK-2860 Søborg, Denmark
* Correspondence: amfritzen@nexs.ku.dk; Tel.: +45-42633359

Received: 4 June 2020; Accepted: 9 July 2020; Published: 10 July 2020

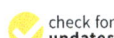

Abstract: Aging is related to an inevitable loss of muscle mass and strength. The mechanisms behind age-related loss of muscle tissue are not fully understood but may, among other things, be induced by age-related differences in myogenic regulatory factors. Resistance exercise training and deconditioning offers a model to investigate differences in myogenic regulatory factors that may be important for age-related loss of muscle mass and strength. Nine elderly (82 ± 7 years old) and nine young, healthy persons (22 ± 2 years old) participated in the study. Exercise consisted of six weeks of resistance training of the quadriceps muscle followed by eight weeks of deconditioning. Muscle biopsy samples before and after training and during the deconditioning period were analyzed for MyoD, myogenin, insulin-like growth-factor I receptor, activin receptor IIB, smad2, porin, and citrate synthase. Muscle strength improved with resistance training by 78% (95.0 ± 22.0 kg) in the elderly to a similar extent as in the young participants (83.5%; 178.2 ± 44.2 kg) and returned to baseline in both groups after eight weeks of deconditioning. No difference was seen in expression of muscle regulatory factors between elderly and young in response to exercise training and deconditioning. In conclusion, the capacity to gain muscle strength with resistance exercise training in elderly was not impaired, highlighting this as a potent tool to combat age-related loss of muscle function, possibly due to preserved regulation of myogenic factors in elderly compared with young muscle.

Keywords: resistance exercise training; muscle regulatory factors; sarcopenia; muscle strength; deconditioning; skeletal muscle; elderly; hypertrophy

1. Introduction

Sarcopenia means loss of flesh. The term is used to describe the pathological age-related loss of muscle mass, function, and strength that inevitable occurs in humans [1]. From the age of 50 to 85, humans lose 50% of their muscle mass, which is mainly a result of loss of type II muscle fibers [2]. Age-related loss of muscle mass and strength is associated with increasing risk of falling and disability, and thus impairment of basic daily activities.

It is well established that resistance exercise training can counteract the age-related changes in contractile function, strength, hypertrophy, and morphology of aging skeletal muscle [3]. However, whether the potential to adapt to resistance exercise training is completely preserved in skeletal muscles of elderly has been debated. [3]. Although 6–10 weeks of exercise training increased skeletal muscle strength to a similar extent in young and elderly in some studies [4,5], others report greater improvements in young individuals [6,7]. The rate of decline in muscle strength with age is 2–5 times greater than declines in muscle size [8] and strength loss is highly associated with both mortality and physical disability, even when adjusting for sarcopenia, indicating that muscle mass loss may be secondary to the effects of strength loss [9]. It is thus of key interest to elucidate whether increased muscle strength after a period of resistance exercise training occurs to a similar or blunted extent in old compared to young muscle. Moreover, although an aged-associated loss of muscle mass or strength [10,11] appears improved with resistance training in elderly individuals [12–16], several studies find a blunted muscle hypertrophy response [17–19].

Mechanisms responsible for resistance exercise-induced muscle hypertrophy are numerous, but some of the key factors include MyoD, myogenin, and insulin-like growth factor-I (IGF-I) [20–22]. The myogenic regulatory factors (MRF) are transcription factors that promote and regulate the expression of muscle-specific genes, which are essential to the hypertrophic and regenerative response following resistance exercise [23–26]. As MyoD is highly involved in muscle adaptation to resistance exercise, this has been a key factor in studies investigating potential differences in age-related muscle loss [27–29]. Differences in MRFs between young and elderly could be crucial mechanisms behind differences in muscle mass and strength [22,23,30] and in the response to resistance training and deconditioning. Previous studies found elevated levels of MyoD, myogenin, and IGF-I-R mRNA in elderly both at rest [17,31–34] and in response to one bout of resistance exercise [11]. Moreover, 16 weeks of resistance training increased muscle myoD mRNA levels to a similar extent in young and elderly, whereas the training-induced increase in mRNA levels of myogenin was impaired in the elderly [17].

Proteins responsible for negative muscle mass regulation, e.g., actRIIB and smad2, could be upregulated in inactive, aged muscle and be attenuated in response to resistance exercise, resulting in decreased muscle mass. In support, the mRNA level of actRIIB was downregulated after 21 weeks of resistance exercise in elderly [35,36]. The regulation of these molecular pathways involved in negative muscle mass regulation in response to resistance training in young and old muscle is unknown.

Mitochondrial dysfunction is another suggested key contributor loss of muscle mass with age [30]. Resistance exercise training has been found to affect mitochondrial function [37] evidenced by improved mitochondrial respiration and complex protein content after 12 weeks of resistance exercise training in young men [38]. However, whether resistance exercise training induces markers of mitochondrial content in elderly to a similar extent seems not clear.

In the present study, we therefore investigated the effect of resistance exercise training on strength and the protein expression or phosphorylation of factors important for upregulating (MyoD, myogenin, and IGF-I-R) and downregulating (activin receptor IIB (actRIIB) and smad2) skeletal muscle mass and mitochondrial markers in elderly compared to young individuals. In addition, we aimed at elucidating whether subsequent deconditioning affected these parameters in young and elderly similarly.

2. Materials and Methods

2.1. Subjects

Young and elderly volunteers were recruited with the criteria that for the elderly group age should be ≥74 years old and for the younger group age <30 years old. Exclusion criteria were non-sedentary status, illness requiring medical treatment other than treatment for hypertension and antithrombotic treatment, severe back or musculoskeletal pain, rheumatologic or neurological disorders, traumatic musculoskeletal and/or joint injuries, smoking, cardiovascular disease, attendance rate below 80% of total exercise sessions, additional exercise during the exercise phase, or failure to comply with instructions of inactivity during the deconditioning phase. Sedentary was defined as performing a maximum of three kilometers of cycling for transportation a day.

Twenty-two healthy, sedentary participants participated in the study; four were excluded due to noncompliance. Nine elderly, healthy persons—five men and four women (82 ± 7 year old)—fulfilled the inclusion criteria, and completed the resistance exercise training and deconditioning interventions. Data were compared to those found in nine young, healthy persons, also five men and four women (23 ± 3 yrs. of age). All participants completed a detailed medical history and had a normal neurological examination before entering the study. Demographic data of participants are shown in Table 1.

Table 1. General demographic data.

	Young Group		Elderly Group	
Age, years	22.4 ± 2.2		82.3 ± 6.8 ***	
Height, cm	174.8 ± 10.4		167.5 ± 8.6	
Weight, kg	70.9 ± 15.1		64.7 ± 9.7	
BMI, kg/m^2	22.9 ± 2.4		23.5 ± 2.9	
	Pre training	Post training	Pre training	Post training
Body fat (%)	26.2 ± 8.6	26.3 ± 9.5	27.9 ± 4.8	27.1 ± 5.8
LBM (%)	74.5 ± 8.9	74.5 ± 8.8	73.9 ± 6.6	73.7 ± 6.9
LLM (kg)	16.7 ± 4.2	17.0 ± 4.2	14.0 ± 2.9	14.2 ± 2.4

BMI, Body Mass Index; LBM, Lean Body Mass, LLM, lean leg mass. Age, height, weight, and BMI are presented at baseline pre intervention. Body fat, LBM, and LLM was measured before and after six weeks of resistance exercise training in elderly and young men and women. Data are shown as means ± SD. $n = 9$ in both groups. *** Significantly different ($p < 0.001$) from young group.

The study was approved by the Health Research Ethics Committee of the Capital Region of Copenhagen (No. KF-293615) and complied with the guidelines set out in the Declaration of Helsinki. The subjects were all informed about the nature and risks of the study and gave written consent to participate before inclusion.

2.2. Study Design

Nine young and 9 elderly participants completed a six-week resistance exercise training intervention of the lower body (two-legged knee extension) followed by eight weeks of deconditioning (Figure 1). Muscle strength was evaluated by a three-repetition max test before and after resistance exercise training. Skeletal muscle biopsies were taken from the vastus lateralis muscle before and after resistance exercise training and after two, four, six, and eight weeks of deconditioning for measurement of myogenic regulatory factors and mitochondrial markers. DEXA scanning of body composition was performed before and after resistance training.

2.3. DEXA Scanning

A whole-body Dual-Energy X-ray Absorptiometry (DEXA) scan (GE Medical Systems, Lunar, Prodigy, Chicago, IL, USA) was performed prior to the intervention and after the resistance exercise training intervention. The images were analyzed using enCORE™2004 Software (v.8.5) (GE Medical Systems). Reliability of this DEXA scanning was recently described [39].

2.4. Exercise Equipment and Protocol

Testing and exercise training intervention were carried out in a two-legged knee extension resistance exercise model using standard strength exercise equipment machines (Nordic Gym, Technogym, Cesena, Italy). Furthermore, to compensate for muscle imbalances during the selective exercise of the quadriceps, the exercise decline leg press (Nordic Gym) was incorporated into the exercise regimen.

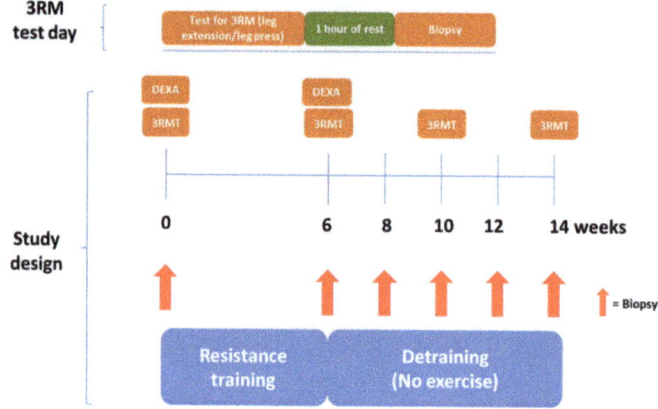

Figure 1. Study design overview. Eighteen participants completed a six-week resistance exercise training intervention followed by eight weeks of deconditioning (detraining—no exercise). Muscle strength was evaluated by a three-repetition max test before and after resistance exercise training. Skeletal muscle biopsies were taken from the vastus lateralis muscle on each test day. Furthermore, a biopsy was taken after two, four, and six weeks of deconditioning.

2.5. Strength Testing

Strength testing was performed using a three-repetition maximum (RM) test-protocol. Before initial testing, participants were familiarized with the equipment and test protocol on a separate occasion to reduce the impact that skill learning has on strength performance. The estimated measure of bilateral knee extension muscle strength was recently found to be applicable for monitoring adaptations promoted by physical exercise for older adults with and without sarcopenia [40].

Three repetition maximum test (3RMT): Prior to the 3RMT, participants warmed up using five minutes of low intensity (60–80 watt and 30–50 watt for young and elderly, respectively) cycling ergometer exercise. Afterwards, participants were instructed to execute four repetitions in each attempt. Full range of motion (ROM) for three consecutive repetitions and failure to complete a 4th repetition across a full-ROM was set as a criterion for a successful 3RM estimate. Participants rested 3 min after warm-up, and 1.5 min between all other attempts. After 10 min of rest, the validity of the estimate was evaluated by trying to outperform the current 3RM estimate. 1RM was calculated using Brzycki's formula [41]. 3RMT was measured before and after the resistance training intervention (Figure 1).

2.6. Resistance Exercise Training and Deconditioning Interventions

The resistance exercise training intervention lasted for six weeks and consisted of 16 supervised resistance exercise sessions. Resistance exercise followed a progressive protocol in weekly exercise sessions from two to three sessions per week after the first two weeks of exercise. Sessions were divided into three sessions of different load carried on a two-legged knee extension and a decline leg press machine to voluntary failure, and each set was separated by three minutes of rest. The first session encompassed three sets of 10–12 repetitions with 10–12 RM load, followed by three sets of 6–8 repetitions with 6–8 RM load, ending with three sets of 4–6 repetitions with 4–6 RM load. Each session was separated by approximately 48 h of rest.

In addition to and following knee extension resistance exercise, participants exercised in the decline leg press with the same exercise protocol (e.g., three sets of 10–12 reps with 10–12 RM in both exercises in the same session). After six weeks of resistance exercise training, participants stopped the exercise program and returned to their habitual sedentary lifestyle and were instructed not to initiate any new form of exercise the following eight weeks. This was ensured by participants wearing accelerometers and weekly interviews of the participants.

2.7. Skeletal Muscle Biopsy

A skeletal muscle biopsy was performed in vastus lateralis right leg muscle before and after the six weeks resistance exercise training intervention, and after two, four, six, and eight weeks of deconditioning (post2w, post4w, post6w, and post8w) approximately one hour post the acute 3RMT on the experimental days. The biopsy was performed as previously described using a 5 mm percutaneous Bergström needle [42]. Needle entry was at least three centimeters away from the previous insertion to avoid scar tissue and interference with data due to post-biopsy edema, regeneration, and cellular infiltration. Muscle samples were immediately frozen in isopentane cooled by liquid nitrogen before storage at −80 °C for later analysis.

2.8. Western Blotting Analysis

Western blot analysis was performed as previously described [43]. Biopsies were sectioned on a cryostat at −20 °C and homogenized in ice-cold lysis buffer with protease and phosphatase inhibitors (10 mM Tris, pH 7.4, 0.1% Triton-X 100, 0.5% sodium deoxycholate, 0.07 U/mL aprotinin, 20 M leupeptin, 20 M pepstatin, 1 mM phenylmethanesulfonyl fluoride (PMSF), 1 mM EDTA, 1 mM EGTA, 1 mM DTT, 5 mM β-glycerophosphate, 1 mM sodium fluoride, 1.15 mM sodium molybdate, 2 mM sodium pyrophosphate decahydrate, 1 mM sodium orthovanadate, 4 mM sodium tartrate, 2 mM imidazole, 10 nM calyculin, and 5 mM cantharidin; Sigma-Aldrich, St. Louis, MO, USA) using a Bullet Blender bead-mill at 4 °C (Next Advance, Averill, NY, USA). The homogenate was directly centrifuged at 15,000× g for 5 min at 4 °C. The supernatant was immediately transferred to new Eppendorf tubes and added 4× sample buffer including beta mercapto-ethanol. Equal amounts of extracted muscle proteins (10 µL) were separated on 4–15% polyacrylamide gels (Bio-Rad, Hercules, CA, USA) at 200 V for 40–50 min along with molecular weight markers (Bio-Rad). Proteins were transferred to PVDF membranes at 2.5 A for 5 min using a Trans-Blot Turbo (Bio-Rad) and blocked in Bailey's Irish cream (R. J. Bailey & Co, Dublin, Ireland) for 30 min and washed in TBS-T to remove excess Bailey's (3 × 10 min). The study investigated the expression and/or phosphorylation of proteins involved in muscle development/regeneration (IGF-I-R, MyoD, myogenin) and negative regulators of muscle mass (actRIIB and smad2) as well as porin [44], a mitochondrial membrane protein, to assess any changes in mitochondrial content. Thus, to investigate MRFs, antibodies against MyoD (45 kDa; diluted 1:1000; host: mouse; Thermo Fisher Scientific, Waltham, MA, USA) and myogenin (F5D) (40/25 kDa; diluted 1:1000; host: mouse; Developmental Studies Hybridoma Bank (DSHB), University of Iowa, IA, USA) were used. Antibodies against phosphorylated insulin-like growth factor 1 receptor (p-IGF-IR beta Y1135/1136; 95 kDa; diluted 1:500; host: rabbit; Cell Signaling Technology, Danvers, MA, USA), activin IIB receptor (58 kDa; diluted 1:1000; host: rabbit; ab180185, Abcam, Cambridge, UK), and phospho-smad2/3 (pSer250; 58 kDa; diluted 1:1000; host rabbit; Cell Signaling Technology) were used to investigate if muscle growth regulation had changed. Antibodies against porin (30–33 kDa; diluted 1:50,000; host: mouse; Thermo Fisher Scientific) were used to investigate a marker of mitochondrial content.

Antibodies against glyceraldehyde-3-phosphate dehydrogenase (GAPDH) were used at 1:5000 (ab22555; Abcam, Cambridge, UK) as loading control. Secondary goat anti-rabbit and goat anti-mouse antibodies coupled with horseradish peroxidase at concentration 1:10,000 were used to detect primary antibodies (DAKO, Glostrup, Denmark). Immunoreactive bands were detected by chemiluminescence using Clarity Max, (BioRad), quantified using a GBox XT16 darkroom, and GeneTools software was used to measure the intensities of immunoreactive bands (Syngene, Cambridge, UK). Immunoreactive band intensities were normalized to the intensity of the GAPDH bands for each subject to correct for differences in total muscle protein loaded on the gel.

2.9. Muscle Histology and Immunohistochemistry

Cryosections (10 µm) were cut from biopsies mounted in Tissue-Tek (Sakura Finetek Europe B.V., AJ Alphen aan den Rijn Netherlands), mounted on glass slides, and stored at −20 °C until stained. To assess myosin heavy chain (MHC) muscle fiber type distribution, sections were stained with MHC antibody clone BA-D5 (DSHB) for MHC type I, and a secondary goat anti-mouse antibody was used (GAM IgG2b Alexa Fluor 594, Thermo Fisher Scientific). For MHC type II assessment, sections were stained with MHC antibody clone A4.74 (DSHB), and a secondary goat anti-mouse antibody (GAM IgG1 Alexa Fluor 488) was used. All sections were observed at room temperature using a Nikon 20× Plan Apo VC N/A 0.75 mounted on a Nikon Ti-E epifluorescence microscope (Nikon Instruments, Melville, NY, USA). Images of the entire sections were acquired at 20× with a 5-Mpixel Andor Neo camera for fluorescence imaging (Andor, Belfast, Northern Ireland), using NIS-Elements Advanced Research (AR) software (Nikon Instruments) and merged in software.

2.10. Mitochondrial Citrate Synthase Enzyme Activity

Citrate synthase enzyme activity was investigated in muscle biopsies pre-exercise, post-exercise, and after 8 weeks of deconditioning. In short, skeletal muscle tissue (~200 mg) was sectioned on a cryostat (Microm HM550, Thermo Fisher, by, stat) at −20 °C and homogenized in ice-cold CelLytic MT (Mammalian tissue lysis/extraction reagent) containing protease inhibitor cocktail. The tissue was homogenized using a Bullet Blender bead-mill at 4 °C (Next Advance, Averill, NY, USA). The homogenate was directly centrifuged at 15,000× g for 5 min at 4 °C. The supernatant was transferred to new Eppendorf tubes and used for subsequent analysis. The assay was carried out according to the manufacturer's instructions (#CS0720, Sigma-Aldrich). Briefly, the assay solutions were heated at 25 °C. A master mix consisting of 1× assay buffer, 30 mM Acetyl-CoA solution, and 10 mM DTNB solution were mixed and added in the lysate to perform triple measurements per sample. Citrate synthase was measured by reading absorbance at 412 nm every 10th second for 1.5 min, and thereafter adding 10 mM OAA solution and then remeasured again every 10 s for 1.5 min at 412 nm.

2.11. Statistical Analysis

All statistical analyses were carried out using Excel 2010 (Microsoft®, Redmond, WA, USA) and GraphPad PRISM 8 (GraphPad, San Diego, CA, USA). A Shapiro–Wilkinson test was performed to test for normal distribution of data. Baseline subject characteristics were evaluated with unpaired *t*-tests between young and elderly groups and by a repeated measures two-way ANOVA for DEXA data before and after training (Table 1).The differences among groups were analyzed by a three-way repeated measures ANOVA in Figure 2A and a two-way repeated measures ANOVA in Figure 2B, Figure 3, and Table 2, followed by Tukey's multiple comparison tests when ANOVA revealed significant interactions. Prior to this, an additional two-way ANOVA was performed to ensure no gender differences prior to pooling data for male and females.). Correlation analyses were performed with the Pearson's product-moment correlation coefficient. All data are presented as means ± standard deviation (SD). Differences were considered to be statistically significant when $p < 0.05$.

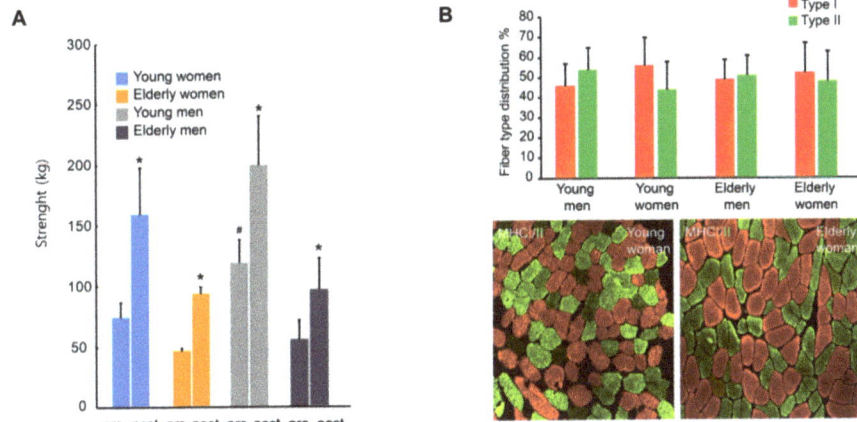

Figure 2. Muscle strength and muscle fiber type composition. (**A**) Quadriceps muscle strength measured in a three repetition maximum test before and after six weeks of resistance exercise training in elderly and young men and women. (**B**) Pre-intervention muscle fiber type distribution shown as bar graph and by representative cross-sectional images of m. vastus lateralis in a younger and older woman showing fiber type distribution of myosin heavy chain (MHC) type I (red) and type II (green). * $p < 0.05$, post-exercise vs. pre-exercise within the same group. # $p < 0.05$, pre-exercise, young men vs. young women. $n = 5$ elderly men, $n = 4$ elderly women, $n = 5$ young men, and $n = 4$ young women. All data are presented as means ± SD.

Table 2. Mitochondrial markers.

	Young Group			Elderly Group		
	Pre Training	Post Training	Post Deconditioning	Pre Training	Post Training	Post Deconditioning
Porin protein content relative to young pre training (AU)	1.00 ± 0.4	0.98 ± 1.1	1.60 ± 1.3	1.19 ± 1.2	1.53 ± 1.3	2.40 ± 1.9
CS activity, µmol/min/mg w.w.	1.7 ± 1.0	2.2 ± 1.3	2.0 ± 0.6	1.0 ± 0.6	1.7 ± 1.9	1.4 ± 0.9

Porin protein content and maximal muscle citrate synthase (CS) activity measured pre-training, following six weeks of resistance exercise training (post training), and after eight weeks of subsequent deconditioning (post decondition). Porin protein content is expressed relative to young pre training. Data are shown as means ± SD. $n = 9$ in both groups.

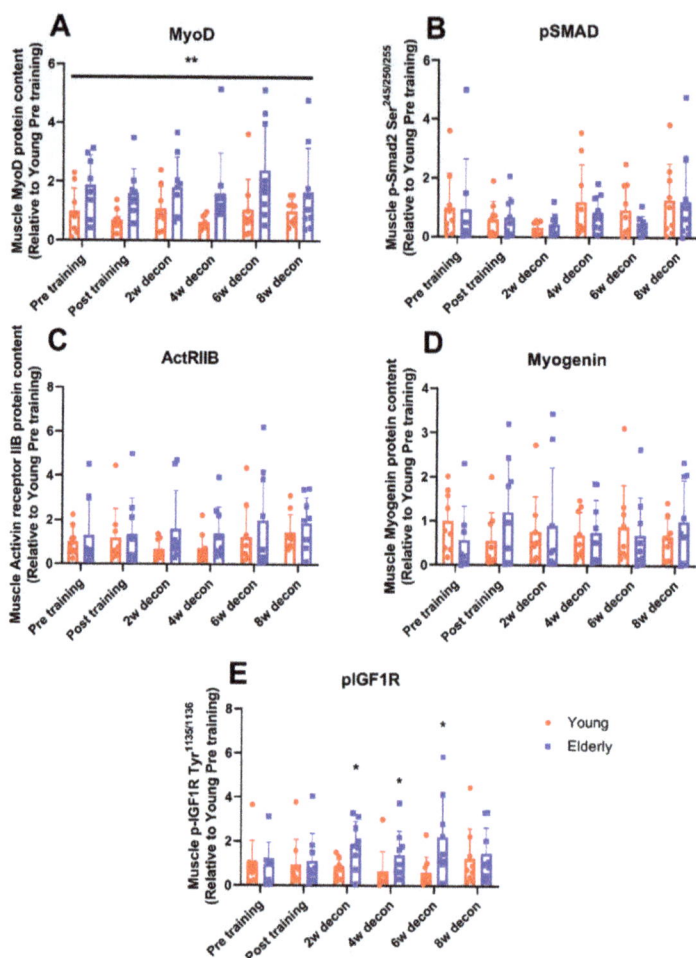

Figure 3. Muscle regulatory factors. Muscle regulatory factors measured in skeletal muscle pre and post six weeks of resistance exercise training and during 2, 4, 6, and 8 weeks into a subsequent deconditioning period in young (red bars) and elderly (blue bars) individuals. (**A**) Protein expression of activin receptor IIB, (**B**). Phosphorylation level of smad2 at Ser245/250/255. (**C**) Protein expression of MyoD. (**D**) Protein expression of myogenin. (**E**) Phosphorylation level of IGF-I-R at Tyr1135/1136. Measurements have been performed as single determinations by Western blotting. Representative Western blots are shown in Supplementary Figure S1. $n = 9$ in young group and $n = 9$ in the elderly group. Values are arbitrary units (means ± SD) and expressed relative to young group pre training. * $p < 0.05$, young vs. elderly group, ** $p < 0.01$, main effect of age independently of training and deconditioning. ANOVA F-values ($F_{time}/F_{age}/F_{time \times age}$): (**A**) 1.08/11.62/0.32; (**B**) 0.76/0.58/0.49; (**C**) 0.77/2.97/0.23; (**D**) 0.09/0.15/1.20; (**E**) 0.54/8.62/1.41.

3. Results

3.1. Anthropometry

Total body weight, body mass index (BMI), body fat %, and lean body mass % were similar between the young and the elderly group (Table 1). Six weeks of resistance exercise training did not lead to changes in whole body fat %, lean body mass %, or lean leg mass, as a read out for muscle mass, in the trained legs in neither the young nor the elderly individuals.

3.2. Muscle Strength

Six weeks of resistance exercise training increased quadriceps muscle strength in the elderly group by 78% (53.4 ± 14.3 kg (pre-exercise) vs. 95.0 ± 22.0 kg (post-exercise); $p < 0.05$), which was similar to that found in the young healthy persons (83.5%; 97.1 ± 27.5 kg (pre-exercise) vs. 178.2 ± 44.2 kg (post-exercise); $p < 0.05$) (Figure 2A). Pre-exercise, the elderly men did not have a significantly greater muscle strength compared to elderly women (56.2 ± 16.1 kg vs. 46.5 ± 2.5 kg), whereas a gender difference in muscle strength was observed in the younger group, in which the younger men had a 59% greater muscle strength at pre-training compared to younger women (119.2 ± 19.5 kg vs. 75 ± 12.6 kg; $p < 0.05$) (Figure 2A). No significant differences in strength between genders were observed post-exercise within the elderly or young group (Figure 2A).

3.3. Muscle Fiber Type Composition

No pre-exercise fiber type differences were seen between gender, young, and elderly participants (Figure 2B).

3.4. Myogenic Regulatory Factors

Six weeks of resistance exercise training and 8 weeks of deconditioning did not change the protein expression of MyoD, actRIIB, and myogenin and phosphorylation of Smad2 and IGF-I- receptor in the elderly and the young group (Figure 3A–E).

MyoD protein expression were overall higher ($p < 0.01$) in muscles of elderly compared with young individuals (Figure 3A).

No differences in total protein expression of actRIIB and myogenin and phosphorylation of Smad2 and IGF-I-R were observed pre-training or after six weeks following resistance training in young versus elderly participants (Figure 3B–E). IGF-I receptor phosphorylation at Tyr1135/1136 was lower in the younger group of healthy persons compared to the elderly group two weeks post-exercise (post2w) (0.7 ± 0.5 vs. 1.9 ± 1.1, $p < 0.05$), four weeks post-exercise (post4w) (0.6 ± 0.9 vs. 1.4 ± 1.1, $p < 0.05$) and six weeks post-exercise (post6w) (0.6 ± 0.7 vs. 2.6 ± 2.7, $p < 0.05$) (Figure 3E). There was no difference between genders at all time points in both groups in all protein and phosphorylation levels investigated, why these data were pooled in the data shown.

3.5. Mitochondrial Markers: Porin and Citrate Synthase

The protein expression of porin did not change with six weeks of resistance exercise training and remained unchanged after deconditioning in both the young and the elderly and was not significantly different between the groups (Table 2).

The maximal muscle enzyme activity of citrate synthase in the elderly was not significantly different from that found in the young participants (Table 2). Maximal muscle enzyme activity of citrate synthase in the elderly group remained unchanged with resistance exercise training and subsequent deconditioning, which was similar to that found in the young group (Table 2). There was no difference in the citrate synthase activity among genders in the elderly and young groups, which is why these data were pooled (Table 2).

3.6. Correlation between Myogenic and Mitochondrial Factors and Muscle Strength

There was no association between any of the studied MRFs (MyoD, myogenin, actRIIB protein expression, and IGF-I-R and smad2 phosphorylation) or mitochondrial factors (citrate synthase activity and porin protein expression) and absolute or relative change in muscle strength after six weeks of resistance exercise training in the elderly or the young group.

4. Discussion

Resistance exercise training and deconditioning offer a unique opportunity to investigate differences in myogenic regulatory factors that may be crucial in the age-related loss of muscle mass and strength. The aim of this study was to investigate regulation of myogenic factors prior and in response to resistance exercise training and deconditioning in elderly (74–92 years of age) versus young, healthy, gender-matched individuals. The primary findings were (1) six weeks of intensive resistance exercise training induced the same increase in muscle strength in young and older individuals, (2) the key myogenic regulating factors (MyoD, myogenin, and IGF-I-R) were similar in muscles of young and elderly individuals and not differently regulated by six weeks of resistance exercise training or subsequent eight weeks of deconditioning, and (3) no change was found in markers of oxidative capacity and mitochondrial content after six weeks of resistance exercise training in either elderly or young healthy persons.

Age-related loss of muscle strength is inevitable and cannot be explained by age-related decreased physical activity level alone [45]. It has been suggested that elderly persons have a blunted muscle hypertrophy response to resistance exercise training [17–19]. Thus, it could be that differences in muscle mass and function between young and elderly are driven by age-related changes in the ability to gain and/or maintain muscle strength with age. However, the present study showed that six weeks of intensive resistance exercise training resulted in the same increase in quadriceps muscle strength in elderly compared to that found in young, gender-matched, sedentary individuals. Therefore, skeletal muscle of elderly has the same capacity to increase strength in response to resistance training as in young healthy individuals. This finding is important in a translational perspective, emphasizing that resistance exercise training benefits elderly as much as in young persons and therefore seems to be a valid tool to combat loss of muscle function and strength in aging.

Myogenic regulatory factors promote and regulate the expression of muscle-specific genes after muscle injury or strenuous resistance exercise leading to muscle hypertrophy [46]. It has been hypothesized that the inevitably age-related muscle strength loss may relate to downregulation of MRFs, and thus skeletal muscle atrophy, which we were unable to corroborate. With the same levels of MRFs in elderly compared to young persons in the present study, our findings contrast the majority of previous studies measuring on mRNA levels. Previous studies found elevated levels of MyoD, myogenin, and IGF-I-R mRNA in elderly both at rest [17,31–34] and in response to exercise training compared to younger individuals [17,47–50]. This suggests that the increase in MRF mRNA levels represented a continuous compensatory mechanism to preserve muscle protein and mass with aging [17]. The present study is the first to investigate protein levels of MRFs, obviating the issues with changes in mRNA levels that may not translate into similar changes in protein expression due to post-translational regulation [51]. The present study suggests that the myogenic program is intact in the elderly, as the levels of MyoD, myogenin, and IGF-I-R are activated to the same extent as in younger skeletal muscle. An overall higher level of MyoD protein expression in the elderly compared with the young muscle, and a higher IGF-I-R phosphorylation 2, 4, and 6 weeks into the deconditioning period in the elderly compared with young individuals support that compensatory mechanisms in MRF regulation contribute to preserve muscle protein and mass in aging. Importantly, our study underscores that protein and phosphorylation levels should be measured in favor of mRNA. Our finding further suggests that an intact anabolic muscle response seems able to compensate in part for the loss of muscle.

As the expression of MRFs are time-dependent in relation to external and internal stimuli, it could be hypothesized that lack of differences in MRFs in the present versus other studies (measuring mRNA levels though) investigating this could be related to the timing of the muscle biopsy sampling. In the present study, the muscle biopsy intervention was taken one hour post-exercise. As the expression of the proteins that was investigated in the present study is expected to be stable and not affected by an acute bout of exercise, timing of muscle sample seems not have an impact on the data presented in the present study. This is supported by findings in post-exercise muscle biopsy intervention (3 h post-exercise), in which no increase was found in key myogenic factors (MyoD, myf-6), except for myogenin [52], underscoring that timing of muscle biopsy sampling likely did not impact the protein levels of MRFs in the present study.

Muscle growth is tightly regulated through the myostatin, actRIIB, and smad2 pathway [53]. In response to muscle disuse, this and other pathways mediate a decrease in muscle mass [54]. In line with this, studies have shown that inhibition of myostatin-actRIIB-smad pathway leads to skeletal muscle hypertrophy in mice [55]. Studies by Hulmi et al. [35,36] have indicated that factors downregulating muscle mass in aged muscle could be attenuated in response to resistance exercise, as the mRNA level of actRIIB was downregulated after 21 weeks of resistance exercise in elderly (62.3 ± 6.3 years of age). The findings from that study indicate that proteins responsible for negative muscle mass regulation, e.g., actRIIB and smad2, could be upregulated in inactive aged muscle, resulting in decreased muscle mass and thus strength. However, our results did not support that finding. Instead, our data demonstrate that skeletal muscles of elderly have the same dynamics of MRF-mediated hypo- and hypertrophy, indicating that resistance exercise and deconditioning regulatory effects on skeletal muscle anabolism is the same irrespective of age.

Citrate synthase is a key mitochondrial matrix enzyme and a strong indicator of oxidative capacity in skeletal muscle [56–59] and maximal citrate synthase activity was also found to strongly correlate with mitochondrial volume measured by electron microscopy in skeletal muscles of healthy, young men [58]. Porin (also known as voltage dependent anion channel, VDAC1) is a pore-forming protein localized in the outer membrane of mitochondria, and is used as a marker of mitochondrial content [60,61]. Alterations in mitochondrial function and content has been proposed to be a factor underlying sarcopenia and muscle atrophy [62,63]. In order to investigate whether age-related decline in muscle strength was accompanied by muscle mitochondrial impairments in response to resistance training, muscle citrate synthase activity, and porin protein expression were measured before and after six weeks of resistance exercise training and eight weeks of deconditioning. Data showed that there was no change in oxidative capacity and indices of mitochondrial content after six weeks of resistance exercise training in either elderly or young healthy individuals, indicating that the gain in muscle strength was not associated with any changes in mitochondrial content.

It has been hypothesized that change in age-related muscle mass is driven by loss of muscle fiber type II number with age. However, findings regarding age-related changes in muscle fiber type II number have been ambiguous [64–67]. In the present study, the elderly individuals were older than those previously studied (+74 years old), and despite an age difference of 60 years between the young and elderly participants, there was no difference in number of type I and II fibers between elderly and younger persons. In the present study, we did not measure fiber type composition after training and deconditioning. Fiber type composition is in most studies not changed with exercise training [68] especially not within 6 weeks of resistance training. However, we cannot exclude that fiber type composition was mildly affected by exercise training in the present study. Furthermore, it was not within the scope of the present investigation to evaluate fiber size changes with resistance exercise training and deconditioning and it remains to be established, whether muscle fiber sizes are affected by 6 weeks of resistance training and subsequent 8 weeks of deconditioning in skeletal muscle of young and elderly.

5. Conclusions

Despite the fact that aging is associated with substantial loss of muscle mass resulting in a net loss of muscle strength and function, our study showed that elderly (aged 74+ years old) are remarkably capable of gaining muscle strength compared to younger participants in response to resistance exercise training. This underlines the applicability of resistance exercise training as an important instrument to diminish age-related loss of muscle function. Interestingly, the preserved ability to gain muscle strength with resistance exercise training was associated with a similar interaction between myogenic factors for up- and downregulation of skeletal muscle in elderly and young individuals. Thus, our data suggests that the entire myogenic regulatory program is not impaired in aged relative to younger skeletal muscle.

Supplementary Materials: The following are available online at http://www.mdpi.com/2077-0383/9/7/2188/s1, Figure S1: Representative Western blots.

Author Contributions: Conceptualization, F.D.T. and T.D.J.; methodology, T.K., K.A.N.Q.; formal analysis, K.A.N.Q., A.M.F.; investigation, A.M.F., F.D.T., K.A.N.Q., T.K., M.-L.S., T.D.J.; resources, J.V.; data curation, A.M.F., F.D.T., K.A.N.Q.; writing—original draft preparation, A.M.F., K.A.N.Q., T.D.J.; writing—review and editing A.M.F., F.D.T., K.A.N.Q., T.K., M.-L.S., J.V., T.D.J.; visualization, A.M.F., K.A.N.Q., T.D.J.; supervision, T..K., J.V., T.D.J.; project administration, F.D.T., T.D.J.; funding acquisition, J.V. All authors have read and agree to the published version of the manuscript.

Funding: A.M.F. was supported by a research grant from the Danish Diabetes Academy (grant number NNF17SA0031406), which was funded by the Novo Nordisk Foundation. A.M.F. was further supported by the Alfred Benzon Foundation.

Acknowledgments: We thank Tessa Munkeboe Hornsyld and Danuta Goralska-Olsen for excellent technical assistance.

Conflicts of Interest: The authors declare no conflict of interest.

References

1. Fuggle, N.; Shaw, S.; Dennison, E.; Cooper, C. Sarcopenia. *Best Pract. Res. Clin. Rheumatol.* **2017**, *31*, 218–242. [CrossRef] [PubMed]
2. Drey, M. Sarcopenia—Pathophysiology and clinical relevance. *Wien Med. Wochenschr.* **2011**, *161*, 402–408. [CrossRef] [PubMed]
3. Fragala, M.S.; Cadore, E.L.; Dorgo, S.; Izquierdo, M.; Kraemer, W.J.; Peterson, M.D.; Ryan, E.D. Resistance Training for Older Adults: Position Statement from the National Strength and Conditioning Association. *J. Strength Cond. Res.* **2019**, *33*, 2019–2052. [CrossRef]
4. Newton, R.U.; Hakkinen, K.; Hakkinen, A.; McCormick, M.; Volek, J.; Kraemer, W.J. Mixed-methods resistance training increases power and strength of young and older men. *Med. Sci. Sports Exerc.* **2002**, *34*, 1367–1375. [CrossRef]
5. HÃkkinen, K.; Newton, R.U.; Gordon, S.E.; McCormick, M.; Volek, J.S.; Nindl, B.C.; Gotshalk, L.A.; Campbell, W.W.; Evans, W.J.; HÃ¤kkinen, A.; et al. Changes in muscle morphology, electromyographic activity, and force production characteristics during progressive strength training in young and older men. *J. Gerontol. A Biol. Sci. Med. Sci.* **1998**, *53*, B415–B423. [CrossRef] [PubMed]
6. Lemmer, J.T.; Hurlbut, D.E.; Martel, G.F.; Tracy, B.L.; Ivey, F.M.; Metter, E.J.; Fozard, J.L.; Fleg, J.L.; Hurley, B.F. Age and gender responses to strength training and detraining. *Med. Sci. Sports Exerc.* **2000**, *32*, 1505–1512. [CrossRef] [PubMed]
7. Macaluso, A.; De Vito, G.; Felici, F.; Nimmo, M.A. Electromyogram changes during sustained contraction after resistance training in women in their 3rd and 8th decades. *Eur. J. Appl. Physiol.* **2000**, *82*, 418–424. [CrossRef] [PubMed]
8. Delmonico, M.J.; Harris, T.B.; Visser, M.; Park, S.W.; Conroy, M.B.; Velasquez-Mieyer, P.; Boudreau, R.; Manini, T.M.; Nevitt, M.; Newman, A.B.; et al. Longitudinal study of muscle strength, quality, and adipose tissue infiltration. *Am. J. Clin. Nutr.* **2009**, *90*, 1579–1585. [CrossRef]
9. Clark, B.C.; Manini, T.M. Functional consequences of sarcopenia and dynapenia in the elderly. *Curr. Opin. Clin. Nutr. Metab. Care* **2010**, *13*, 271–276. [CrossRef]
10. Karlsen, A.; Bechshoft, R.L.; Malmgaard-Clausen, N.M.; Andersen, J.L.; Schjerling, P.; Kjaer, M.; Mackey, A.L. Lack of muscle fibre hypertrophy, myonuclear addition, and satellite cell pool expansion with resistance training in 83-94-year-old men and women. *Acta Physiol.* **2019**, *227*, e13321. [CrossRef]
11. Snijders, T.; Verdijk, L.B.; Smeets, J.S.; McKay, B.R.; Senden, J.M.; Hartgens, F.; Parise, G.; Greenhaff, P.; van Loon, L.J. The skeletal muscle satellite cell response to a single bout of resistance-type exercise is delayed with aging in men. *Age* **2014**, *36*, 9699. [CrossRef]
12. Verdijk, L.B.; Gleeson, B.G.; Jonkers, R.A.; Meijer, K.; Savelberg, H.H.; Dendale, P.; van Loon, L.J. Skeletal muscle hypertrophy following resistance training is accompanied by a fiber type-specific increase in satellite cell content in elderly men. *J. Gerontol. A Biol. Sci. Med. Sci.* **2009**, *64*, 332–339. [CrossRef] [PubMed]

13. Leenders, M.; Verdijk, L.B.; van der Hoeven, L.; van Kranenburg, J.; Nilwik, R.; van Loon, L.J. Elderly men and women benefit equally from prolonged resistance-type exercise training. *J. Gerontol. A Biol. Sci. Med. Sci.* **2013**, *68*, 769–779. [CrossRef] [PubMed]
14. Snijders, T.; Nederveen, J.P.; Joanisse, S.; Leenders, M.; Verdijk, L.B.; van Loon, L.J.; Parise, G. Muscle fibre capillarization is a critical factor in muscle fibre hypertrophy during resistance exercise training in older men. *J. Cachexia Sarcopenia Muscle* **2017**, *8*, 267–276. [CrossRef] [PubMed]
15. Karlsen, A.; Soendenbroe, C.; Malmgaard-Clausen, N.M.; Wagener, F.; Moeller, C.E.; Senhaji, Z.; Damberg, K.; Andersen, J.L.; Schjerling, P.; Kjaer, M.; et al. Preserved capacity for satellite cell proliferation, regeneration, and hypertrophy in the skeletal muscle of healthy elderly men. *FASEB J.* **2020**, *34*, 6418–6436. [CrossRef] [PubMed]
16. Blocquiaux, S.; Gorski, T.; Van Roie, E.; Ramaekers, M.; Van Thienen, R.; Nielens, H.; Delecluse, C.; De Bock, K.; Thomis, M. The effect of resistance training, detraining and retraining on muscle strength and power, myofibre size, satellite cells and myonuclei in older men. *Exp. Gerontol.* **2020**, *133*, 110860. [CrossRef] [PubMed]
17. Kosek, D.J.; Kim, J.S.; Petrella, J.K.; Cross, J.M.; Bamman, M.M. Efficacy of 3 days/wk resistance training on myofiber hypertrophy and myogenic mechanisms in young vs. older adults. *J. Appl. Physiol.* **2006**, *101*, 531–544. [CrossRef] [PubMed]
18. Mero, A.A.; Hulmi, J.J.; Salmijarvi, H.; Katajavuori, M.; Haverinen, M.; Holviala, J.; Ridanpaa, T.; Hakkinen, K.; Kovanen, V.; Ahtiainen, J.P.; et al. Resistance training induced increase in muscle fiber size in young and older men. *Eur. J. Appl. Physiol.* **2013**, *113*, 641–650. [CrossRef]
19. Brook, M.S.; Wilkinson, D.J.; Mitchell, W.K.; Lund, J.N.; Phillips, B.E.; Szewczyk, N.J.; Greenhaff, P.L.; Smith, K.; Atherton, P.J. Synchronous deficits in cumulative muscle protein synthesis and ribosomal biogenesis underlie age-related anabolic resistance to exercise in humans. *J. Physiol.* **2016**, *594*, 7399–7417. [CrossRef]
20. Hwa, V.; Fang, P.; Derr, M.A.; Fiegerlova, E.; Rosenfeld, R.G. IGF-I in human growth: Lessons from defects in the GH-IGF-I axis. *Nestle Nutr. Inst. Workshop Ser.* **2013**, *71*, 43–55. [CrossRef]
21. Stilling, F.; Wallenius, S.; Michaelsson, K.; Dalgard, C.; Brismar, K.; Wolk, A. High insulin-like growth factor-binding protein-1 (IGFBP-1) is associated with low relative muscle mass in older women. *Metabolism* **2017**, *73*, 36–42. [CrossRef] [PubMed]
22. Zanou, N.; Gailly, P. Skeletal muscle hypertrophy and regeneration: Interplay between the myogenic regulatory factors (MRFs) and insulin-like growth factors (IGFs) pathways. *Cell. Mol. Life Sci.* **2013**, *70*, 4117–4130. [CrossRef] [PubMed]
23. Hernandez-Hernandez, J.M.; Garcia-Gonzalez, E.G.; Brun, C.E.; Rudnicki, M.A. The myogenic regulatory factors, determinants of muscle development, cell identity and regeneration. *Semin. Cell Dev. Biol.* **2017**, *72*, 10–18. [CrossRef]
24. Seward, D.J.; Haney, J.C.; Rudnicki, M.A.; Swoap, S.J. bHLH transcription factor MyoD affects myosin heavy chain expression pattern in a muscle-specific fashion. *Am. J. Physiol. Cell Physiol.* **2001**, *280*, C408–C413. [CrossRef] [PubMed]
25. Mozdziak, P.E.; Greaser, M.L.; Schultz, E. Myogenin, MyoD, and myosin heavy chain isoform expression following hindlimb suspension. *Aviat. Space Environ. Med.* **1999**, *70*, 511–516. [PubMed]
26. Mozdziak, P.E.; Greaser, M.L.; Schultz, E. Myogenin, MyoD, and myosin expression after pharmacologically and surgically induced hypertrophy. *J. Appl. Physiol.* **1998**, *84*, 1359–1364. [CrossRef] [PubMed]
27. Steffl, M.; Bohannon, R.W.; Sontakova, L.; Tufano, J.J.; Shiells, K.; Holmerova, I. Relationship between sarcopenia and physical activity in older people: A systematic review and meta-analysis. *Clin. Interv. Aging* **2017**, *12*, 835–845. [CrossRef]
28. Schoene, D.; Kiesswetter, E.; Sieber, C.C.; Freiberger, E. Musculoskeletal factors, sarcopenia and falls in old age. *Z. Gerontol. Geriatr.* **2019**, *52*, 37–44. [CrossRef]
29. Distefano, G.; Goodpaster, B.H. Effects of Exercise and Aging on Skeletal Muscle. *Cold Spring Harb. Perspect. Med.* **2018**, *8*, a029785. [CrossRef]
30. Tieland, M.; Trouwborst, I.; Clark, B.C. Skeletal muscle performance and ageing. *J. Cachexia Sarcopenia Muscle* **2018**, *9*, 3–19. [CrossRef] [PubMed]
31. Haddad, F.; Adams, G.R. Aging-sensitive cellular and molecular mechanisms associated with skeletal muscle hypertrophy. *J. Appl. Physiol.* **2006**, *100*, 1188–1203. [CrossRef] [PubMed]

32. Hameed, M.; Orrell, R.W.; Cobbold, M.; Goldspink, G.; Harridge, S.D. Expression of IGF-I splice variants in young and old human skeletal muscle after high resistance exercise. *J. Physiol.* **2003**, *547*, 247–254. [CrossRef] [PubMed]
33. Kim, J.S.; Kosek, D.J.; Petrella, J.K.; Cross, J.M.; Bamman, M.M. Resting and load-induced levels of myogenic gene transcripts differ between older adults with demonstrable sarcopenia and young men and women. *J. Appl. Physiol.* **2005**, *99*, 2149–2158. [CrossRef]
34. Raue, U.; Slivka, D.; Jemiolo, B.; Hollon, C.; Trappe, S. Myogenic gene expression at rest and after a bout of resistance exercise in young (18–30 yr) and old (80–89 yr) women. *J. Appl. Physiol.* **2006**, *101*, 53–59. [CrossRef] [PubMed]
35. Hulmi, J.J.; Ahtiainen, J.P.; Kaasalainen, T.; Pollanen, E.; Hakkinen, K.; Alen, M.; Selanne, H.; Kovanen, V.; Mero, A.A. Postexercise myostatin and activin IIb mRNA levels: Effects of strength training. *Med. Sci. Sports Exerc.* **2007**, *39*, 289–297. [CrossRef] [PubMed]
36. Hulmi, J.J.; Kovanen, V.; Selanne, H.; Kraemer, W.J.; Hakkinen, K.; Mero, A.A. Acute and long-term effects of resistance exercise with or without protein ingestion on muscle hypertrophy and gene expression. *Amino Acids* **2009**, *37*, 297–308. [CrossRef]
37. Groennebaek, T.; Vissing, K. Impact of Resistance Training on Skeletal Muscle Mitochondrial Biogenesis, Content, and Function. *Front. Physiol.* **2017**, *8*, 713. [CrossRef]
38. Porter, C.; Reidy, P.T.; Bhattarai, N.; Sidossis, L.S.; Rasmussen, B.B. Resistance Exercise Training Alters Mitochondrial Function in Human Skeletal Muscle. *Med. Sci. Sports Exerc.* **2015**, *47*, 1922–1931. [CrossRef]
39. Dordevic, A.L.; Bonham, M.; Ghasem-Zadeh, A.; Evans, A.; Barber, E.; Day, K.; Kwok, A.; Truby, H. Reliability of Compartmental Body Composition Measures in Weight-Stable Adults Using GE iDXA: Implications for Research and Practice. *Nutrients* **2018**, *10*, 1484. [CrossRef]
40. Abdalla, P.P.; Carvalho, A.D.S.; Dos Santos, A.P.; Venturini, A.C.R.; Alves, T.C.; Mota, J.; Machado, D.R.L. One-repetition submaximal protocol to measure knee extensor muscle strength among older adults with and without sarcopenia: A validation study. *BMC Sports Sci. Med. Rehabil.* **2020**, *12*, 29. [CrossRef]
41. Abdul-Hameed, U.; Rangra, P.; Shareef, M.Y.; Hussain, M.E. Reliability of 1-repetition maximum estimation for upper and lower body muscular strength measurement in untrained middle aged type 2 diabetic patients. *Asian J. Sports Med.* **2012**, *3*, 267–273. [CrossRef] [PubMed]
42. Bergstrom, J. Percutaneous needle biopsy of skeletal muscle in physiological and clinical research. *Scand. J. Clin. Lab. Invest.* **1975**, *35*, 609–616. [CrossRef] [PubMed]
43. Fritzen, A.M.; Thogersen, F.B.; Thybo, K.; Vissing, C.R.; Krag, T.O.; Ruiz-Ruiz, C.; Risom, L.; Wibrand, F.; Hoeg, L.D.; Kiens, B.; et al. Adaptations in Mitochondrial Enzymatic Activity Occurs Independent of Genomic Dosage in Response to Aerobic Exercise Training and Deconditioning in Human Skeletal Muscle. *Cells* **2019**, *8*, 237. [CrossRef]
44. Ben-Hail, D.; Shoshan-Barmatz, V. VDAC1-interacting anion transport inhibitors inhibit VDAC1 oligomerization and apoptosis. *Biochim. Biophys. Acta* **2016**, *1863*, 1612–1623. [CrossRef] [PubMed]
45. Brioche, T.; Pagano, A.F.; Py, G.; Chopard, A. Muscle wasting and aging: Experimental models, fatty infiltrations, and prevention. *Mol. Aspects Med.* **2016**, *50*, 56–87. [CrossRef]
46. Kopantseva, E.E.; Belyavsky, A.V. Key regulators of skeletal myogenesis. *Mol. Biol. (Mosk.)* **2016**, *50*, 195–222. [CrossRef] [PubMed]
47. Agergaard, J.; Reitelseder, S.; Pedersen, T.G.; Doessing, S.; Schjerling, P.; Langberg, H.; Miller, B.F.; Aagaard, P.; Kjaer, M.; Holm, L. Myogenic, matrix, and growth factor mRNA expression in human skeletal muscle: Effect of contraction intensity and feeding. *Muscle Nerve* **2013**, *47*, 748–759. [CrossRef]
48. Heinemeier, K.M.; Olesen, J.L.; Schjerling, P.; Haddad, F.; Langberg, H.; Baldwin, K.M.; Kjaer, M. Short-term strength training and the expression of myostatin and IGF-I isoforms in rat muscle and tendon: Differential effects of specific contraction types. *J. Appl. Physiol.* **2007**, *102*, 573–581. [CrossRef] [PubMed]
49. Luo, L.; Lu, A.M.; Wang, Y.; Hong, A.; Chen, Y.; Hu, J.; Li, X.; Qin, Z.H. Chronic resistance training activates autophagy and reduces apoptosis of muscle cells by modulating IGF-1 and its receptors, Akt/mTOR and Akt/FOXO3a signaling in aged rats. *Exp. Gerontol.* **2013**, *48*, 427–436. [CrossRef]
50. Mathers, J.L.; Farnfield, M.M.; Garnham, A.P.; Caldow, M.K.; Cameron-Smith, D.; Peake, J.M. Early inflammatory and myogenic responses to resistance exercise in the elderly. *Muscle Nerve* **2012**, *46*, 407–412. [CrossRef]

51. Myers, J.; Prakash, M.; Froelicher, V.; Do, D.; Partington, S.; Atwood, J.E. Exercise capacity and mortality among men referred for exercise testing. *N. Engl. J. Med.* **2002**, *346*, 793–801. [CrossRef] [PubMed]
52. Bamman, M.M.; Ragan, R.C.; Kim, J.S.; Cross, J.M.; Hill, V.J.; Tuggle, S.C.; Allman, R.M. Myogenic protein expression before and after resistance loading in 26- and 64-yr-old men and women. *J. Appl. Physiol.* **2004**, *97*, 1329–1337. [CrossRef] [PubMed]
53. Marcotte, G.R.; West, D.W.; Baar, K. The molecular basis for load-induced skeletal muscle hypertrophy. *Calcif. Tissue Int.* **2015**, *96*, 196–210. [CrossRef] [PubMed]
54. Schiaffino, S.; Dyar, K.A.; Ciciliot, S.; Blaauw, B.; Sandri, M. Mechanisms regulating skeletal muscle growth and atrophy. *FEBS J.* **2013**, *280*, 4294–4314. [CrossRef]
55. Bogdanovich, S.; Krag, T.O.; Barton, E.R.; Morris, L.D.; Whittemore, L.A.; Ahima, R.S.; Khurana, T.S. Functional improvement of dystrophic muscle by myostatin blockade. *Nature* **2002**, *420*, 418–421. [CrossRef]
56. Cai, Q.; Zhao, M.; Liu, X.; Wang, X.; Nie, Y.; Li, P.; Liu, T.; Ge, R.; Han, F. Reduced expression of citrate synthase leads to excessive superoxide formation and cell apoptosis. *Biochem. Biophys. Res. Commun.* **2017**, *485*, 388–394. [CrossRef]
57. Kadenbach, B. Introduction to mitochondrial oxidative phosphorylation. *Adv. Exp. Med. Biol.* **2012**, *748*, 1–11. [CrossRef]
58. Larsen, S.; Nielsen, J.; Hansen, C.N.; Nielsen, L.B.; Wibrand, F.; Stride, N.; Schroder, H.D.; Boushel, R.; Helge, J.W.; Dela, F.; et al. Biomarkers of mitochondrial content in skeletal muscle of healthy young human subjects. *J. Physiol.* **2012**, *590*, 3349–3360. [CrossRef]
59. Proctor, D.N.; Joyner, M.J. Skeletal muscle mass and the reduction of VO2max in trained older subjects. *J. Appl. Physiol.* **1997**, *82*, 1411–1415. [CrossRef]
60. Meierhofer, D.; Mayr, J.A.; Foetschl, U.; Berger, A.; Fink, K.; Schmeller, N.; Hacker, G.W.; Hauser-Kronberger, C.; Kofler, B.; Sperl, W. Decrease of mitochondrial DNA content and energy metabolism in renal cell carcinoma. *Carcinogenesis* **2004**, *25*, 1005–1010. [CrossRef]
61. Van Moorsel, D.; Hansen, J.; Havekes, B.; Scheer, F.A.; Jorgensen, J.A.; Hoeks, J.; Schrauwen-Hinderling, V.B.; Duez, H.; Lefebvre, P.; Schaper, N.C.; et al. Demonstration of a day-night rhythm in human skeletal muscle oxidative capacity. *Mol. Metab.* **2016**, *5*, 635–645. [CrossRef]
62. Calvani, R.; Joseph, A.M.; Adhihetty, P.J.; Miccheli, A.; Bossola, M.; Leeuwenburgh, C.; Bernabei, R.; Marzetti, E. Mitochondrial pathways in sarcopenia of aging and disuse muscle atrophy. *Biol. Chem.* **2013**, *394*, 393–414. [CrossRef] [PubMed]
63. Romanello, V.; Sandri, M. Mitochondrial Quality Control and Muscle Mass Maintenance. *Front. Physiol.* **2016**, *6*, 422. [CrossRef] [PubMed]
64. Green, H.; Goreham, C.; Ouyang, J.; Ball-Burnett, M.; Ranney, D. Regulation of fiber size, oxidative potential, and capillarization in human muscle by resistance exercise. *Am. J. Physiol.* **1999**, *276*, R591–R596. [CrossRef]
65. Hiatt, W.R.; Regensteiner, J.G.; Wolfel, E.E.; Carry, M.R.; Brass, E.P. Effect of exercise training on skeletal muscle histology and metabolism in peripheral arterial disease. *J. Appl. Physiol.* **1996**, *81*, 780–788. [CrossRef]
66. Kirkendall, D.T.; Garrett, W.E., Jr. The effects of aging and training on skeletal muscle. *Am. J. Sports Med.* **1998**, *26*, 598–602. [CrossRef]
67. Miljkovic, N.; Lim, J.Y.; Miljkovic, I.; Frontera, W.R. Aging of skeletal muscle fibers. *Ann. Rehabil. Med.* **2015**, *39*, 155–162. [CrossRef]
68. Wilson, J.M.; Loenneke, J.P.; Jo, E.; Wilson, G.J.; Zourdos, M.C.; Kim, J.S. The effects of endurance, strength, and power training on muscle fiber type shifting. *J. Strength Cond. Res.* **2012**, *26*, 1724–1729. [CrossRef]

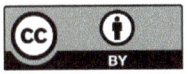

© 2020 by the authors. Licensee MDPI, Basel, Switzerland. This article is an open access article distributed under the terms and conditions of the Creative Commons Attribution (CC BY) license (http://creativecommons.org/licenses/by/4.0/).

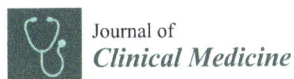 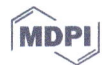

Article

Comparison of Three Nutritional Screening Tools with the New Glim Criteria for Malnutrition and Association with Sarcopenia in Hospitalized Older Patients

Francesco Bellanti [1,*], Aurelio Lo Buglio [1], Stefano Quiete [1], Giuseppe Pellegrino [1], Michał Dobrakowski [2], Aleksandra Kasperczyk [2], Sławomir Kasperczyk [2] and Gianluigi Vendemiale [1]

[1] Department of Medical and Surgical Sciences, University of Foggia, viale Pinto 1, 71122 Foggia, Italy; aurelio.lobuglio@unifg.it (A.L.B.); stefanoquiete@gmail.com (S.Q.); giuseppe_pellegrino.539013@unifg.it (G.P.); gianluigi.vendemiale@unifg.it (G.V.)
[2] Department of Biochemistry, Faculty of Medical Sciences in Zabrze, Medical University of Silesia in Katowice, Jordana 19, 41-808 Zabrze, Poland; michal.dobrakowski@poczta.fm (M.D.); olakasp@poczta.onet.pl (A.K.); kaslav@mp.pl (S.K.)
* Correspondence: francesco.bellanti@unifg.it

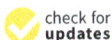

Received: 25 May 2020; Accepted: 16 June 2020; Published: 17 June 2020

Abstract: The integrated assessment of nutritional status and presence of sarcopenia would help improve clinical outcomes of in-hospital aged patients. We compared three common nutritional screening tools with the new Global Leadership Initiative on Malnutrition (GLIM) diagnostic criteria among hospitalized older patients. To this, 152 older patients were assessed consecutively at hospital admission by the Malnutrition Universal Screening Tool (MUST), the Subjective Global Assessment (SGA), and the Nutritional Risk Screening 2002 (NRS-2002). A 46% prevalence of malnutrition was reported according to GLIM. Sensitivity was 64%, 96% and 47%, and specificity was 82%, 15% and 76% with the MUST, SGA, and NRS-2002, respectively. The concordance with GLIM criteria was 89%, 53% and 62% for the MUST, SGA, and NRS-2002, respectively. All the screening tools had a moderate value to diagnose malnutrition. Moreover, patients at high nutritional risk by MUST were more likely to present with sarcopenia than those at low risk (OR 2.5, CI 1.3-3.6). To conclude, MUST is better than SGA and NRS-2002 at detecting malnutrition in hospitalized older patients diagnosed by the new GLIM criteria. Furthermore, hospitalized older patients at high risk of malnutrition according to MUST are at high risk of presenting with sarcopenia. Nutritional status should be determined by MUST in older patients at hospital admission, followed by both GLIM and the European Working Group on Sarcopenia in Older People (EWGSOP2) assessment.

Keywords: nutritional status; sarcopenia; nutritional screening tools; hospitalized older patients

1. Introduction

The average population age is increasing in developed countries, causing a rise in older subjects with consequently greater need of hospitalization [1]. In such scenario, the association between hospitalization and malnutrition is increasingly reported, with a negative impact on treatment response, functional recovery, hospital length-of-stay and costs, and quality of life [2,3]. Hospitalization is also linked to loss of muscle mass and strength, which define sarcopenia [4]. Malnutrition is strongly associated with sarcopenia, and the presence of both conditions is related to several adverse outcomes [5]. The concomitant occurrence of malnutrition and sarcopenia is defined as malnutrition-sarcopenia syndrome (MSS), which represents a prognostic factor for hospitalized older adults [6]. The integrated assessment of nutritional status and presence of sarcopenia would help improve clinical outcomes of such patients.

Diagnosis of malnutrition or risk of malnutrition requires a comprehensive nutritional assessment, which is frequently difficult to perform on all in-hospital patients due to both time and financial restraints [7]. To overcome this limitation, the Global Leadership Initiative on Malnutrition (GLIM) recommends a two-step model in which diagnosis assessment is preceded by risk screening using any validated tool [8]. Nevertheless, despite several tools for rapid identification of malnutrition in older adults [9], patients are not consistently screened for nutritional status at hospital admission [10,11].

The Mini Nutritional Assessment (MNA) is considered one of the most validated tools for the identification of malnutrition or risk of malnutrition, and it is particularly used in older people [12–14]. However, the MNA has disadvantages such as subjective questions unsuitable to hospitalized older people, inability to be used in patients with cognitive impairment, and 10 to 15 min to be performed [7,15]. Several nutritional screening tools have been applied to rapidly identify malnutrition in older patients in hospital settings, and each present with improvements and weaknesses [7]. Very recently, a systematic review evaluated the available studies which considered malnutrition and sarcopenia simultaneously, resulting in methodological unpredictability [16].

First, this study aimed to compare different tools for nutritional screening, such as the Malnutrition Universal Screening Tool (MUST), the Subjective Global Assessment (SGA), and the Nutritional Risk Screening 2002 (NRS-2002) in hospitalized older patients, in order to define their sensitivity, specificity, and rapidity with respect to the GLIM consensus, chosen as the reference method. Furthermore, the present investigation evaluated the association between the alteration of nutritional status identified by these tools and the presence of sarcopenia.

2. Experimental Section

2.1. Study Design and Participants

We collected and analyzed data from older patients hospitalized at the Internal and Aging Medicine clinic of the "Ospedali Riuniti", a teaching hospital in Foggia (Italy). We recruited consecutive patients aged 65 years or older, admitted to our ward from March 2019 to February 2020. Frequency of the main causes for hospital admission is reported in Table 1. The exclusion criteria were the following: dysphagia, active cancer, severe cognitive impairment (assessed with a Mini Mental State Examination score ≤ 9 points), inability to comply with the study protocol or to provide written informed consent. Further exclusion criteria were chronic bedridden conditions, physical handicap, severe neuromuscular disease, and use of drugs affecting body composition (such as glucocorticoids, statins, active vitamin D metabolites, anabolic steroids, selective estrogen receptor modulators). The study was approved by our Institutional Review Board at the Ospedali Riuniti in Foggia and performed according to the Declaration of Helsinki. All patients gave written informed consent.

2.2. Biochemical Analysis, Anthropometric Measurements and Body Composition Evaluation

A blood sample was taken at the time of admission for the determination of hemoglobin (Hb) and lymphocytes in whole blood, and total proteins, albumin, total cholesterol, and iron in the serum. Height, body weight, and waist, arm, and hip circumference, as well as tricipital, bicipital, subscapular, and supra-iliac skinfold thicknesses were measured according to standardized procedures. Body mass index (BMI) was calculated as the ratio between weight in kilograms and the square of height in meters. Body composition was assessed within 24 h from admission by bioelectrical impedance using a BIA 101-F device (Akern/RJL, Florence, Italy), as previously reported [17]. The BIA analyzer underwent calibration by the manufacturer, and the measurements were validated according to previously published equations [18].

Table 1. Baseline demographic, clinical, anthropometric, and biochemical characteristics of patients, stratified according to the Global Leadership Initiative on Malnutrition consensus.

Characteristic	No Malnutrition $n = 82$ (54%)	Malnutrition $n = 70$ (46%)	p
Age (years)	77.8 ± 7.8	78.7 ± 7.3	0.4664
Genre M/F (n, %)	47/35 (57/43)	40/30 (57/43)	0.9827
Education (n, %)			
None	0 (0)	0 (0)	
Primary School	45 (55)	40 (57)	
Secondary School	17 (21)	17 (24)	0.8812
High School	17 (21)	10 (14)	
University	3 (3)	3 (5)	
Co-morbidities > 3 (n, %)	37 (45)	32 (46)	0.9417
MMSE score	21.4 ± 6.6	19.9 ± 5.8	0.1420
Weight (kg)	76.7 ± 14.2	71.8 ± 16.0	**0.0473**
Height (m)	1.63 ± 0.1	1.62 ± 0.08	0.5021
BMI (kg/m^2)	28.9 ± 5.9	27.4 ± 5.5	0.1091
Arm circumference (cm)	28.6 ± 4.0	27.2 ± 4.4	**0.0417**
Waist circumference (cm)	104.2 ± 10.7	99.7 ± 13.0	**0.0206**
Hip circumference (cm)	100.6 ± 10.5	99.2 ± 11.6	0.4159
Waist-to-Hip ratio	1.04 ± 0.11	1.00 ± 0.08	**0.0126**
Tricipital skinfold thickness (cm)	13.2 ± 4.7	12.6 ± 5.4	0.4651
Bicipital skinfold thickness (cm)	11.5 ± 4.6	9.8 ± 5.7	**0.0437**
Subscapular skinfold thickness (cm)	16.5 ± 6.2	14.0 ± 5.2	**0.0085**
Supra-iliac skinfold thickness (cm)	18.4 ± 7.0	13.7 ± 5.2	**<0.0001**
Total proteins (g/dL)	6.4 ± 0.6	6.0 ± 0.8	**0.0006**
Albumin (g/dL)	3.3 ± 0.5	3.1 ± 0.6	**0.0265**
Total Cholesterol (mg/dL)	147 ± 36	116 ± 52	**<0.0001**
Lymphocytes (n × 10^3/mm^3)	1.9 ± 2.5	2.6 ± 3.9	0.1837
Hemoglobin (g/dL)	11.8 ± 2.9	9.6 ± 1.9	**<0.0001**
Iron (mg/dL)	53.4 ± 32.7	47.3 ± 36.0	0.0839

Data are expressed as mean ± SD (continuous variables) or frequency and percentage (categorical variables). Statistical differences were assessed by Student's t-test (continuous variables) or by Pearson's Chi-squared test and Fisher's exact test (categorical variables). M, male; F, female; MMSE, Mini-Mental State Examination. Bold: statistically significant.

2.3. Tools for Screening of Nutritional Status

The MUST, SGA, and NRS-2002 tools were used for nutritional screening, and the time (in seconds) required to complete each test was recorded. To avoid any interindividual variance, all tools were performed by an experienced operator.

The MUST includes three clinical parameters and rates each parameter as 0, 1 or 2 as follows: (a) BMI > 20 kg/m^2 = 0; 18.5–20.0 kg/m^2 = 1; <18.5 kg/m^2 = 2; (b) weight loss in the past 3–6 months < 5% = 0; 5–10% = 1; >10% = 2; (c) acute disease: absent = 0; if present = 2. Overall risk of malnutrition is established as follows: 0 = low risk; 1 = medium risk; 2 = high risk [19].

The SGA questionnaire includes patient history (weight loss, changes in dietary intake, gastrointestinal symptoms and functional capacity), physical examination (muscle, subcutaneous fat, sacral and ankle edema, ascites) and the clinician's overall judgment of the patient status ((a) well nourished; (b) suspected malnourished or moderately malnourished; (c) severely malnourished) [20].

The NRS-2002 consists of a nutritional score and a severity of disease score and an age adjustment for patients aged > 70 years (+1). Nutritional score: weight loss 45% in 3 months or food intake below 50–75% in the preceding week = 1; weight loss 45% in 2 months or BMI 18.5–20.5 kg/m^2 and impaired general condition or food intake 25–60% in the preceding week = 2; weight loss 45% in 1 months or >15% in 3 months or BMI < 18.5 kg/m^2 and impaired general condition or food intake 0–25% in the preceding week = 3. Severity of disease score: hip fracture, chronic patients with acute complications = 1; major abdominal surgery, stroke, severe pneumonia, hematological malignancies = 2; head injury, bone marrow transplantation, intensive care patients with APACHE > 10 = 3. NRS-2002 score is the total of the nutritional score, severity of disease score and age adjustment. Patients are classified at no risk = 0, low risk = 0–1, medium risk = 3–4, and high risk = ≥ 5 [21].

2.4. Diagnostic Criteria for Malnutrition and Sarcopenia

Following the new GLIM diagnostic criteria, malnutrition was diagnosed when the patients met 1 phenotypic criterion (among non-volitional weight loss, low body mass index, and reduced muscle mass) and 1 etiologic criterion (among reduced food intake or assimilation, and disease burden/inflammatory condition), according to Table 2 [8].

Table 2. Bioelectrical impedance analysis parameters in patients stratified according to the Global Leadership Initiative on Malnutrition consensus.

Parameter	No Malnutrition $n = 82$ (54%)	Malnutrition $n = 70$ (46%)	p
Body Cell Mass (kg)	18.8 ± 6.6	10.4 ± 9.2	**<0.0001**
Total Body Water (L)	37.5 ± 5.5	41.2 ± 9.4	**0.003**
Extracellular water (L)	22.4 ± 3.9	28.9 ± 10.1	**<0.0001**
Fat-Free Mass (%)	63.2 ± 9.4	58.2 ± 11.4	**0.0035**
Fat Mass (%)	36.8 ± 9.4	41.8 ± 11.4	**0.0035**
Skeletal Muscle Index	8.2 ± 1.3	7.3 ± 1.9	**0.0007**
Appendicular Skeletal Muscle Mass (kg)	19.4 ± 3.7	16.5 ± 4.4	**<0.0001**
Appendicular Skeletal Muscle Mass (kg/m^2)	7.32 ± 2.6	6.30 ± 2.0	**0.0083**

Data are expressed as mean ± SD. Statistical differences were assessed by Student's t-test. Bold: statistically significant.

Sarcopenia was diagnosed on admission according to the European Working Group on Sarcopenia in Older People updated recommendation (EWGSOP2) [22]. Particularly, sarcopenia was first assessed by gait speed or grip strength, and then, confirmed in subjects presenting with a relative skeletal muscle index (RSMI) < 7.25 kg/m^2 (men) or <5.67 kg/m^2 (women).

2.5. Statistical Analysis

Data were expressed as mean ± standard deviation of the mean (SDM) for quantitative variables, and as count and percentages for qualitative values. Gaussian distribution of the samples was evaluated by the Kolgomorov–Smirnov test. The significance of differences between 2 groups was assessed by Student's t-test (continuous variables) or in contingency tables by Pearson's Chi-squared test and Fisher's exact test (categorical variables). The significance of differences between more than 2 groups was assessed by the one-way analysis of variance (ANOVA) after ascertaining normality by the Kolgomorov–Smirnov test; Tukey–Kramer was applied as post hoc test. To determine the diagnostic concordance between the three screening tools and the GLIM diagnostic criteria for malnutrition, Cohen's statistic was calculated. The coefficient reflects the consistency of qualitative variables: = 1 indicates complete consistency between the variables, and = 0 indicates no consistency among the variables. Positive likelihood ratios and negative likelihood ratios were calculated for all three tools. Sensitivity and specificity values for the three nutritional screening tools with the GLIM diagnostic criteria for malnutrition were calculated. To determine the diagnostic concordance, consistency, accuracy, likelihood ratio, sensitivity, and specificity, medium and high-risk categories for the three nutritional assessment tools were combined, according to previous publications [23,24]. Receiver operating characteristic (ROC) curves of the three screening tools were also used to evaluate the ability to accurately distinguish malnourished patients. The Youden Index was calculated as (sensitivity + specificity) − 1 for each cut-off point. The odds ratio (OR) and the 95% confidence interval (CI) were calculated. Univariate binary logistic regression analysis was used to analyze the association between nutritional status and the presence of sarcopenia.

All tests were 2-sided, and p values <0.05 were considered statistically significant. Statistical analysis was performed with the Statistical Package for Social Sciences version 23.0 (SPSS, Inc., Chicago, IL, USA) and the package GraphPad Prism 6.0 for Windows (GraphPad Software, Inc., San Diego, CA, USA).

3. Results

3.1. Patients Characteristics

In total, 689 consecutive patients were evaluated for enrolment; of these, 152 met the inclusion criteria and did not present any of the exclusion criteria. According to the GLIM criteria, malnutrition was diagnosed in 70 patients (46%) at admission (Figure 1, Supplementary Table S3).

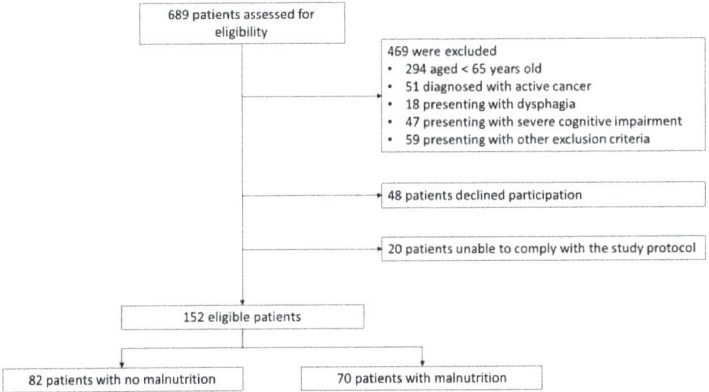

Figure 1. Participant flowchart. Other exclusion criteria were chronic bedridden conditions, physical handicap, severe neuromuscular disease, and use of drugs affecting body composition (such as glucocorticoids, statins, active vitamin D metabolites, anabolic steroids, selective estrogen receptor modulators). Diagnosis of malnutrition was performed according to the new criteria of the Global Leadership Initiative on Malnutrition.

Baseline demographic, clinical, anthropometric, and biochemical characteristics of patients presenting with malnutrition or not malnourished are represented in Table 1. Of note, we reported lower weight, arm and waist circumference, waist-to-hip ratio, bicipital, subscapular and supra-iliac skinfold thickness, serum total proteins, serum albumin, serum total cholesterol and blood hemoglobin in the group of patients with malnutrition with respect to the group with no malnutrition.

Interestingly, significant differences in body composition parameters were observed between the two groups (Table 2). In detail, patients with malnutrition were observed with reduced Body Cell Mass, Fat-Free Mass, Skeletal Muscle Index and Appendicular Skeletal Muscle Mass, and increased Total Body Water, Extracellular Water and Fat Mass as compared with not malnourished patients.

3.2. Rapidity, Sensitivity, Specificity, Accuracy, and Diagnostic Value of Nutritional Screening Tools

All patients were subjected to three nutritional screening tools (MUST, SGA, and NRS-2002) at admission. As shown in Figure 2, MUST was the less rapid tool as compared to SGA and NRS-2002.

The MUST misclassified 18%, the SGA 47%, and the NRS-2002 38% of patients. Sensitivity was 64.3% with the MUST, 95.7% with the SGA, and 47.1% with the NRS-2002, while specificity was 81.7%, 14.6% and 75.6% with the MUST, SGA and NRS-2002, respectively; MUST accuracy was 73.7%, while accuracy resulted 52% for SGA and 62.5% for NRS-2002 (Table 3).

Finally, the area under the curve (AUC) calculated by the ROC indicated that all three screening tools had a moderate value to diagnose malnutrition in hospitalized older patient (AUC of MUST, SGA, and NRS-2002 were found to be 0.80, 0.77 and 0.69, respectively; Figure 3). The highest Youden indexes were 0.461 for a MUST score ≥ 0.5 (sensitivity 0.643, specificity 0.818), 0.461 for a SGA score ≥ 8.5 (sensitivity 0.643, specificity 0.818), and 0.257 for a NRS-2002 score ≥ 2.5 (sensitivity 0.464, specificity 0.758).

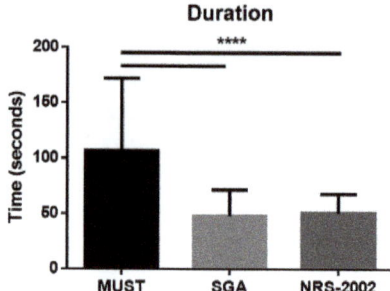

Figure 2. Duration of the nutritional screening tools (time expressed in seconds), performed in all the 152 hospitalized patients enrolled in this study. Data are expressed as mean ± SD. Statistical differences were assessed by one-way ANOVA and Tukey as post hoc test. MUST, Malnutrition Universal Screening Tool; SGA, Subjective Global Assessment; NRS-2002, Nutritional Risk Screening 2002. ****: $p < 0.0001$ vs. MUST.

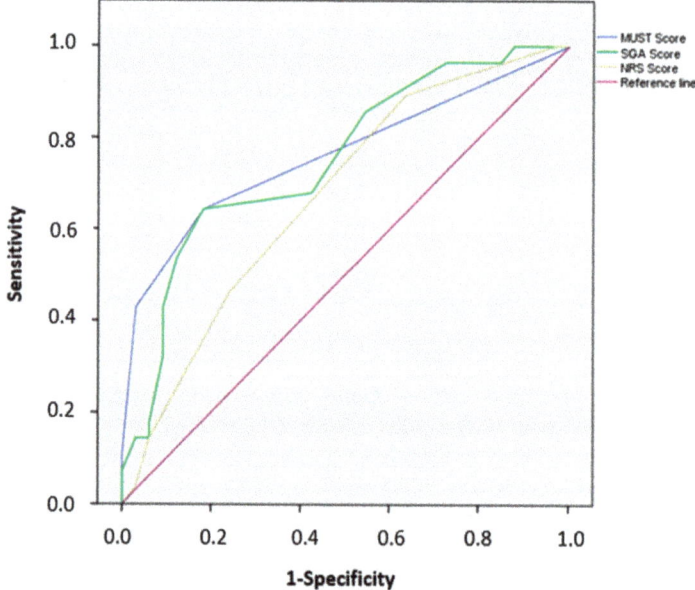

Figure 3. Receiver Operating Characteristic (ROC) curve for prediction of malnutrition based on the score obtained by the Malnutrition Universal Screening Tool (MUST, blue line), the Subjective Global Assessment (SGA, green line), and the Nutritional Risk Screening 2002 (NRS-2002, yellow line).

3.3. Malnutrition and Sarcopenia

According to the EWGSOP2 recommendation, sarcopenia was diagnosed in 77 (50.6%) patients; of these, 45 (64.3%) were also diagnosed with malnutrition according to the GLIM criteria, and 32 (39.0%) were not malnourished ($X_2 = 9.641$, $p = 0.0019$). We did not find any difference between genders with respect to the diagnosis of sarcopenia. Malnutrition diagnosed according to the GLIM criteria increased the risk of presenting with sarcopenia 2.7-fold (95% CI 1.4–4.9, $p = 0.0029$). There was a significant association between sarcopenia and nutritional status at high risk of malnutrition detected by MUST, but not by other nutritional screening tools (Table 4).

Table 3. Statistical comparison of nutritional diagnosis and screening tools values at hospital admission.

GLIM	MUST			SGA			NRS-2002		
	Low Risk	Medium/High Risk	Total	Well Nourished	Moderately/Severely Malnourished	Total	Low Risk	Medium/High Risk	Total
Well nourished	67	15	82	12	70	82	62	20	82
Malnutrition	25	45	70	3	67	70	37	33	70
Total	92	60	152	15	137	152	99	53	152
	%	95% CI		%	95% CI		%	95% CI	
Sensitivity	64.3	51.9–75.4		95.7	88.0–99.1		47.1	35.1–59.4	
Specificity	81.7	71.6–89.3		14.6	7.8–24.1		75.6	64.9–84.4	
Positive predictive value	75.0	62.1–85.3		48.9	40.3–57.6		62.3	47.9–75.2	
Negative predictive value	72.8	62.5 81.6		80.0	51.9–95.7		62.6	52.3–72.1	
Accuracy	73.7	66.7–80.7		52.0	44.1–59.9		62.5	54.8–70.2	
	0.89			0.53			0.62		

Malnutrition Universal Screening Tool (MUST), Subjective Global Assessment (SGA) and Nutritional Risk Screening 2002 (NRS-2002) versus Global Leadership Initiative on Malnutrition (GLIM) criteria. CI, confidence interval; statistic, percent of agreement.

Table 4. Association between nutritional status and presence of sarcopenia on admission.

Tool	Outcome	No Sarcopenia n (%)	Sarcopenia n (%)	OR (95% CI)	p
GLIM	No malnutrition	50 (61.0)	32 (39.0)	1	
	Malnutrition	25 (35.7)	45 (64.3)	2.7 (1.4–4.9)	**0.0029**
MUST	Low risk	60 (65.2)	32 (34.8)	1	
	Medium risk	8 (34.8)	15 (65.2)	0.6 (0.3–1.2)	0.459
	High risk	7 (18.9)	30 (81.1)	2.5 (1.3–3.6)	**0.0068**
SGA	Well nourished	9 (60.0)	6 (40.0)	1	
	Moderately malnourished	44 (51.8)	41 (48.2)	1.4 (0.3–4.1)	0.516
	Severely malnourished	22 (42.3)	30 (57.7)	2.7 (0.2–9.4)	0.414
NRS-2002	Low risk	53 (53.5)	46 (46.5)	1	
	Medium risk	12 (57.1)	9 (42.9)	0.1 (0.0–1.1)	0.059
	High risk	16 (47.0)	18 (53.0)	1.2 (0.2–5.8)	0.835

Incidence and odds ratio (OR; 95% confidence interval, CI), adjusted for age, gender, and education, between Global Leadership Initiative on Malnutrition (GLIM) diagnosis of malnutrition or nutritional screening tools and presence of sarcopenia. MUST, Malnutrition Universal Screening Tool; SGA, Subjective Global Assessment; NRS-2002, Nutritional Risk Screening 2002. Bold: statistically significant.

4. Discussion

This is the first study which compared the diagnostic reliability of different nutritional screening tools to the GLIM criteria in a population of hospitalized older patients. According to the GLIM framework, 46% of patients were identified as malnourished when using combinations of two criteria. This prevalence could be apparently high as compared with previous studies which used the GLIM criteria for the diagnosis of malnutrition [5,25–27]. Nevertheless, this investigation focused on a special population that presented with a high prevalence of etiologic GLIM criteria for malnutrition. Indeed, the prevalence of malnutrition is close to 50% when diagnosed in critically ill patients [28]. Furthermore, even though this study was not designed to validate the diagnosis of malnutrition in hospitalized older subjects according to the GLIM consensus, our data show that patients with malnutrition presented with alterations in anthropometry, biochemical parameters, and bioelectrical impedance analysis results, compatible with their impaired nutritional status.

Nutritional screening tools detect features associated with alterations of nutritional status to distinguish persons presenting with risk of malnutrition. These tools play an important role in providing a standardized and systematic approach to identifying malnutrition [29]. Considering the utility of such tools in a daily routine, they should be easy to use, rapid, sensitive, and specific, to be included in a defined clinical protocol [30]. In this study, we compared the MUST, created to identify malnutrition in care settings [31]; the SGA, considered by several Authors as the most validated tool in hospital settings [25]; the NRS-2002, a tool used in hospital settings to detect patients who would benefit from nutritional therapy [21]. We first considered the rapidity of each tool in our special population, concluding that the MUST requires longer time with respect to both SGA and NRS-2002. Medium and high nutritional risk was 39.5% by MUST, 90.1% by SGA, and 34.9% by NRS-2002, compared to 46% of patients being malnourished by GLIM consensus. Concordance of the three screening tools with respect to GLIM criteria resulted dissimilar. These data are similar to other comparisons between different nutritional screening tools applied to hospitalized older patients [32]. Overall, the three screening tools misclassified 11–47% of patients, the MUST having the highest concordance with GLIM framework compared with SGA and NRS-2002. Furthermore, the MUST showed higher specificity than SGA and NRS-2002, meaning that more hospitalized older patients presenting with no malnutrition were correctly identified as at a low risk of malnutrition than malnourished patients being at high risk. On the contrary, the SGA showed higher sensitivity with respect to MUST and NRS-2002, properly identifying hospitalized older patients with malnutrition as at high risk than well-nourished ones at low risk. A previous study analyzed the validity of GLIM criteria with respect to SGA, describing a higher sensitivity when weight loss was combined with high C-reactive protein values, and a higher specificity with the combination of a low BMI and low food intake [25]. Both reduced food intake and increased C-reactive protein were registered very frequently in our population of hospitalized older patients, however, weight loss was more prevalent than low BMI, partially explaining the high sensitivity (but low specificity) of SGA. Finally, even though the ROC curve showed a moderate value to identify malnutrition by all three nutritional screening tools, MUST was found to have the greatest AUC with respect to SGA and NRS-2002. Based on the results of this study, the time spared in the administration of SGA or NRS-2002 is not well matched with accuracy or diagnostic value of these tools in hospitalized older patients. Further investigations are needed to confirm this observation.

This study reported a significant prevalence of sarcopenia diagnosed with the EWGSOP2 criteria, with malnutrition diagnosed with the GLIM criteria (64.3%). Malnutrition is considered as a determinant factor for the onset of sarcopenia, and the presence of malnutrition-sarcopenia syndrome (MSS) is associated with a four times higher risk of mortality in hospitalized older patients [6]. A recent longitudinal study investigated the incidence of sarcopenia (identified through the EWGSOP2 criteria) during a four-year follow-up in community-dwelling older individuals diagnosed with malnutrition at baseline according to both the European Society of Clinical Nutrition and Metabolism (ESPEN) and the GLIM criteria [5]. This report registered a threefold higher risk of developing sarcopenia in malnourished patients based on the GLIM [5]. Even though the present investigation is not designed as a prospective longitudinal study, our analysis shows that the risk of MSS is almost threefold in hospitalized older patients presenting with malnutrition at admission. Moreover, amongst the three screening tools applied, MUST is the only to identify older hospitalized patients at high risk of malnutrition with a significant 2.5 times higher risk of having MSS.

The strengths of this study consist in the use of standardized diagnostic criteria for the diagnosis of malnutrition or sarcopenia, and a rigorous statistical analysis. Nevertheless, this study presents several main limitations. First, it is a single center study with a small sample size, which restricted the subgroup analysis. Moreover, this study did not investigate the association between nutritional status and the underlying disease that led to hospitalization. The three nutritional screening tools were not compared with MNA, because of biased questions inappropriate to hospitalized older people even with mild or moderate cognitive impairment, and longer time to be performed. Muscle mass was evaluated by bioelectrical impedance, which could be influenced by fluid distribution changes. A further limitation of the study is that information about the dietary regimens or the pharmacological treatments potentially affecting the nutritional status of single participants was not registered. Moreover, in our study, we did not estimate other confounding factors, such as socioeconomic and family status, which could partially impact the results.

In conclusion, the present study reports a prevalence of malnutrition of 46% in hospitalized older patients, according to the GLIM framework criteria. The comparison of three different nutritional screening tools indicates that MUST is better at detecting malnutrition in hospitalized older patients diagnosed by the new GLIM criteria despite being less rapid, with respect to SGA and NRS-2002. Furthermore, there is a significant association between the presence of sarcopenia in hospitalized older patients at high risk of malnutrition according to MUST. This evidence confirms the importance of routine nutritional assessment in hospitalized older patients. We suggest that nutritional status should be determined by MUST in older patients at hospital admission, followed by both GLIM and EWGSOP2 assessment. The choice of this diagnostic tool could allow on-time nutritional intervention, thus preventing the worsening of negative caloric balance and loss of muscle mass. Furthermore, an early and valuable recognition of malnutrition and sarcopenia would be beneficial to plan individualized treatment during hospitalization and at discharge.

Supplementary Materials: The following are available online at http://www.mdpi.com/2077-0383/9/6/1898/s1, Table S1: Main causes for hospital admission in patients stratified according to the Global Leadership Initiative on Malnutrition consensus. Table S2: Assessment criteria of malnutrition according to the Global Leader Initiative on Malnutrition (GLIM). Table S3: Prevalence of criteria of the Global Leader Initiative on Malnutrition (GLIM) registered in the study population.

Author Contributions: Conceptualization, F.B. and A.L.B.; methodology, F.B.; validation, F.B., A.L.B., S.Q., and G.P.; formal analysis, F.B., M.D., A.K. and S.K.; investigation, F.B., A.L.B., S.Q., G.P., M.D., A.K., and S.K.; resources, G.V.; data curation, F.B. and G.V.; writing—original draft preparation, F.B.; writing—review and editing, A.L.B., M.D., A.K., S.K. and G.V.; supervision, S.K. and G.V.; project administration, F.B. and G.V. All authors have read and agreed to the published version of the manuscript.

Funding: This research received no external funding.

Acknowledgments: Authors are grateful to Martina Valentino, Debora Testa and Emma Finamore for their technical assistance and support.

Conflicts of Interest: The authors declare no conflict of interest.

References

1. Wittenberg, R.; Sharpin, L.; McCormick, B.; Hurst, J. The ageing society and emergency hospital admissions. *Health Policy* **2017**, *121*, 923–928. [CrossRef]
2. Lim, S.L.; Ong, K.C.; Chan, Y.H.; Loke, W.C.; Ferguson, M.; Daniels, L. Malnutrition and its impact on cost of hospitalization, length of stay, readmission and 3-year mortality. *Clin. Nutr.* **2012**, *31*, 345–350. [CrossRef]
3. Ruiz, A.J.; Buitrago, G.; Rodriguez, N.; Gomez, G.; Sulo, S.; Gomez, C.; Partridge, J.; Misas, J.; Dennis, R.; Alba, M.J.; et al. Clinical and economic outcomes associated with malnutrition in hospitalized patients. *Clin. Nutr.* **2019**, *38*, 1310–1316. [CrossRef]
4. Bellanti, F.; Buglio, A.L.; De Stasio, E.; di Bello, G.; Tamborra, R.; Dobrakowski, M.; Kasperczyk, A.; Kasperczyk, S.; Vendemiale, G. An open-label, single-center pilot study to test the effects of an amino acid mixture in older patients admitted to internal medicine wards. *Nutrition* **2020**, *69*, 110588. [CrossRef]
5. Beaudart, C.; Sanchez-Rodriguez, D.; Locquet, M.; Reginster, J.Y.; Lengele, L.; Bruyere, O. Malnutrition as a Strong Predictor of the Onset of Sarcopenia. *Nutrients* **2019**, *11*, 2883. [CrossRef] [PubMed]
6. Hu, X.; Zhang, L.; Wang, H.; Hao, Q.; Dong, B.; Yang, M. Malnutrition-sarcopenia syndrome predicts mortality in hospitalized older patients. *Sci. Rep.* **2017**, *7*, 3171. [CrossRef] [PubMed]
7. Dent, E.; Hoogendijk, E.O.; Visvanathan, R.; Wright, O.R.L. Malnutrition Screening and Assessment in Hospitalised Older People: A Review. *J. Nutr. Health Aging* **2019**, *23*, 431–441. [CrossRef] [PubMed]
8. Cederholm, T.; Jensen, G.L.; Correia, M.I.T.D.; Gonzalez, M.C.; Fukushima, R.; Higashiguchi, T.; Baptista, G.; Barazzoni, R.; Blaauw, R.; Coats, A.J.S.; et al. GLIM criteria for the diagnosis of malnutrition—A consensus report from the global clinical nutrition community. *J. Cachexia Sarcopenia Muscle* **2019**, *10*, 207–217. [CrossRef]
9. Power, L.; Mullally, D.; Gibney, E.R.; Clarke, M.; Visser, M.; Volkert, D.; Bardon, L.; de van der Schueren, M.A.E.; Corish, C.A. A review of the validity of malnutrition screening tools used in older adults in community and healthcare settings—A MaNuEL study. *Clin. Nutr. ESPEN* **2018**, *24*, 1–13. [CrossRef]
10. Campbell, S.E.; Avenell, A.; Walker, A.E. Assessment of nutritional status in hospital in-patients. *QJM* **2002**, *95*, 83–87. [CrossRef] [PubMed]
11. Frank, M.; Sivagnanaratnam, A.; Bernstein, J. Nutritional assessment in elderly care: A MUST! *BMJ Qual. Improv. Rep.* **2015**, *4*, u204810.w2031. [CrossRef]
12. Guigoz, Y. The Mini Nutritional Assessment (MNA) review of the literature–What does it tell us? *J. Nutr. Health Aging* **2006**, *10*, 466–485. [PubMed]
13. Cereda, E. Mini nutritional assessment. *Curr. Opin. Clin. Nutr. Metab Care* **2012**, *15*, 29–41. [CrossRef] [PubMed]
14. Ghazi, L.; Fereshtehnejad, S.M.; Abbasi, F.S.; Sadeghi, M.; Shahidi, G.A.; Lokk, J. Mini Nutritional Assessment (MNA) is Rather a Reliable and Valid Instrument to Assess Nutritional Status in Iranian Healthy Adults and Elderly with a Chronic Disease. *Ecol. Food Nutr.* **2015**, *54*, 342–357. [CrossRef]
15. Vellas, B.; Villars, H.; Abellan, G.; Soto, M.E.; Rolland, Y.; Guigoz, Y.; Morley, J.E.; Chumlea, W.; Salva, A.; Rubenstein, L.Z.; et al. Overview of the MNA–Its history and challenges. *J. Nutr. Health Aging* **2006**, *10*, 456–463. [PubMed]
16. Juby, A.G.; Mager, D.R. A review of nutrition screening tools used to assess the malnutrition-sarcopenia syndrome (MSS) in the older adult. *Clin. Nutr. ESPEN* **2019**, *32*, 8–15. [CrossRef] [PubMed]
17. Buglio, A.L.; Bellanti, F.; Capurso, C.; Paglia, A.; Vendemiale, G. Adherence to Mediterranean Diet, Malnutrition, Length of Stay and Mortality in Elderly Patients Hospitalized in Internal Medicine Wards. *Nutrients* **2019**, *11*, 790. [CrossRef]

18. Scafoglieri, A.; Clarys, J.P.; Bauer, J.M.; Verlaan, S.; Van, M.L.; Vantieghem, S.; Cederholm, T.; Sieber, C.C.; Mets, T.; Bautmans, I. Predicting appendicular lean and fat mass with bioelectrical impedance analysis in older adults with physical function decline—The PROVIDE study. *Clin. Nutr.* **2017**, *36*, 869–875. [CrossRef]
19. Elia, M. *Screening for Malnutrition: A Multidisciplinary Responsibility. Development and Use of the Malnutrition Universal Screening Tool ('MUST') for Adults*; BAPEN: Redditch, UK, 2003.
20. Detsky, A.S.; McLaughlin, J.R.; Baker, J.P.; Johnston, N.; Whittaker, S.; Mendelson, R.A.; Jeejeebhoy, K.N. What is subjective global assessment of nutritional status? *JPEN J. Parenter. Enter. Nutr.* **1987**, *11*, 8–13. [CrossRef]
21. Kondrup, J.; Rasmussen, H.H.; Hamberg, O.; Stanga, Z. Nutritional risk screening (NRS 2002): A new method based on an analysis of controlled clinical trials. *Clin. Nutr.* **2003**, *22*, 321–336. [CrossRef]
22. Cruz-Jentoft, A.J.; Bahat, G.; Bauer, J.; Boirie, Y.; Bruyere, O.; Cederholm, T.; Cooper, C.; Landi, F.; Rolland, Y.; Sayer, A.A.; et al. Sarcopenia: Revised European consensus on definition and diagnosis. *Age Ageing* **2019**, *48*, 16–31. [CrossRef] [PubMed]
23. Kyle, U.G.; Kossovsky, M.P.; Karsegard, V.L.; Pichard, C. Comparison of tools for nutritional assessment and screening at hospital admission: A population study. *Clin. Nutr.* **2006**, *25*, 409–417. [CrossRef]
24. Ye, X.J.; Ji, Y.B.; Ma, B.W.; Huang, D.D.; Chen, W.Z.; Pan, Z.Y.; Shen, X.; Zhuang, C.L.; Yu, Z. Comparison of three common nutritional screening tools with the new European Society for Clinical Nutrition and Metabolism (ESPEN) criteria for malnutrition among patients with geriatric gastrointestinal cancer: A prospective study in China. *BMJ Open* **2018**, *8*, e019750. [CrossRef]
25. Allard, J.P.; Keller, H.; Gramlich, L.; Jeejeebhoy, K.N.; Laporte, M.; Duerksen, D.R. GLIM criteria has fair sensitivity and specificity for diagnosing malnutrition when using SGA as comparator. *Clin. Nutr.* **2019**. [CrossRef] [PubMed]
26. Yilmaz, M.; Atilla, F.D.; Sahin, F.; Saydam, G. The effect of malnutrition on mortality in hospitalized patients with hematologic malignancy. *Supportive Care Cancer* **2020**, *28*, 1441–1448. [CrossRef]
27. Matsumoto, Y.; Iwai, K.; Namikawa, N.; Matsuda, S.; Wakano, C.; Heya, H.; Yamanaka, M. The relationship between existing nutritional indicators and Global Leadership Initiative on Malnutrition (GLIM) criteria: A one-institution cross-sectional analysis. *Clin. Nutr.* **2020**. [CrossRef]
28. Rattanachaiwong, S.; Zribi, B.; Kagan, I.; Theilla, M.; Heching, M.; Singer, P. Comparison of nutritional screening and diagnostic tools in diagnosis of severe malnutrition in critically ill patients. *Clin. Nutr.* **2020**. [CrossRef] [PubMed]
29. Bauer, J.M.; Kaiser, M.J.; Sieber, C.C. Evaluation of nutritional status in older persons: Nutritional screening and assessment. *Curr. Opin. Clin. Nutr. Metab. Care* **2010**, *13*, 8–13. [CrossRef]
30. Reber, E.; Gomes, F.; Vasiloglou, M.F.; Schuetz, P.; Stanga, Z. Nutritional Risk Screening and Assessment. *J. Clin. Med.* **2019**, *8*, 1065. [CrossRef]
31. Weekes, C.E.; Elia, M.; Emery, P.W. The development, validation and reliability of a nutrition screening tool based on the recommendations of the British Association for Parenteral and Enteral Nutrition (BAPEN). *Clin. Nutr.* **2004**, *23*, 1104–1112.
32. Diekmann, R.; Winning, K.; Uter, W.; Kaiser, M.J.; Sieber, C.C.; Volkert, D.; Bauer, J.M. Screening for malnutrition among nursing home residents—A comparative analysis of the mini nutritional assessment, the nutritional risk screening, and the malnutrition universal screening tool. *J. Nutr. Health Aging* **2013**, *17*, 326–331. [CrossRef] [PubMed]

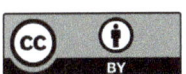

© 2020 by the authors. Licensee MDPI, Basel, Switzerland. This article is an open access article distributed under the terms and conditions of the Creative Commons Attribution (CC BY) license (http://creativecommons.org/licenses/by/4.0/).

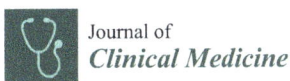

Article

Effects of Physical Exercises and Verbal Stimulation on the Functional Efficiency and Use of Free Time in an Older Population under Institutional Care: A Randomized Controlled Trial

Agnieszka Wiśniowska-Szurlej [1,*], Agnieszka Ćwirlej-Sozańska [1], Natalia Wołoszyn [1], Bernard Sozański [1] and Anna Wilmowska-Pietruszyńska [2]

1 Institute of Health Sciences, Medical College of Rzeszow University, 35-310 Rzeszow, Poland; sozanska@ur.edu.pl (A.Ć.-S.); natalia.woloszyn@op.pl (N.W.); benieks@poczta.onet.pl (B.S.)
2 Faculty of Medicine, Lazarski University, 02-662 Warsaw, Poland; anna.wilmowska@autograf.pl
* Correspondence: wisniowska@vp.pl; Tel.: +48-604181162

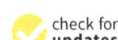

Received: 18 January 2020; Accepted: 6 February 2020; Published: 9 February 2020

Abstract: Older people in institutional care are, for the most part, physically inactive and do not interact with each other or medical staff. Therefore, reducing sedentary behaviour is a new, important, and modifiable lifestyle variable that can improve the health of elderly people. The aim of the project was to assess the degree of improvement in functional performance and the possibility of changing habitual, free time behaviour among elderly people under institutional care by applying physical training with verbal stimulation. The study covered older people, aged 65–85 years, who are living a sedentary lifestyle in care homes in Southeastern Poland. Those who met the eligibility criteria were enrolled in the study and were assigned, at random, to one of four parallel groups: basic exercises ($n = 51$), basic exercises combined with verbal stimulation ($n = 51$), functional exercise training ($n = 51$), and functional exercise training with verbal stimulation ($n = 51$). No statistically significant differences in baseline characteristics were observed across the groups. Data were collected at baseline and at 12 and 24-weeks following the completion of the intervention. In the group with functional exercise training with verbal stimulation, in comparison to the group with basic exercises, the greatest positive short-term impact of intervention was demonstrated in terms of functional fitness (increased by 1.31 points; 95% confidence interval (CI) = 0.93–1.70), gait speed (improved by 0.17 m/s, 95% CI = 0.13–0.22), hand grip strength (by over 4 kg; 95% CI = 2.51–4.95), and upper-limb flexibility (by 10 cm; 95% CI = 5.82–12.65). There was also a significant increase in the level of free-time physical activity and an improvement in the quality of life, especially as expressed in the domain of overall physical functioning. Our study showed that a functional exercise program, combined with verbal stimulation, is effective at improving physical fitness and raising the level of free-time physical activity.

Keywords: sedentary behaviour; aged; exercise; motivation

1. Introduction

In recent years, there has been a slowdown in the demographic development of people in Europe and Poland. At the end of 2017, the number of people aged 65 and older in Poland amounted to six million, of which over 105,000 were covered by institutional care [1,2]. While changes in care and health policies and services have propagated alternative, long-term care methods, around 25% of older people spent the last years of their lives in a care home [3].

A low level of physical activity (PA) is one of the most serious health problems facing older people [4]. A lack of PA increases the incidence of cardiovascular diseases, reduces cardiovascular and respiratory function, and increases the risk of falling, osteoporotic fractures and disability [5]. According to a report published by the American Journal of Clinical Nutrition, a sedentary lifestyle accounts for twice as many deaths in Europe as obesity. Moreover, increasing PA levels among Europeans would reduce the deaths in Europe by 7.5%, as reported by Ekelund et al. [6]. Encouraging even a slight increase in activity, with reference to inactive people, can be beneficial to public health.

An insufficient level of PA is one of the main behavioural burdens in the world [7]. From 60% to 70% of older people do not meet the World Health Organization's recommendations, with respect to PA, to achieve health benefits [8]. The nationwide Polish data compiled by Kozdroń show that only 7% of people aged 60–64 and 0.6% aged 80 years and more undertake regular physical activity [9]. Research conducted in nursing homes indicates that their residents are physically inactive most of the time and do not interact with each other or medical personnel [10].

There are a number of factors in the daily life of older people that can hinder PA. These include, among other things, a negative exercise history, lack of exercise skills, low social and cultural support, and a low level of motivation and self-efficacy [11]. According to Resnick et al. [12], interventions that focus on teaching older people about the benefits of PA, setting goals for exercise program implementation, and reducing unpleasant exercise-related sensations can improve regular participation in exercises and functional performance [13]. Another important element influencing whether an older person is able and willing to participate in physical activity and a model of healthy behaviours is motivation. Motivation is a term that defines the process regulating behaviour that is designed to control the engagement, maintenance, and termination of activities.

Despite the publication of several systematic reviews concerning the effectiveness of exercise programs for older people, the most effective of them has not been clearly identified yet. A systematic review of Carode et al. [14] showed that a multi-component intervention is the best strategy to improve the functional state of older people. Marcos-Pardo et al. developed a motivational resistance-training program and demonstrated the positive effect of training on motivational variables and the body composition of older people. However, the described results concern a preliminary study with a small number of people affected by the intervention [15]. In a systematic review, Farrance et al. indicated that programs for group exercises that used social support proved to be an effective way to improve physical fitness and to increase the level of PA for older people [16]. The authors noted that incorporating education about exercise benefits, social ties, and professional advice on enhancing health behaviours, with reference to exercise programs, could provide guidelines for designing innovative interventions in order to improve the health of older people. The International Association of Gerontology and Geriatrics (IAGG) Global Aging Research Network and the IAGG European Region Clinical Section have developed recommendations regarding motivation and pleasure as key factors to increase the level of PA in people receiving long-term care [17]. Experts have argued for the development and implementation of long-term care improvement strategies to improve the health of residents. Therefore, the aim of the project was to assess the degree of improvement in functional performance and the possibility of changing habitual ways of spending free time among elderly people under institutional care, by applying physical training with verbal stimulation. We hypothesized that the biggest changes regarding the functional efficiency and use of free time will be observed in the group with functional exercise training connected to verbal stimulation.

2. Materials and Methods

2.1. Trial Design

Our study contained a controlled, randomized trial with four open-label parallel groups. The study was conducted from March 2016 to December 2018. Data were collected at baseline and at 12 and 24-weeks. This procedure was established according to the "CONSORT" statement [18]. The study was registered in the Sri Lanka Clinical Trials Registry (SLCTR / 2016/004).

Availability of data and materials: All data used in this study were stored at https://repozytorium.ur.edu.pl/handle/item/5094.

Ethics approval and consent to participate: The research project was accepted by the Bioethics Committee of the University of Rzeszow (Resolution No. 6/06/2015). In accordance with the Declaration of Helsinki, the participants were provided with information about the aim and the course of the study, and expressed their written and informed consent to participate. The older persons were informed about the possibility of withdrawing from the study at any point during the study procedures.

2.2. Participants

The study was conducted in nine randomly selected nursing homes for older people and the chronically physically ill in Southeastern Poland. The management department of the centers were informed about the objectives and conduct of the study. After obtaining permission to implement the project in individual centers, the recruitment of participants began. To promote the exercise programs, information was posted, leaflets were distributed, and residents were orally informed about the details. The initial qualification for participants in the study was made by a physiotherapist working in the center. Participants who were eligible for the trial were required to comply with the following criteria: age 65–85 years, Mini-Mental State Examination (MMSE) score >19, Geriatric Depression Scale (GDS) score <11 points, physical fitness without serious restrictions, Short Physical Performance Battery score >5, and spending free time sitting for at least 4 h/day, 6 to 7 days/week (the Physical Activity Scale for the Elderly questionnaire). Exclusion criteria were: symptoms of cardiovascular diseases, severe systemic disease, severe circulatory or organic insufficiency, severe neurological disorder, injuries of the lower limbs during the last 6 months, use of medication significantly affecting the body's balance and participation in improvement exercise programs in the 3 months prior to the trial. Subsequently, an interview was conducted with a physician employed in the nursing home to eliminate the health contraindications in performing physical exercise by selected residents. After taking into account the inclusion criteria and obtaining written consent from the physician and residents to participate in the study, 204 people were included in the exercise program

2.3. Interventions

The subjects were assigned, at random, to one of four groups:
Group BE: Basic exercises without verbal stimulation
Group BE + VS: Basic exercises combined with verbal stimulation
Group FET: Functional exercise training without verbal stimulation
Group FET + VS: Functional exercise training with verbal stimulation

Exercise Program

All study participants took part in a 12-week exercise program, with or without verbal stimulation. Exercises were conducted in groups of 4–8 people, twice a week for 30 min. Each session was adapted to the functional capabilities of the subjects and was supplemented with breathing exercises. The exercise intensity was moderate, at 11–13 points, according to the Borg scale. The load during resistance training was up to 60% of one repetition maximum. Participants exercised with the music preferred by the subgroup (low volume level of 60 dB, moderate tempo). Exercise programs were performed by 9 physiotherapists (one physiotherapist per care home) with at least 2 years of experience working with older people. Each therapist was trained in the field of exercise programs and verbal stimulation before starting the program. They also dealt with the assessment of participants in the exercise programs, and monitored possible pain or other complications resulting from the performed exercises. Their observations were noted in activity diaries prepared for each group. In the case of health problems, such as malaise—a pain caused by excessive effort—the physician supervising the research made the decision to exclude participants from the study. Furthermore, the blood pressure and pulse of the older people were monitored before and after exercise. In addition, the study director was in contact with all physiotherapists in the course of the intervention in order to ensure that the exercise was of high quality and consistent in all care homes.

Basic exercises: the program included exercises performed in a sitting position. The exercises contained elements of aerobic fitness, stretching and equivalent exercises.

Functional exercise training: the program was divided into two sessions. Session I contained strengthening and stretching, with exercises performed in a sitting position using a Thera-Band and gymnastic sticks. Lower-limb strengthening exercises included tasks such as dorsi flexion and plantar flexion of the ankle joints, flexion and extension of the knee joints, flexion, extension and abduction in the hip joints, standing up and sitting down on a chair, and lifting objects from the floor. Upper-body exercises included stretching and strengthening of the shoulder girdle. Session II contained equivalent and functional training, using exercises performed in a seated or standing position, using chairs as stabilizing aids. Functional exercises included complex motor tasks, such as head rotation when sitting and standing, changing the body position, and lifting objects from the floor and keeping them. Balance exercises included exercises performed with and without visual control; static and dynamic balance of the elderly people was practiced (physical support was provided by a physiotherapist and auxiliary aids). The progression of the balance exercises was achieved by reducing the support plane, or by eliminating the visual control. Exercises were oriented towards achieving the goals of functional activity established by the elderly people.

Verbal stimulation: a model physical exercise program that incorporates the use of verbal stimulation. The model is focused on studying the achievements of participant's in regard to (objective) functional goals, and altering his/her (subjective) perception of the intensity of the training program and their individual aims. Before starting the intervention, a systematic review was performed to assess which elements had the greatest impact on health benefits among older people. The next step was to determine the baseline assessment; therefore, both the short- and long-term objectives of exercise participation were established. Short-term objectives assessed what a person is able to perform while exercising daily (e.g., perform 20 sit-ups, which improves lower extremity strength), whereas long-term objectives determined the "ultimate goal" (e.g., walking to the shop unaided or generally obtaining an improved level of mobility). Furthermore, specified objectives were helpful in achieving individual goals, as well as in persevering with these new health behaviours. According to the results of the studies carried out by Park et al., setting functional goals is an important motivating factor for PA performed by older people [19].

The program uses:

- Generating extrinsic motivation: the participants were informed about a small reward at the end of the program. Seniors were involved in a given activity to achieve extrinsic consequences. After performing physical exercises, a meeting was organized, at which diplomas for participation in the exercises and commemorative photos were handed out.
- Generating intrinsic motivation: a model for class management was developed, which assumed that the participants would achieve the set goals (challenges). The subjective feelings associated with performing physical exercises and independent steps towards a goal were strengthened. In accordance with the assumptions of the theory of competence-based models of intrinsic motivation [20], the examined person best estimates, depending on individual beliefs based on the significance of the goals established by them, the possibilities of motivation

In addition, informative materials were provided to the subjects:

- Explanation of the importance of physical activity in order to maintain independence and health;
- illustrations of exercises that older people could perform on their own after completing the program;
- description of fears and barriers appearing while physical activity is undertaken by older people and a description of the necessary ways to overcome them.

According to Locke, education and discussion about the anxiety connected to physical activity allows an older person to feel the need to participate in exercises [21].

The verbal stimulation program was included in the individual exercise programs.

2.4. Outcome Measures

Outcome assessments were performed at the baseline and at 12 and 24-weeks. The study was divided into two stages. On the first day, sociodemographic data and questionnaire interviews were collected; on the second day, anthropometric measurements and functional activity tests were performed.

Data regarding age, sex, education, marital status, and years in a nursing home were gathered on the basis of the records kept by care homes and by interviews with the individuals researched. Data related to chronic diseases and the number of drugs were collected from medical records kept by physicians in care homes. Cognitive status was also assessed by MMSE [22] and depression symptoms were assessed by the use of GDS [23].

2.4.1. Main Outcome

The Short Physical Performance Battery (SPPB) test was used to assess the functional status of the participants. The test comprised the assessment of three physical sequences: maintaining balance in three positions, gait speed over a short distance and attempting to stand up from a chair five times without the use of the upper limbs [24].

2.4.2. Secondary Outcomes

Physical Activity Assessment

Physical activity was assessed by means of the Physical Activity Scale for the Elderly (PASE) [25]. It is based on the evaluation of how free time was spent, as well as the work-related activities or voluntary work performed within 7 days of the survey, taking into account the frequency, duration and the level of intensity of these activities.

Functional Assessment

The performance of basic and complex everyday activities was assessed using the activities of daily living and instrumental activities of daily living (ADL-IADL) scale [26].

Muscular Strength Assessments

Hand grip strength (HGS) was carried out by the use of a hand dynamometer (JAMAR PLUS + Digital Hand Dynamometer, Patterson Medical). The values were obtained from measurements carried out on the participants while seated on a chair without armrests, with their feet rested flat on the floor—In pursuance to the recommendations of the American Society of Hand Therapists [27]. The average of the three measurements was recorded. The 5× Sit to Stand Test (5× STS) was used to assess the strength of the lower limbs. The participants were required to stand up 5 times from a sitting position as fast as possible without using their upper extremities [28].

Mobility Assessment

Mobility was assessed using the Timed Up and Go test (TUG) without a cognitive task and with a cognitive task (TUG cog) [29]. The TUG test was performed as follows: the participant will stand (from a sitting position on a chair), walk a distance of 3 m, turn around (180°), walk the 3 m back to the starting position, and resume the sitting position. The final result was the average time of the three attempts. Gait speed was assessed using the 10-Meter Walk Test [30]. Participants were asked to walk a distance, marked with an adhesive tape, of 10 m.

Flexibility Assessment

The elasticity of the upper and lower limbs was assessed using the back stretch test (BS) and the chair sit and reach test (CSR) [31]. BS estimates the elasticity of the girdle of the upper limb, which is necessary in the course of performing such activities as rubbing and washing the back. The test consisted of griping the hand of one limb from above with the other hand from below and behind the subject's back. The distance between the fingertips of the middle fingers was measured. CSR assessed the elasticity of the lower body, which was necessary in order to maintain the correct pattern of walking, getting out of the bathtub or dressing socks. The test was to bend the body in a seated position towards the outstretched lower limb. The distance between fingertips and toes was measured.

Body Balance Assessment

Balance was assessed using the Berg balance scale (BBS) [32]. The scale included 14 simple tasks, including: changing body position, maintaining a sitting position, maintaining a standing position under visual control and without it, watching, standing in a tandem position, standing on one leg, rotation around the axis, reaching forward, lifting objects from the floor, transferring, and going up a step.

2.5. Other Outcomes

2.5.1. Postural Stability Assessment

The assessment of the postural stability was performed by the use of a two-plate stability platform CQ Stab 2P (CQ Elektronik System, Czernica, Poland). Each of the platform plates had 3 force sensors that determined the displacement of the center of pressure on the support plane. During the measurements, the values describing the static balance were recorded. Platform plates were placed parallel, 2 m from the wall of the room where there was a marker to fix eyesight during the test with open eyes. Before each set of measurements was taken, the device was calibrated. The test included a 30 s sample performed with eyes open and eyes closed. The participants were instructed to remove their shoes and take a free-standing position on the platform plates with their arms set adjacent to the torso [33].

All testing procedures were fully explained and presented prior to assessment.

2.5.2. Quality of Life Assessment

Quality of life (QoL) was examined using the SF-36v2 questionnaire, consisting of 36 questions, which analysed the functional profile of health, well-being and psychometric assessment based on the subject's mental state of health. The quality of life established with respect to physical health was measured using two main domains: functioning in the physical dimension, i.e., general physical health (physical component summary: PCS), and functioning in the mental dimension, i.e., general mental health (mental component summary: MCS) [34].

2.6. Sample Size

The sample size was estimated from an a priori power analysis to detect the statistically significant effects of exercise [35]. The sample size was chosen according to the Cohen method, using standard assumptions: 0.05 for significance level, 0.8 for power of test, and 0.5 for effect size, accounting for, according to Cohen, a medium effect size [36]. The sample size calculation for the main outcome measure was based on changes in SPPB scores. The sample size calculation was based on 80% power to detect a one-point change in the SPPB score with an alpha level of 0.05. It was calculated that, based on the final analysis, the total number of people surveyed should amount to 39 people in each group. Therefore, 51 people were recruited to individual groups in order to allow for a 20% dropout rate from the study.

2.7. Randomization and Blinding

Randomization that implemented the stratified method by the use of the statistical package R 3.2.2 (The R Foundation for Statistical Computing, Vienna, Austria) was carried out. Four-in-one blocks were randomized, which made it possible to obtain an even distribution of elderly people in the studied groups. The order of randomization was determined by using a computerized schedule of random numbers. An independent biostatistician implemented randomization, hid the block size from the executive module and used randomly mixed block sizes. He was responsible for the confidentiality of the list of people included in the study. Outcome assessors were blind to the group division and did not take part in implementing interventions. Due to the ensemble nature of care homes, participants in the study were not blinded after being assigned to groups.

2.8. Statistical Methods

Descriptive characteristics were presented as a mean and standard deviations, or a number and percent when appropriate. A one-way ANOVA test was used to assess the differences between groups. The mean difference between treatment groups and the confidence intervals for quantitative variables was also determined. Post-hoc analysis for the quantitative variables analysis was conducted with t-tests with Bonferroni correction. The significance of changes in the examined variables, between two time points, were assessed with paired t-tests. Standard intention-to-treat analysis was performed for each outcome. Missing data were deemed to be missing at random and were calculated using the imputation technique according to the protocol study [37]. Analyses were conducted at a 0.05 level of significance. R software version 3.6.1 (The R Foundation for Statistical Computing, Vienna, Austria) was used.

3. Results

After the initial test was performed and the inclusion and exclusion criteria were taken into account, the older people were randomly assigned to four exercising groups: BE group, 51 people; BE + VS group, 51 people; FET group, 51 people; and FET + VS group, 51 people (Figure 1). The withdrawal rate from the study was: BE group, 10 people; BE + VS, 12 people; and FET, 10 people and FET + VS, 9 people. The main reasons for withdrawal from the study were: moving house, influenza diagnosed by a physician, refusal to participate without any reason given, and the death of a participant. The analysis included people whose attendance at exercises was over 80%.

In the studied groups, baseline parameters did not differ across the groups in terms of sociodemographic features and clinical parameters, including: cognitive status, mood, functional state, mobility, muscle strength, flexibility, body balance, postural stability with and without visual control, quality of life and level of physical activity. The average age of the study groups fluctuated between 73 and 74 years. Baseline scores of the research variables are presented in Table 1. Postural balance characteristics of the participants can be found in Supplementary Materials, Table S1.

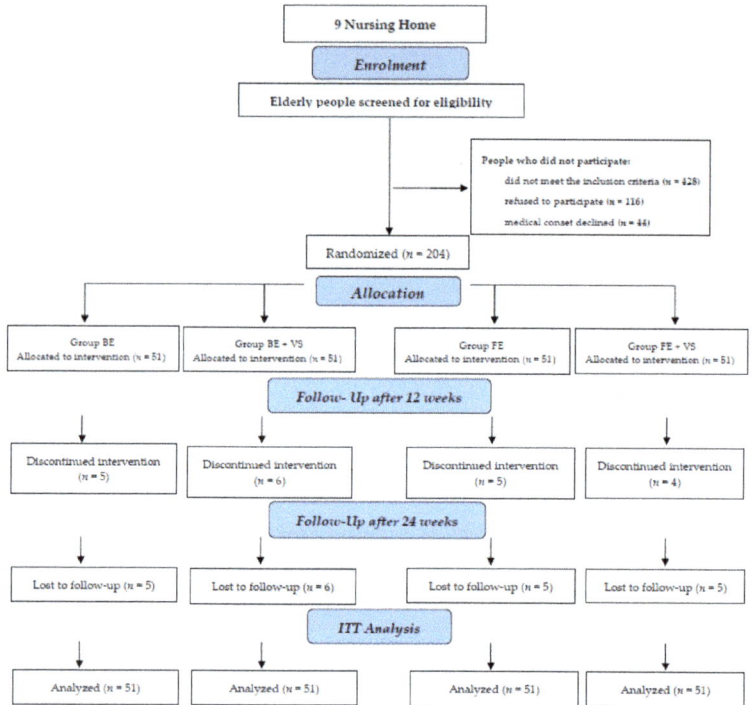

Figure 1. Flow diagram of the intervention study. ITT, intention-to-treat.

Table 1. Sociodemographic and clinical characteristics of the participants.

		BE (n = 51)	BE + VS (n = 51)	FET (n = 51)	FET+VS (n = 51)	p-Value
		Number (%) Mean (SD)				
Sociodemographic						
Sex	Female	32 (62.75)	29 (56.86)	29 (56.86)	28 (54.90)	p = 0.868
	Male	19 (37.25)	22 (43.14)	22 (43.14)	23 (45.10)	
BMI (kg/m^2)	Underweight	1 (1.96)	3 (5.88)	0 (0.00)	1 (1.96)	p = 0.266
	Normal body weight	22 (43.14)	20 (39.22)	19 (37.25)	20 (39.22)	
	Overweight	19 (37.25)	11 (21.57)	18 (35.29)	21 (41.18)	
	Obesity	9 (17.65)	17 (33.33)	14 (27.45)	9 (17.65)	
Marital status	Married	6 (11.76)	6 (11.76)	6 (11.76)	3 (5.88)	p = 0.570
	Widow/widower	21 (41.18)	13 (25.49)	22 (43.14)	22 (43.14)	
	Divorced	7 (13.73)	6 (11.76)	5 (9.80)	8 (15.69)	
	Single	17 (33.33)	26 (50.98)	18 (35.29)	18 (35.29)	
Education	Basic	23 (45.10)	16 (31.37)	18 (35.29)	21 (41.18)	p = 0.411
	Vocational	11 (21.57)	22 (43.14)	17 (33.33)	15 (29.41)	
	Secondary	14 (27.45)	13 (25.49)	15 (29.41)	14 (27.45)	
	Higher	3 (5.88)	0 (0.00)	1 (1.96)	1 (1.96)	
Chronic disease	Cardiovascular	45 (88.24)	42 (82.35)	47 (92.16)	42 (82.35)	p = 0.395
	Musculoskeletal	31 (60.78)	32 (62.75)	33 (64.71)	28 (54.90)	p = 0.765
	Neurological	10 (19.61)	11 (21.57)	16 (31.37)	9 (17.65)	p = 0.354
	Pulmonary	25 (49.02)	24 (47.06)	25 (49.02)	27 (52.94)	p = 0.946
	Urinary system	6 (11.76)	8 (15.69)	8 (15.69)	14 (27.45)	p = 0.183
GDS	No depression	36 (70.59)	33 (64.71)	35 (68.63)	34 (66.67)	p = 0.930
	Moderate depression	15 (29.41)	18 (35.29)	16 (31.37)	17 (33.33)	
MMSE	No cognitive impairment	16 (31.37)	22 (43.14)	18 (35.29)	17 (33.33)	p = 0.805
	Cognitive impairment without dementia	13 (25.49)	12 (23.53)	14 (27.45)	17 (33.33)	
	Mild dementia	22 (43.14)	17 (33.33)	19 (37.25)	17 (33.33)	

Table 1. Sociodemographic and clinical characteristics of the participants.

		BE (n = 51)	BE + VS (n = 51)	FET (n = 51)	FET+VS (n = 51)	p-Value
		Number (%) Mean (SD)				
	Age (years)	74.37 (8.36)	73.22 (7.33)	74.88 (7.54)	73.76 (7.58)	p = 0.717
	Body mass (kg)	70.59 (16.5)	71.81 (20.74)	71.81 (16.15)	71.56 (16.00)	p = 0.982
	Height (cm)	163.2 (10.11)	163.24 (11.61)	161.82 (11.19)	164.67 (9.02)	p = 0.603
	Years in nursing home	4.18 (3.51)	4.43 (4.11)	3.92 (4.66)	4.10 (3.90)	p = 0.937
	Number of drugs	4.16 (1.50)	4.27 (1.73)	4.27 (1.56)	4.25 (1.49)	p = 0.978
	Number of falls	0.71 (1.27)	0.88 (1.14)	0.88 (1.42)	0.76 (1.27)	p = 0.867
Main Outcome						
	SPPB	9.00 (2.20)	9.25 (2.06)	9.22 (2.09)	9.04 (2.24)	p = 0.912
Secondary Outcomes						
Physical Activity Assessment	Total PASE	23.35 (13.61)	23.91 (13.56)	22.92 (13.69)	23.49 (13.07)	p = 0.987
	Leisure time activity	6.19 (3.68)	6.26 (3.42)	6.25 (3.68)	6.33 (3.31)	p = 0.998
	Household activity	17.16 (11.72)	17.65 (11.50)	16.67 (11.9)	17.16 (11.72)	p = 0.981
Functional Assessment	ADL	5.29 (0.86)	5.18 (0.89)	5.25 (0.93)	5.35 (0.84)	p = 0.782
	IADL	8.61 (2.07)	8.59 (2.5)	8.67 (2.45)	8.78 (2.28)	p = 0.974
Muscular Strength Assessments	HGS_P (kg)	18 (8.77)	19.12 (9.77)	19.96 (10.88)	18.65 (9.04)	p = 0.773
	HGS_L (kg)	15.82 (9.25)	17.99 (9.06)	17.03 (9.03)	17.93 (8.71)	p = 0.584
	5× STS (s)	22.83 (10.54)	23.87 (8.5)	23.80 (10.90)	23.96 (11.17)	p = 0.940
Mobility Assessment	TUG (s)	21.07 (9.88)	20.2 (9.87)	21.32 (10.72)	20.99 (10.72)	p = 0.952
	TUG_{cog} (s)	25.17 (11.58)	24.33 (11.19)	25.00 (11.08)	24.88 (12.25)	p = 0.985
	Gait speed (m/s)	0.59 (0.27)	0.62 (0.32)	0.57 (0.27)	0.60 (0.27)	p = 0.828
Flexibility Assessment	BS_R (cm)	−32.82 (16.74)	−31.59 (16.31)	−33.57 (13.46)	−31.39 (13.40)	p = 0.868
	BS_L (cm)	−34.18 (17.41)	−34.22 (16.79)	−34.9 (13.41)	−31.20 (18.47)	p = 0.681
	CSR_R (cm)	−14.06 (14.8)	−13.98 (16.04)	−11.29 (12.69)	−11.59 (13.82)	p = 0.649
	CSR_L (cm)	−14.59 (15.2)	−14.88 (15.21)	−11.59 (12.5)	−12.53 (13.83)	p = 0.589
Body Balance Assessment	BBS	33.96 (13.15)	33.10 (13.20)	32.67 (14.40)	33.00 (13.94)	p = 0.969
Other Outcomes						
Quality of Life Assessment	Physical Component Summary	52.01 (15.74)	51.61 (14.80)	54.06 (15.44)	54.51 (3.34)	p = 0.693
	Mental Health Component Summary	58.09 (15.42)	59.24 (19.07)	61.48 (14.71)	62.75 (14.89)	p = 0.456

SD, Standard Deviation; BMI, body mass index; GDS, Geriatric Depression Scale; MMSE, Mini-Mental State Examination; SPPB, Short Physical Performance Battery; PASE, Physical Activity for Elderly; ADL, Activity of Daily Living; IADL, Instrumental Activity of Daily Living; HGS, Handgrip Strength; 5× STS, 5× Sit to Stand; TUG, Timed Up and Go; TUG cog, Timed Up and Go cognitive; BS, Back Stretch; CSR, Chair Sit and Reach; BBS, Berg Balance Scale.

Regarding the BE group, after 12 weeks of exercises, a statistically significant improvement was noticed in the following areas: functional fitness, muscle strength of lower limbs, mobility and gait speed, and flexibility of the lower limbs. The observed improvement was only maintained for the following 12 weeks in terms of lower-limb flexibility.

In the BE + VS group, after 12 weeks of exercises, a statistically significant improvement was shown in regard to functional fitness, performing complex everyday activities, hand grip and lower-limb strength, flexibility of the upper and lower limbs, body balance, as well as the quality of life of the people studied. The obtained change was maintained in most of the aforementioned parameters until 24 weeks after the exercises began.

The largest positive changes were observed in the groups with FET and FET + VS. In the group FET + VS, the greatest positive short-term impact of intervention was demonstrated in terms of functional fitness (SPPB increased by 1.31 points; 95% CI = 0.93–1.70), gait speed improved by 0.17 m/s (95% CI = 0.13–0.22), hand grip strength enhanced over 3.5 kg (95% CI = 2.51–4.95) and flexibility of the upper limbs developed by 10 cm (95% CI = 5.82–12.65). There was also a significant increase in the level of physical activity spent in free time (an increase by 6.91 PASE score; 95% CI = 4.58–9.24) and an improvement in the quality of life, especially in the domain of overall physical functioning (an increase by 11.79 score; 95% CI = 8.64–14.95).

The groups exercising with a verbal stimulation element were characterized by maintaining improvement in most of the studied parameters for a period of 24 weeks from the beginning of the study (Table 2). A mean difference scores for each group across time in terms of postural balance can be found in Supplementary Materials, Table S2.

In order to assess the differences between the four groups (BE, BE + VS, FET, and FET + VS), a one-way ANOVA analysis was applied. After 12 weeks of exercises, there was a statistically significant difference between the BE and FET + VS groups. In the FET + VS group, functional fitness, mobility without a cognitive task, flexibility of the upper and lower limbs, hand grip and lower-limb strength, balance and quality of life in the physical domain significantly improved, in comparison to the BE group (SPPB 0.25 vs. 1.27; TUG −0.91 vs. −3.89; HGS $_R$ −0.65 vs. 3.63; 5× STS −2.55 vs. −6.36; BS $_R$ 1.57 vs. 9.27; and BBS 1.18 vs. 7.27). All the studied groups after the intervention improved, in a similar way, their ability to perform basic and complex everyday activities, mobility with a cognitive task, and quality of life in the mental domain (Table 3). No statistically significant difference between groups was observed in body balance parameters after 12 weeks of exercise (Supplementary Materials, Table S3).

After 24 weeks of commencing exercises, the greatest effects were noted in the FET + VS group, in comparison to the BE group in most of the studied parameters besides lower-limb flexibility and quality of life in the mental domain. A significantly stronger short-term impact of interventions in the FET + VS group was demonstrated in the range of improvement of functional fitness and changes in the habit of spending free time among older people ($p < 0.001$). In the FET + VS group, compared to the other exercising groups (BE, BE + VS, FET), there were statistically significant, larger positive changes in the functional fitness, leisure-time activity, performance of complex daily activities, mobility, gait speed, and quality of life in the physical domain ($p < 0.001$) (Table 4). No statistically significant difference between groups was observed in body balance parameters after 24 weeks follow-up (Supplementary Materials, Table S4).

Table 2. Mean difference scores for each group across time.

		BE	BE + VS	FET	FET+ VS	BE	BE + VS	FE	FE + VS
		Baseline—12 weeks				Baseline—24 weeks			
		Mean change from baseline (95% CI)							
Main Outcome									
	SPPB	0.25 (0.10–0.41) *	0.51 (0.27–0.75) *	0.73 (0.47–0.98) *	1.27 (0.88–1.67) *	−0.04 (−0.23–0.15)	0.41 (0.17–0.66) *	0.53 (0.28–0.78) *	1.31 (0.93–1.70) *
Secondary Outcomes									
Physical Activity Assessment	Total PASE	5.50 (4.85–6.14) *	4.83 (3.33–6.32) *	4.02 (1.78–6.27) *	5.46 (4.89–6.02) *	1.44 (0.70–2.19) *	5.59 (2.98–8.20) *	4.14 (0.94–7.34) *	6.91 (4.58–9.24) *
	Leisure time activity	5.50 (4.85–6.14) *	5.42 (4.84–5.99) *	5.40 (4.84–5.95) *	5.50 (4.98–6.02) *	1.44 (0.70–2.19) *	3.73 (2.77–4.68) *	2.57 (1.64–3.51) *	5.77 (4.32–7.22) *
	Household activity	0.00 (0.00–0.00)	0.00 (0.00–0.00)	0.00 (0.00–0.00)	0.00 (0.00–0.00)	0.00 (0.00–0.00)	2.45 (0.34–4.56) *	2.94 (0.65–5.23) *	1.18 (−0.50–2.85)
Functional Assessment	ADL	0.06 (−0.07–0.19)	0.04 (−0.13–0.21)	0.25 (0.10–0.41) *	0.31 (0.13–0.50) *	−0.16 (−0.27—0.04) *	−0.08 (−0.20–0.05)	0.10 (0.01–0.18) *	0.29 (0.09–0.50) *
	IADL	0.73 (0.34–1.12) *	0.80 (0.39–1.22) *	0.94 (0.52–1.36) *	1.51 (1.08–1.94) *	0.16 (0.03–0.29) *	0.37 (0.13–0.62) *	0.53 (0.24–0.82) *	1.33 (0.87–1.80) *
Muscular Strength Assessments	HGS $_P$ (kg)	0.65 (−0.30–1.60)	2.51 (1.18–3.83) *	3.08 (0.98–5.18) *	3.63 (2.21–5.06) *	−0.13 (−1.08–0.81)	2.14 (0.86–3.42) *	2.07 (0.43–3.70) *	3.73 (2.51–4.95) *
	HGS $_L$ (kg)	0.71 (−0.04–1.46)	1.77 (0.63–2.91) *	2.85 (1.29–4.40) *	3.27 (1.92–4.63) *	0.16 (−0.87–1.18)	1.10 (0.02–2.19) *	2.17 (0.58–3.76) *	3.41 (2.20–4.62) *
	5× STS (s)	−2.55 (−3.80—1.30) *	−3.98 (−5.72—2.23) *	−4.46 (−6.20—2.71) *	−6.36 (−8.43—4.29) *	−0.73 (−1.83–0.36)	−2.86 (−4.35—1.38) *	−3.75 (−5.47—2.03) *	−6.30 (−8.40—4.19) *
Mobility Assessment	TUG (s)	−0.91 (−1.60—0.23) *	−1.63 (−2.93—0.33) *	−3.32 (−5.16—1.48) *	−3.89 (−5.82—1.97) *	0.25 (−0.72–1.23)	−0.24 (−1.37–0.88)	−0.71 (−2.04–0.62)	−4.13 (−6.09—2.18) *
	TUG $_{cog}$ (s)	−1.29 (−2.42—0.16) *	−1.85 (−3.18—0.51) *	−2.79 (−3.87—1.72) *	−3.61 (−5.87—1.36) *	0.08 (−1.30–1.47)	−0.10 (−1.45–1.26)	−0.70 (−2.21–0.80)	−3.88 (−6.66—1.10) *
	Gait speed (m/s)	0.07 (0.04–0.09) *	0.09 (0.05–0.13) *	0.09 (0.05–0.14) *	0.17 (0.13–0.21) *	−0.02 (−0.04–0.01)	0.01 (−0.02–0.05)	0.04 (0.01–0.07) *	0.17 (0.13–0.22) *
Flexibility Assessment	BS $_R$ (cm)	1.57 (−0.74–3.88)	7.16 (4.49–9.82) *	6.41 (4.76–8.06) *	9.27 (5.94–12.61) *	0.82 (−1.45–3.10)	5.14 (2.53–7.75) *	5.31 (3.20–7.42) *	9.24 (5.82–12.65) *
	BS $_L$ (cm)	1.63 (−0.44–3.70)	7.18 (4.57–9.78) *	8.31 (5.67–10.96) *	7.53 (3.00–12.06) *	0.59 (−1.49–2.66)	4.49 (1.98–7.00) *	6.41 (4.24–8.58) *	8.80 (4.01–13.59) *
	CSR $_R$ (cm)	4.16 (2.18–6.14) *	7.90 (3.96–11.85) *	10.02 (6.94–13.10) *	11.43 (7.96–14.90) *	2.22 (0.29–4.14) *	5.55 (2.16–8.94) *	6.78 (3.93–9.64) *	10.86 (7.67–14.06) *
	CSR $_L$ (cm)	3.90 (1.52–6.29) *	8.76 (6.18–11.35) *	10.73 (7.75–13.70)	10.94 (7.99–13.89) *	2.10 (0.49–3.70) *	6.80 (4.21–9.40) *	8.41 (5.60–11.23) *	10.84 (7.82–13.87) *

Table 2. Mean difference scores for each group across time.

		BE	BE + VS	FET	FET+ VS	BE	BE + VS	FE	FE + VS
Body Balance Assessment	BBS	1.18	4.27	5.82	7.27	0.20	2.78	4.39	7.31
		(−0.47–2.83)	(2.82–5.73) *	(3.65–8.00) *	(5.27–9.28) *	(−1.64–2.03)	(1.67–3.90) *	(2.29–6.49) *	(5.40–9.23) *
Other Outcomes									
Quality of Life Assessment	Physical Component Summary	0.97	6.46	5.46	12.10	−0.21	4.80	2.78	11.79
		(−1.94–3.87)	(3.24–9.67) *	(3.00–7.92) *	(9.33–14.86) *	(−2.22–1.80)	(2.04–7.56) *	(0.23–5.32) *	(8.64–14.95) *
	Mental Health Component Summary	2.28	7.88	5.18	7.28	0.04	6.34	4.27	5.01
		(−1.44–5.99)	(3.30–12.45) *	(2.35–8.01) *	(3.50–11.07) *	(−2.43–2.50)	(2.04–10.63) *	(1.55–6.99) *	(1.22–8.79) *

* statistically significant result. SPPB, Short Physical Performance Battery; PASE, Physical Activity for Elderly; ADL, Activity of Daily Living; IADL, Instrumental Activity of Daily Living; HGS, Handgrip Strength; 5× STS, 5× Sit to Stand; TUG, Timed Up and Go; TUG cog, Timed Up and Go cognitive; BS, Back Stretch; CSR, Chair Sit and Reach; BBS, Berg Balance Scale.

Table 3. Between-group comparisons at 12 weeks.

		Post hoc (Bonferroni) Analysis					ANOVA p Value
		BE vs. BE + VS	BE vs. FET	BE vs. FET + VS	FET vs. BE + VS	BE + VS vs. FET + VS	FET vs. FET + VS	
Main Outcome	SPPB	p = 0.387	p = 0.051	p < 0.001 *	p = 0.387	p = 0.001 *	p = 0.022 *	p < 0.001 *
Secondary Outcomes								
Functional Assessment	ADL	p = 1.000	p = 0.255	p = 0.127	p = 0.233	p = 0.097	p = 1.000	p = 0.033 *
	IADL	p = 1.000	p = 1.000	p = 0.047 *	p = 1.000	p = 0.082	p = 0.210	p = 0.034 *
Muscular Strength Assessments	HGS P (kg)	p = 0.330	p = 0.116	p = 0.033 *	p = 1.000	p = 0.871	p = 1.000	p = 0.033 *
	HGS L (kg)	p = 0.657	p = 0.075	p = 0.022 *	p = 0.657	p = 0.346	p = 0.657	p = 0.017 *
	5× STS (s)	p = 0.483	p = 0.474	p = 0.012 *	p = 0.695	p = 0.257	p = 0.474	p = 0.020 *
Mobility Assessment	TUG (s)	p = 1.000	p = 0.129	p = 0.036 *	p = 0.349	p = 0.144	p = 1.000	p = 0.018 *
	TUG cog (s)	p = 1.000	p = 0.655	p = 0.191	p = 1.000	p = 0.509	p = 1.000	p = 0.144
	Gait speed (m/s)	p = 0.935	p = 0.935	p = 0.001 *	p = 0.935	p = 0.021 *	p = 0.027 *	p = 0.002 *
Flexibility Assessment	BS R (cm)	p = 0.011 *	p = 0.032 *	p < 0.001 *	p = 0.680	p = 0.484	p = 0.343	p < 0.001 *
	BS L (cm)	p = 0.048 *	p = 0.015 *	p = 0.038 *	p = 1.000	p = 1.000	p = 1.000	p = 0.010 *
	CSR R (cm)	p = 0.393	p = 0.050 *	p = 0.009 *	p = 0.697	p = 0.393	p = 0.697	p = 0.009 *
	CSR L (cm)	p = 0.050 *	p = 0.002 *	p = 0.002 *	p = 0.780	p = 0.780	p = 0.911	p = 0.001 *
Body Balance Assessment	BBS	p = 0.071	p = 0.002 *	p < 0.001 *	p = 0.468	p = 0.071	p = 0.468	p < 0.001 *
Other Outcomes								
Quality of Life Assessment	Physical Component Summary	p = 0.022 *	p = 0.052	p < 0.001 *	p = 0.620	p = 0.022 *	p = 0.006 *	p < 0.001 *
	Mental Health Component Summary	p = 0.218	p = 1.000	p = 0.306	p = 1.000	p = 1.000	p = 1.000	p = 0.146

* statistically significant result. SPPB, Short Physical Performance Battery; ADL, Activity of Daily Living; IADL, Instrumental Activity of Daily Living; HGS, Handgrip Strength; 5× STS, 5× Sit to * statistically significant result. SPPB, Short Physical Performance Battery; ADL, Activity of Daily Living; IADL, Instrumental Activity of Daily Living; HGS, Handgrip Strength; 5× STS, 5× Sit to Stand; TUG, Timed Up and Go; TUG cog, Timed Up and Go cognitive; BS, Back Stretch; CSR, Chair Sit and Reach; BBS, Berg Balance Scale.

Table 4. Between-group comparisons at 24 weeks.

				Post hoc (Bonferroni) Analysis				ANOVA p Value
		BE vs. BE + VS	BE vs. FET	BE vs. FET + VS	FET vs. BE + VS	BE + VS vs. FET + VS	FET vs. FET + VS	
Main Outcome								
	SPPB	$p = 0.044$ *	$p = 0.012$ *	$p < 0.001$ *	$p = 0.547$	$p < 0.001$ *	$p < 0.001$ *	$p < 0.001$ *
Secondary Outcomes								
Physical Activity Assessment	Total PASE	$p = 0.075$	$p = 0.413$	$p = 0.009$ *	$p = 0.787$	$p = 0.787$	$p = 0.413$	$p = 0.010$ *
	Leisure time activity	$p = 0.010$ *	$p = 0.245$	$p < 0.001$ *	$p = 0.245$	$p = 0.019$ *	$p < 0.001$ *	$p < 0.001$ *
	Household activity	$p = 0.252$	$p = 0.115$	$p = 0.922$	$p = 0.922$	$p = 0.922$	$p = 0.632$	$p = 0.083$
Functional Assessment	ADL	$p = 0.427$	$p = 0.042$ *	$p < 0.001$ *	$p = 0.150$	$p = 0.001$ *	$p = 0.144$	$p < 0.001$ *
	IADL	$p = 0.640$	$p = 0.260$	$p < 0.001$ *	$p = 0.640$	$p < 0.001$ *	$p < 0.001$ *	$p < 0.001$ *
Muscular Strength Assessments	HGS $_P$ (kg)	$p = 0.066$	$p = 0.066$	$p < 0.001$ *	$p = 0.933$	$p = 0.208$	$p = 0.208$	$p < 0.001$ *
	HGS $_L$ (kg)	$p = 0.479$	$p = 0.092$	$p = 0.002$ *	$p = 0.479$	$p = 0.047$ *	$p = 0.479$	$p = 0.002$ *
	5× STS (s)	$p = 0.134$	$p = 0.039$ *	$p < 0.001$ *	$p = 0.444$	$p = 0.017$ *	$p = 0.087$	$p < 0.001$ *
Mobility Assessment	TUG (s)	$p = 1.000$	$p = 0.989$	$p < 0.001$ *	$p = 1.000$	$p = 0.001$ *	$p = 0.002$ *	$p < 0.001$ *
	TUG $_{cog}$ (s)	$p = 1.000$	$p = 1.000$	$p = 0.016$ *	$p = 1.000$	$p = 0.021$ *	$p = 0.063$	$p = 0.008$ *
	Gait speed (m/s)	$p = 0.366$	$p = 0.045$ *	$p < 0.001$ *	$p = 0.366$	$p < 0.001$ *	$p < 0.001$ *	$p < 0.001$ *
Flexibility Assessment	BS $_R$ (cm)	$p = 0.087$	$p = 0.085$	$p < 0.001$ *	$p = 0.925$	$p = 0.088$	$p = 0.088$	$p < 0.001$ *
	BS $_L$ (cm)	$p = 0.224$	$p = 0.040$ *	$p < 0.001$ *	$p = 0.546$	$p = 0.196$	$p = 0.546$	$p = 0.002$ *
	CSR $_R$ (cm)	$p = 0.208$	$p = 0.105$	$p < 0.001$ *	$p = 0.546$	$p = 0.049$ *	$p = 0.141$	$p < 0.001$ *
	CSR $_L$ (cm)	$p = 0.04$ *	$p = 0.003$ *	$p < 0.001$ *	$p = 0.375$	$p = 0.080$	$p = 0.360$	$p < 0.001$ *
Body Balance Assessment	BBS	$p = 0.080$	$p = 0.004$ *	$p < 0.001$ *	$p = 0.201$	$p = 0.002$ *	$p = 0.062$	$p < 0.001$ *
Other Outcomes								
Quality of Life Assessment	Physical Component Summary	$p = 0.024$ *	$p = 0.222$	$p = 0.001$ *	$p = 0.280$	$p = 0.001$ *	$p < 0.001$ *	$p < 0.001$ *
	Mental Health Component Summary	$p = 0.055$	$p = 0.313$	$p = 0.195$	$p = 1.000$	$p = 1.000$	$p = 1.000$	$p = 0.054$

* statistically significant result. SPPB, Short Physical Performance Battery; PASE, Physical Activity for Elderly; ADL, Activity of Daily Living; IADL, Instrumental Activity of Daily Living; HGS, Handgrip Strength; 5× STS, 5× Sit to Stand; TUG, Timed Up and Go; TUG cog, Timed Up and Go cognitive; BS, Back Stretch; CSR, Chair Sit and Reach; BBS, Berg Balance Scale.

4. Discussion

Observational studies suggest that 97% of daytime is spent sedentarily by residents of nursing homes, e.g., sitting and watching TV with low levels of interaction with each other and with medical staff [38]. A lack of engagement with PA has a detrimental effect on physical and mental health, quality of life and social isolation [39]. Therefore, reducing sedentary behaviour is an important new modifiable variable of lifestyle that can improve the health of older people [40]. According to the Copenhagen Consensus statement (2019) that considers PA and aging, researchers determined that self-efficacy, intentions, and the perceptions of one's health are related to the person's level of PA and interventions based on the theory that behavioural changes provides greater results. According to this account, they concluded that future research should assess the potential of these factors to promote PA and the good health of seniors [41].

To the best of our knowledge, this is the first intervention that assesses the impact of exercise programs, combined with verbal stimulation, aimed at motivating people to improve physical fitness and at changing habitual ways of spending free time by older people in institutional care. Furthermore, we have observed that the functional exercise program, combined with verbal stimulation, is the most effective in improving functional fitness, mobility, muscle strength and flexibility, as well as increasing the level of physical activity spent in free time and improving quality of life, especially within the physical domain.

Motivational strategies included in a resistance-training program affected psychological needs, motivation and compliance with the physical-activity principles [15]. Findings on interventions that increased the level of PA in free time are of moderate quality and focus mainly on systematic reviews, indicating a number of guidelines for the techniques used in order to change adult behaviour [42,43]. A systematic review by Orrow et al. [44] showed that the promotion of PA used in older people with a "sedentary" lifestyle leads to a small or medium improvement in the level of physical activity over 12 months. Hilldson et al. demonstrated, in their systematic review, that physical exercise programs moderately affect the functional state of older people and cause changes in the level of PA [45]. They suggested that further research should be planned with a view to propagate the long-term involvement in physical exercises by older people. Taking into account the results of the research herein, and the reports of other authors, when further designing an intervention in order to change the habit of older people in free time and to improve the health and quality of life of older people, it is necessary to focus not only on performing physical exercises at a moderate intensity, but also on the use of verbal stimulation based on generating motivation to replace the time spent sitting down with physical activity.

In our study, the effectiveness of four different exercise programs were compared. Despite the publication of several systematic reviews on the effectiveness of exercise programs for older people, as of yet, the most effective has not been clearly identified [14,46,47]. According to the review carried out by Silva et al., although exercise-based interventions have a positive impact on the physical functioning and wellbeing of older people, the most effective exercise program in this population remains unidentified [48]. Crocker also indicates that the physical rehabilitation of residents in nursing homes can be effective; however, there is no evidence regarding improvements in sustainability, cost-effectiveness, or which interventions are the most appropriate [49]. Regarding our study, we have shown that, after 12 weeks of exercise training, both the group with basic exercises and functional exercises, with or without verbal stimulation, have a positive effect on improving the physical fitness and quality of life of older people. Other authors have also confirmed that, regardless of the exercise program used, 12 weeks of physical training has a beneficial effect on the functional state of older people [50]. However, de Vreede et al. indicated that the beneficial effect of exercise is lost after suspending activity [51].

Taking everything into consideration, the implemented functional exercise program with verbal stimulation turned out to be the most effective with respect to the short-term effects of the intervention. The greatest positive changes were noted in the performance of complex daily activities, functional fitness of the lower limbs, gait speed and quality of life in the physical domain. In the FET + VS group, after 24 weeks, 1.31 points of improvement were obtained in the SPPB test; 4.13 s improvement in the TUG test; and 7.31 points in the BBS test. These values are higher than the suggested minimum clinically important difference for these tests [52,53].

Providing residents of nursing homes with group physical interventions is profitable and safe. It affects the reduction of disability—recording rare adverse events [54]. As for the residents of nursing homes, maintaining an adequate level of physical and psychological functions, enabling them to perform basic and complex everyday activities, allows them to have control over their own lives. Complete dependence on the help of others is the cause of emotional suffering and feelings of helplessness. According to Prat and Scheicher [55], the loss of functional independence is one of the main problems of older people, while independence increases their satisfaction and improves their quality of life. Weeks et al. [56] stated that preventing the expansion of functional limitations is a key factor motivating older people to participate in physical exercise. An additional element affecting the functioning of older people in nursing homes is the ensemble nature of the institution. In order to improve interactions with other residents, collective training should be used to strengthen social relationships and help to maintain interpersonal harmony, which is necessary for a peaceful life in the facility.

Our study has some limitations. First, there was no research examination performed 36 weeks after the start of the intervention due to the high drop-out rate caused by the increased incidence of influenza among older residents in the nursing homes. Secondly, the collective nature of the facilities means that it was not possible to implement double-blinding. In the case of further studies, additional measurement points should be added after six and 12 months from the beginning of the intervention.

5. Conclusions

In summary, the short-term evaluation showed that a functional exercise program, combined with verbal stimulation, is effective in improving physical fitness and raising the level of physical activity spent in free time. To accomplish a sustained functional efficiency and PA change, a prolonged follow-up is required. Finally, the group exercise program is safe and can be implemented into routine practice. Therefore, nursing home staff, as well as relatives, should be involved in the development and implementation of changes aimed at reducing the time spent passively by older people in institutional care.

Supplementary Materials: The following are available online at http://www.mdpi.com/2077-0383/9/2/477/s1, Table S1: Postural balance characteristics of the participants, Table S2: Mean difference scores for each group across time, Table S3: Between-group comparisons in postural balance at 12 weeks, Table S4: Between-group comparisons in postural balance at 24 weeks.

Author Contributions: Conceptualization, A.W.-S.; Data curation, A.W.-S.; Formal analysis, A.W.-S. and B.S.; Investigation, A.W.-S. and N.W.; Methodology, A.W.-S. and A.Ć.-S.; Project administration, A.W.-S.; Supervision, A.W.-P.; Writing—original draft, A.W.-S.; Writing—review & editing, A.W.-S.; A.Ć.-S.; N.W.; B.S.; and A.W.-P. All authors have read and agreed to the published version of the manuscript.

Funding: This study was supported by the funds for statutory research of the University of Rzeszow.

Acknowledgments: The authors would like to thank the study participants for their collaboration.

Conflicts of Interest: The authors declare no conflict of interest.

References

1. Ministry of Family, Labour and Social Policy of the Republic of Poland. Available online: http://senior.gov.pl/materialy_i_badania/pokaz/399 (accessed on 25 November 2019).
2. Statistics Poland. Available online: https://stat.gov.pl/obszary-tematyczne/warunki-zycia/ubostwo-pomoc-spoleczna/zaklady-stacjonarne-pomocy-spolecznej-w-2017-roku,18,2.html (accessed on 25 November 2019).

3. Forder, J.; Fernandez, J.-L. Length of stay in care homes. Report commissioned by Bupa Care Services, PSSRU Discussion Paper 2769, Canterbury: PSSRU. Available online: https://eprints.lse.ac.uk/33895/1/dp2769.pdf (accessed on 25 November 2019).
4. Centers for Disease Control and Prevention. Reporting System (WISQARS) National Center for Injury Prevention and Control. Available online: https://www.cdc.gov/injury/wisqars/index.html. (accessed on 25 November 2019).
5. Llamas-Velasco, S.; Villarejo-Galende, A.; Contador, I.; Lora Pablos, D.; Hernández-Gallego, J.; Bermejo-Pareja, F. Physical activity and long-term mortality risk in older adults: A prospective population based study (NEDICES). *Prev. Med. Rep.* **2016**, *4*, 546–550. [CrossRef] [PubMed]
6. Ekelund, U.; Ward, H.A.; Norat, T.; Luan, J.; May, A.M.; Weiderpass, E.; Sharp, S.J.; Overvad, K.; Østergaard, J.N.; Tjønneland, A.; et al. Physical activity and all-cause mortality across levels of overall and abdominal adiposity in European men and women: The European Prospective Investigation into Cancer and Nutrition Study (EPIC). *Am. J. Clin. Nutr.* **2015**, *101*, 613–621. [CrossRef] [PubMed]
7. Das, P.; Horton, R. Rethinking our approach to physical activity. *Lancet* **2012**, *380*, 189–190. [CrossRef]
8. Centers for Disease Control and Prevention. U.S. Physical activity statistics. Available online: https://www.cdc.gov/physicalactivity/data/index.html (accessed on 25 November 2019).
9. Kozdroń, E. *Program Rekreacji Ruchowej Osób Starszych*; Akademia Wychowania Fizycznego: Warszawa, Poland, 2008; pp. 73–75.
10. Douma, J.G.; Volkers, K.M.; Engels, G.; Sonneveld, M.H.; Goossens, R.; Scherder, E. Setting-related influences on physical inactivity of older adults in residential care settings: A review. *BMC Geriatrics* **2017**, *17*, 97. [CrossRef]
11. Zhang, M.; Zhao, Y.; Wang, G.; Zhang, H.; Ren, Y.; Wang, B.; Zhang, L.; Yang, X.; Han, C.; Pang, C.; et al. Body mass index and waist circumference combined predicts obesity-related hypertension better than either alone in a rural Chinese population. *Sci. Rep.* **2016**, *6*, 31935. [CrossRef]
12. Resnick, B.; Spellbring, A.M. Understanding what motivates older adults to exercise. *J. Gerontol. Nurs.* **2000**, *26*, 34–42. [CrossRef]
13. Resnick, B. Geriatric rehabilitation: The influence of efficacy beliefs and motivation. *Rehabil. Nurs.* **2002**, *27*, 152–159. [CrossRef]
14. Cadore, E.L.; Casas-Herrero, A.; Zambom-Ferraresi, F.; Idoate, F.; Millor, N.; Gomez, M. Multicomponent exercises including muscle power training enhance muscle mass, power output, and functional outcomes in institutionalized frail nonagenarians. *Age (Dordr)* **2014**, *36*, 773–785. [CrossRef]
15. Marcos-Pardo, P.J.; Martínez-Rodríguez, A.; Gil-Arias, A. Impact of a motivational resistance-training programme on adherence and body composition in the elderly. *Sci. Rep.* **2018**, *8*, 1370. [CrossRef]
16. Farrance, C.; Tsofliou, F.; Clark, C. Adherence to community based group exercise interventions for older people: A mixed-methods systematic review. *Prev. Med.* **2016**, *87*, 155–166. [CrossRef]
17. de Souto Barreto, P.; Morley, J.E.; Chodzko-Zajko, W.; Pitkala, K.H.; Weening-Djiksterhuis, E.; Rodriguez-Mañas, L.; Barbagallo, M.; Rosendahl, E.; Sinclair, A.; Landi, F.; et al. Recommendations on Physical Activity and Exercise for Older Adults Living in Long-Term Care Facilities: A Taskforce Report. *J. Am. Med. Dir. Assoc.* **2016**, *17*, 381–392. [CrossRef] [PubMed]
18. Schulz, K.F.; Altman, D.G.; Moher, D.; CONSORT Group. CONSORT 2010 Statement: Updated guidelines for reporting parallel group randomised trials. *BMC Med.* **2010**, *8*, 18. [CrossRef] [PubMed]
19. Park, C.H.; Elavsky, S.; Koo, K.M. Factors influencing physical activity in older adults. *J. Exerc. Rehab.* **2014**, *10*, 45–52. [CrossRef] [PubMed]
20. Losier, G.F.; Bourque, P.E.; Vallerand, R.J. A Motivational Model of Leisure Participation in the Elderly. *J. Psychol.* **1993**, *127*, 153–170. [CrossRef]
21. Locke, E.A. Motivation through conscious goal setting. *Appl. Prev. Psychol.* **1996**, *5*, 117–124. [CrossRef]
22. Fryderyk-Łukasik, M. Comprehensive Geriatric Assessment in everyday geriatric and caring practice. *Geriatr. Opieka Długoter.* **2015**, *1*, 1–6.
23. Albiński, R.; Kleszczewska-Albińska, A.; Bedyńska, S. Geriatric Depression Scale (GDS). Validity and reliability of different versions of the scale-review. *Psychiatr. Pol.* **2018**, *45*, 555–562.
24. Guralnik, J.M.; Simonsick, E.M.; Ferrucci, L.; Glynn, R.J.; Berkman, L.F.; Blazer, D.G.; Scherr, P.A.; Wallace, R.B. A short physical performance battery assessing lower extremity function: Association with self-reported disability and prediction of mortality and nursing home admission. *J. Gerontol.* **1994**, *49*, 85–94. [CrossRef]

25. Washburn, R.A.; Smith, K.W.; Jette, A.M.; Janney, C.A. The physical activity scale for the elderly (PASE): Development and evaluation. *J. Clin. Epidemiol.* **1993**, *46*, 153–162. [CrossRef]
26. Rubenstein, L.V.; Calkins, D.R.; Greenfield, S.; Jette, A.M.; Meenan, R.F.; Nevins, M.A.; Rubenstein, L.Z.; Wasson, J.H.; Williams, M.E. Health status assessment for elderly patients. Report of the Society of General Internal Medicine Task Force on Health Assessment. *J. Am. Geriatr. Soc.* **1989**, *37*, 562–569. [CrossRef]
27. Trampisch, U.S.; Franke, J.; Jedamzik, N.; Hinrichs, T.; Platen, P. Optimal Jamar dynamometer handle position to assess maximal isometric hand grip strength in epidemiological studies. *J. Hand Surg. Am.* **2012**, *37*, 2368–2373. [CrossRef] [PubMed]
28. Schaubert, K.L.; Bohannon, R.W. Reliability and validity of three strength measures obtained from community dwelling elderly persons. *J. Strength Cond. Res.* **2005**, *19*, 717–720. [PubMed]
29. Giladi, N.; Herman, T.; Reider-Groswasser, I.I.; Gurevich, T.; Hausdorff, J.M. Clinical characteristics of elderly patients with a cautious gait of unknown origin. *J. Neurol.* **2005**, *252*, 300–306. [CrossRef] [PubMed]
30. Wolf, S.L.; Catlin, P.A.; Gage, K.; Gurucharri, K.; Robertson, R.; Stephen, K. Establishing the reliability and validity of measurements of walking time using the Emory Functional Ambulation Profile. *Phys. Ther.* **1999**, *79*, 1122–1133. [CrossRef]
31. Konopack, J.F.; Marquez, D.X.; Hu, L.; Elavsky, S.; McAuley, E.; Kramer, A.F. Correlates of functional fitness in older adults. *Int. J. Behav. Med.* **2008**, *15*, 311–318. [CrossRef]
32. Berg, K.; Wood-Dauphinee, S.; Williams, J.I.; Gayton, D. Measuring balance in the elderly: Preliminary development of an instrument. *Physiotherapy Canada* **1989**, *41*, 304–311. [CrossRef]
33. Drzal-Grabiec, J.; Rachwał, M.; Trzaskoma, Z.; Rykała, J.; Podgórska-Bednarz, J.; Cichocka, I.; Truszczyńska, A.; Rapała, K. The foot deformity versus postural control in females aged over 65 years. *Acta. Bioeng. Biomech.* **2014**, *16*, 73–80.
34. Maruish, M.E. *User's manual for the SF-36v2 Health Survey*, 3nd ed.; QualityMetric Incorporated: Lincoln, RI, USA, 2009; pp. 55–56.
35. Faul, F.; Erdfelder, E.; Lang, A.G.; Buchner, A. G*Power 3: A flexible statistical power analysis program for the social, behavioral, and biomedical sciences. *Behav. Res. Methods.* **2007**, *39*, 175–191. [CrossRef]
36. Cohen, J. A power primer. *Psychol. Bull.* **1992**, *112*, 155–159. [CrossRef]
37. Wiśniowska-Szurlej, A.; Ćwirlej-Sozańska, A.; Wilmowska-Pietruszyńska, A.; Milewska, N.; Sozański, B. The influence of 3 months of physical exercises and verbal stimulation on functional efficiency and use of free time in an older population under institutional care: Study protocol for a randomized controlled trial. *Trials* **2017**, *18*, 376.
38. Sackley, C.M.; Levin, S.; Cardoso, K.; Hoppitt, T.J. Observations of activity levels and social interaction in a residential care setting. *Int. J. Ther. Rehabil.* **2006**, *13*, 370–373. [CrossRef]
39. National Institute for Health and Care Excellence, Occupational Therapy Interventions and Physical Activity Interventions to Promote the Mental Wellbeing of Older People in Primary Care and Residential Care, London: NICE, 2008. Available online: https://www.nice.org.uk/guidance/ph16/documents/occupational-therapy-and-physical-activity-interventions-to-promote-the-mental-wellbeing-of-older-people-in-primary-care-and-residential-care-review-proposal-consultation-document2 (accessed on 1 December 2019).
40. Wilson, J.J.; Blackburn, N.E.; O'Reilly, R.; Kee, F.; Caserotti, P.; Tully, M.A. Association of objective sedentary behaviour and self-rated health in English older adults. *BMC Res. Notes* **2019**, *12*, 12. [CrossRef] [PubMed]
41. Bangsbo, J.; Blackwell, J.; Boraxbekk, C.J.; Caserotti, P.; Dela, F.; Evans, A.B.; Jespersen, A.P.; Gliemann, L.; Kramer, A.F.; Lundbye-Jensen, J.; et al. Copenhagen Consensus statement 2019: Physical activity and ageing. *Br. J. Sports Med.* **2019**, *53*, 856–858. [CrossRef] [PubMed]
42. Gardner, B.; Smith, L.; Lorencatto, F.; Hamer, M.; Biddle, S.J. How to reduce sitting time? A review of behaviour change strategies used in sedentary behaviour reduction interventions among adults. *Health. Psychol. Rev.* **2016**, *10*, 89–112. [CrossRef]
43. Fitzsimons, C.F.; Kirk, A.; Baker, G.; Michie, F.; Kane, C.; Mutrie, N. Using an individualised consultation and activPAL™ feedback to reduce sedentary time in older Scottish adults: Results of a feasibility and pilot study. *Prev. Med.* **2013**, *57*, 718–720. [CrossRef] [PubMed]
44. Orrow, G.; Kinmonth, A.L.; Sanderson, S.; Sutton, S. Effectiveness of physical activity promotion based in primary care: Systematic review and meta-analysis of randomised controlled trials. *BMJ* **2012**, *344*, e1389. [CrossRef] [PubMed]

45. Hillsdon, M.; Foster, C.; Thorogood, M. Interventions for promoting physical activity. *Cochrane Database Syst. Rev.* **2005**, *1*, CD003180.
46. Chou, C.H.; Hwang, C.L.; Wu, Y.T. Effect of exercise on physical function, daily living activities, and quality of life in the frail older adults: A meta-analysis. *Arch. Phys. Med. Rehabil* **2012**, *93*, 237–244. [CrossRef]
47. de Labra, C.; Guimaraes-Pinheiro, C.; Maseda, A.; Lorenzo, T.; Millán-Calenti, J.C. Effects of physical exercise interventions in frail older adults: A systematic review of randomized controlled trials. *BMC Geriatr.* **2015**, *15*, 154. [CrossRef]
48. Silva, R.B.; Aldoradin-Cabeza, H.; Eslick, G.D.; Phu, S.; Duque, G. The Effect of Physical Exercise on Frail Older Persons: A Systematic Review. *J. Frailty. Aging* **2017**, *6*, 91–96.
49. Crocker, T.; Forster, A.; Young, J.; Brown, L.; Ozer, S.; Smith, J.; Green, J.; Hardy, J.; Burns, E.; Glidewell, E.; et al. Physical rehabilitation for older people in long-term care. *Cochrane Database Syst. Rev.* **2013**, CD004294. [CrossRef] [PubMed]
50. de Oliveira, M.R.; da Silva, R.A.; Dascal, J.B.; Teixeira, D.C. Effect of different types of exercise on postural balance in elderly women: A randomized controlled trial. *Arch. Gerontol. Geriatr.* **2014**, *59*, 506–514. [CrossRef] [PubMed]
51. de Vreede, P.L.; Samson, M.M.; van Meeteren, N.L.; Duursma, S.A.; Verhaar, H.J. Functional-task exercise versus resistance strength exercise to improve daily function in older women: A randomized, controlled trial. *J. Am. Geriatr. Soc.* **2005**, *53*, 2–10. [CrossRef] [PubMed]
52. Donoghue, D. Physiotherapy Research and Older People (PROP) group, Stokes EK. How much change is true change? The minimum detectable change of the Berg Balance Scale in elderly people. *J. Rehabil. Med.* **2009**, *41*, 343–346. [CrossRef] [PubMed]
53. Beauchamp, M.K.; Jette, A.M.; Ward, R.E.; Kurlinski, L.A.; Kiely, D.; Latham, N.K.; Bean, J.F. Predictive validity and responsiveness of patient-reported and performance-based measures of function in the Boston RISE study. *J. Gerontol. A Biol. Sci. Med. Sci.* **2015**, *70*, 616–622. [CrossRef] [PubMed]
54. Forster, A.; Lambley, R.; Hardy, J.; Young, J.; Smith, J.; Green, J.; Burns, E. Rehabilitation for older people in long-term care. *Cochrane Database Syst. Rev.* **2009**, *1*, CD004294.
55. Prata, M.G.; Scheicher, M.E. Correlation between balance and the level of functional independence among elderly people. *Sao Paulo M. J.* **2012**, *130*, 97–101. [CrossRef]
56. Weeks, L.E.; Profit, S.; Campbell, B.; Graham, H.; Chircop, A.; Sheppard-LeMoine, D. Participation in physical activity: Influences reported by seniors in the community and in long-term care facilities. *J. Gerontol. Nurs.* **2008**, *34*, 36–43. [CrossRef]

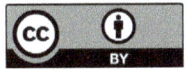 © 2020 by the authors. Licensee MDPI, Basel, Switzerland. This article is an open access article distributed under the terms and conditions of the Creative Commons Attribution (CC BY) license (http://creativecommons.org/licenses/by/4.0/).

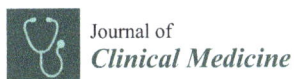
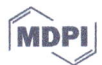

Article

Effects of a Multicomponent Exercise Program in Physical Function and Muscle Mass in Sarcopenic/Pre-Sarcopenic Adults

Hyuma Makizako [1,*], Yuki Nakai [1], Kazutoshi Tomioka [2,3], Yoshiaki Taniguchi [2,4], Nana Sato [2,3], Ayumi Wada [2,3], Ryoji Kiyama [1], Kota Tsutsumimoto [5], Mitsuru Ohishi [6], Yuto Kiuchi [2], Takuro Kubozono [6] and Toshihiro Takenaka [3]

1. Department of Physical Therapy, School of Health Sciences, Faculty of Medicine, Kagoshima University, Kagoshima 890-8544, Japan; nakai@health.nop.kagoshima-u.ac.jp (Y.N.); kiyama@health.nop.kagoshima-u.ac.jp (R.K.)
2. Graduate School of Health Sciences, Kagoshima University, Kagoshima 890-8544, Japan; reha_tommy@yahoo.co.jp (K.T.); p.taniguchi0601@gmail.com (Y.T.); na2.stch.or@gmail.com (N.S.); ayumi0924n.n@gmail.com (A.W.); yuto.kch55@gmail.com (Y.K.)
3. Tarumizu Municipal Medical Center Tarumizu Chuo Hospital, Kagoshima 891-2124, Japan; takenaka@tarumizumh.jp
4. Department of Physical Therapy, Kagoshima Medical Professional College, Kagoshima 891-0133, Japan
5. Center for Gerontology and Social Science, National Center for Geriatrics and Gerontology, Obu 474-5811, Japan; k-tsutsu@ncgg.go.jp
6. Department of Cardiovascular Medicine and Hypertension, Graduate School of Medical and Dental Sciences, Kagoshima University, Kagoshima 890-8520, Japan; ohishi@m2.kufm.kagoshima-u.ac.jp (M.O.); kubozono@m.kufm.kagoshima-u.ac.jp (T.K.)
* Correspondence: makizako@health.nop.kagoshima-u.ac.jp; Tel.: +81-99-275-5111; Fax: +81-99-275-6804

Received: 22 April 2020; Accepted: 6 May 2020; Published: 8 May 2020

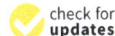

Abstract: This study aimed to assess the effects of a multicomponent exercise program on physical function and muscle mass in older adults with sarcopenia or pre-sarcopenia. Moreover, we aim to standardize the exercise program for easy incorporation in the daily life of community-dwelling older adults as a secondary outcome. A single-blind randomized controlled trial was conducted with individuals (≥60 years) who had sarcopenia or pre-sarcopenia ($n = 72$). Participants were randomly assigned to the exercise and control groups. The exercise program consisted of 12 weekly 60-min sessions that included resistance, balance, flexibility, and aerobic training. Outcome measures were physical function and muscle mass. Assessments were conducted before and immediately after the intervention. Among the 72 participants (mean age: 75.0 ± 6.9 years; 70.8% women), 67 (93.1%) completed the trial. Group-by-time interactions on the chair stand ($p = 0.02$) and timed "up and go" ($p = 0.01$) tests increased significantly in the exercise group. Although the exercise group showed a tendency to prevent loss of muscle mass, no significant interaction effects were observed for cross-sectional muscle area and muscle volume. The 12-week exercise program improved physical function in the intervention group. Although it is unclear whether the program is effective in increasing muscle mass, a multicomponent exercise program would be an effective treatment for physical function among older adults with sarcopenia.

Keywords: muscle strength; sarcopenia; resistance training; randomized controlled trial

1. Introduction

Sarcopenia is defined as a general loss of skeletal muscle mass and strength and is considered a major health problem for older individuals [1,2]. In 2016, sarcopenia was recognized as an independent condition by the International Classification of Disease, Tenth Revision, Clinical Modification (ICD-10-CM), code (i.e., M 62.84) [3].

Over the last decade, several clinical diagnostic criteria for sarcopenia have been reported worldwide [4–9]. In 2010, the European Working Group on Sarcopenia in Older People (EWGSOP) published its recommendations for a clinical definition and consensual diagnosis criteria [4]. Subsequently, many cohort studies identified sarcopenia based on these criteria, which include a combination of muscle mass and strength, and physical function loss [10,11]. In Asia, the most widely utilized criteria for determining sarcopenia are based on the Asia Working Group for Sarcopenia (AWGS) consensus, published in 2014 [8].

According to a previous systematic review that utilized the EWGSOP definition, the prevalence of sarcopenia is 1%–29% in community-dwelling populations and 14%–33% in long-term care populations with regional and age-related variations [12]. In the Asian population (Taiwan), the prevalence of sarcopenia varied from 3.9%–7.3% [13]. According to the AWGS criteria, the prevalence is estimated to range between 4.1% and 11.5% in the general older population [14]. A previous review and meta-analysis showed that the pooled prevalence of sarcopenia based on AWGS criteria among Japanese community-dwelling older individuals is 9.9%; similar prevalence rates were found in older men (9.8%) and women (10.1%) [15]. The numbers of people who had sarcopenia increased to 11%–50% for those aged 80 or above [16]. Community-dwelling older adults with sarcopenia have the worse physical performance [13,17] and are associated with premature mortality [18]. Since almost 10% or more of older individuals may meet the criteria for sarcopenia, effective prevention and improvement strategies are necessary.

Much interest has focused on community-based interventions for treating sarcopenia. A current systematic review and meta-analysis showed positive effects of exercise and nutritional interventions for older individuals [19]. However, there is little evidence of these effects, and the literature concludes that the evidence quality ranges from very low to low [19]. Therefore, well-designed randomized controlled trials (RCTs) to assess the effects of exercise on physical function and body composition, especially muscle mass, should be promoted.

Few well-designed intervention studies with a sufficient sample size have been conducted on the effects of exercise programs on sarcopenia. There is no effective treatment for sarcopenia, but physical exercise seems to be highly effective at counteracting the decline in physical function, muscle mass, and strength associated with ageing. The primary outcome of the present RCT was to investigate the effects of a multicomponent exercise program on physical performance and muscle mass in community-dwelling older adults with sarcopenia or pre-sarcopenia. Furthermore, as a secondary outcome, we aimed to standardize this approach for community-dwelling older adults, which can be easily incorporated into their daily lives.

2. Methods

2.1. Study Design

This community-based intervention study was a single-blind randomized controlled trial (UMIN 000036614). The intervention programs were implemented between June and September 2019. All participants provided written informed consent; after baseline measurements, they were randomly allocated to a 12-week multicomponent exercise program group or a wait-list control group. The study was approved by the Ethics Committee of the Faculty of Medicine, Kagoshima University (#180273).

2.2. Participants and Selection Criteria

We assessed 1151 community-dwelling adults aged 40 years or older who were enrolled in the Tarumizu study in 2018. Each participant was recruited from Tarumizu, a provincial city in Kagoshima Prefecture, Japan, between July and December 2018. Figure 1 presents the study flow. A total of 332 potential participants (≥60 years) with muscle mass loss (e.g., sarcopenia or pre-sarcopenia) were identified. Skeletal muscle mass loss was assessed by multi-frequency bioelectrical impedance analysis using the InBody 470 (InBody Japan, Tokyo, Japan). Appendicular skeletal muscle mass (ASM) was derived as the sum of the muscle mass of the four limbs, and the ASM index (ASMI, kg/m^2) was calculated. Skeletal muscle mass loss was determined based on the AWGS criteria for sarcopenia: ASMI < 7.0 kg/m^2 for men and <5.7 kg/m^2 for women [8]. Participants with skeletal muscle mass loss and low physical function (low grip strength < 26 kg for men or <18 kg for women, and slowness, indicated by normal walking speed < 0.8 m/sec), were determined to have sarcopenia, and those with skeletal muscle mass loss without low physical function were determined as having pre-sarcopenia [20]. Individuals who did not use Japanese long-term care insurance and had a history of hip or knee operations, femoral neck fracture, stroke, Parkinson's disease, Alzheimer's disease, or other severe brain diseases, were excluded from the sample (Figure 1).

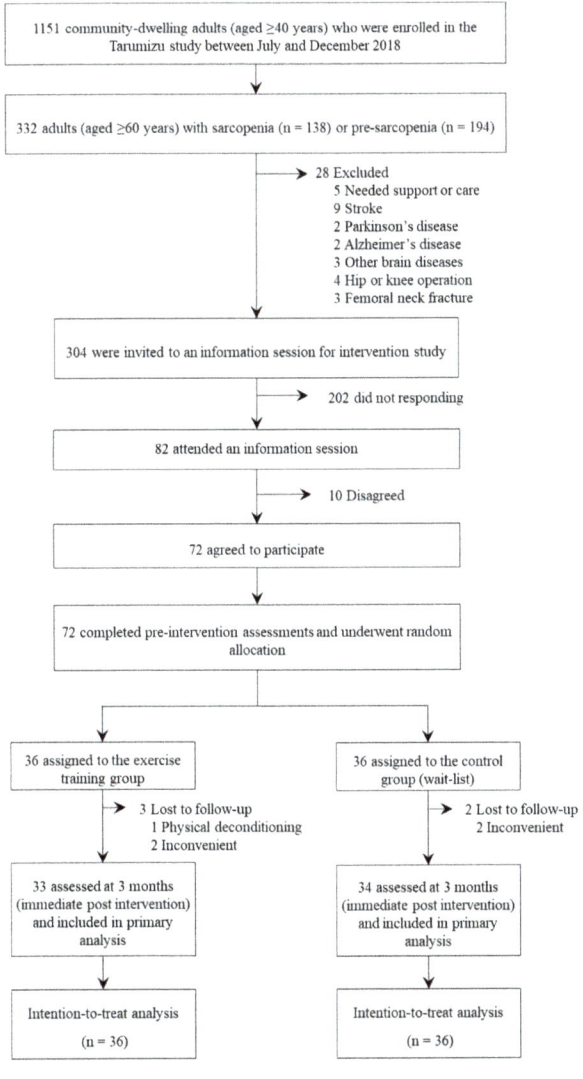

Figure 1. Flow diagram indicating participant progress through the trial.

2.3. Intervention

Following randomization, individuals in the exercise training group participated in a progressive multicomponent exercise program over 12 weeks of supervised 60-min sessions that commenced in June 2019. The intervention consisted of resistance training, balance, flexibility, and aerobic exercises.

Thirty-six participants in the exercise groups were divided into two classes conducted by physiotherapists and instructors at a community center. Before each session, the participants checked their vital signs, including blood pressure, pulse rate, and self-reported physical condition. If vital signs were unsuitable, such as systolic blood pressure ≥ 180 mmHg, diastolic blood pressure ≥ 110 mm Hg, or resting pulse rate ≥ 110 bpm or ≤ 50 bpm, participants were asked to avoid exercise that day. Each session began with a brief warm-up involving stretching, followed by 25 to 30 min of resistance training, 20 to 25 min of balance and aerobic exercises, and 5 min of cool-down. Resistance training used a progressive sequence based on individual strength performance, starting with no resistance load (own weight) for the first two weeks. Progressive resistance was provided by resistance bands (TRIPLE TREE, Carbro Flavor USA Inc., CA, USA) that had five resistance levels. Individuals' strength performance was tested every two weeks to determine the resistance load (intensity of resistance bands) and accordingly increase it for the next two weeks. In the strength performance test, participants determined their suitable resistance load at 12 to 14 on the Borg rate of perceived exertion scale [21], through ten repetitions of knee extensions. For each resistance exercise, participants completed up to ten repetitions of each movement, which included: (1) knee extension (quadriceps), (2) hip flexion (knee raises) (psoas major and iliacus), (3) hip internal rotation (gluteus medius and minimus), (4) elbow flexion and shoulder abduction (trapezius and rhomboid), (5) elbow flexion and trunk rotation (pectoralis major and oblique abdominis), (6) hip extension (gluteus maximus), (7) knee flexion (hamstrings), (8) hip abduction (gluteus medius), and (9) squat (quadriceps, gluteus maximus, and hamstrings). Balance training included a tandem stand, heel-up stand, one-leg stand, weight shifts, and stepping (anterior-posterior and lateral), to improve static and dynamic balance ability. Aerobic exercise consisted of anterior-posterior or lateral stepping repetitions for six minutes. The participants also performed daily home-based exercises, which were self-monitored using booklets, and were encouraged to record an exercise calendar. Exercise class attendance rate was calculated through the 12 exercise sessions as an exercise program adherence.

Participants in the wait-list control group (henceforth referred to as the control group) were asked to maintain their daily activities and attend a 60-min education class once during the trial period. The topic of this class was an irrelevant theme (e.g., preventing billing fraud).

2.4. Outcome Measures

2.4.1. Physical Function

Grip strength and gait speed, performance on the chair stand test and timed "up & go" (TUG) were assessed to determine physical function and sarcopenia status, as recommended by EWGSOP2 and AWGS2 [22,23]. All assessments were administered by well-trained, licensed physical therapists.

Grip strength was measured in kilograms for the participant's dominant hand, using a Smedley-type handheld dynamometer (GRIP-D; Takei Ltd., Niigata, Japan) [24].

Gait speed was measured in seconds using infrared timing gates (YW; Yagami Ltd., Nagoya, Japan). Participants were asked to walk on a flat, straight, 10 m-long walk path, at both usual and maximum gait speeds. Infrared timing gates were positioned at the 2 m mark and at the end of the path.

The chair stand test involved standing up from a sitting position and sitting down five times as quickly as possible without pushing off [25]. Physical therapists recorded the time a participant took to perform this action with their arms folded across their chests. The fifth repetition was recorded in seconds using a stopwatch (timed to 0.1 s).

In the TUG test, the participant rose from a standard chair, walked a distance of 3 m at a normal and safe pace, turned around, walked back, and sat down again [26]. Time was measured once in seconds, using a stopwatch.

2.4.2. Cross-Sectional Muscle Area/Muscle Volume

Cross-sectional muscle area and muscle volume measurements were performed using magnetic resonance imaging (MRI), which was performed using a 1.5T MRI MAGNETOM Essenza (Siemens Healthcare, Germany). Imaging of both thighs was performed before and after the intervention period in a supine position with both legs extended. A total of 120 consecutive T1-weighted axial slices with 1.5 mm slice thickness were acquired from the upper edge of the patella. Three levels of cross-sectional muscle area (m^2), lower, middle, and upper, were calculated from the right thigh. The lower level was calculated using 30 slices from the upper edge of the patella (45 mm proximal along the thigh). The middle and upper levels were determined using 60 (90 mm proximal along the thigh) and 90 slices (135 mm proximal along the thigh) from the upper edge of the patella, respectively. Muscle volume of the right thigh (cm^3) was calculated using 60 consecutive slices between the lower and upper level slices (Figure 2). Image-J (NIH, USA, version 1.3) software was used to analyze the MRI images.

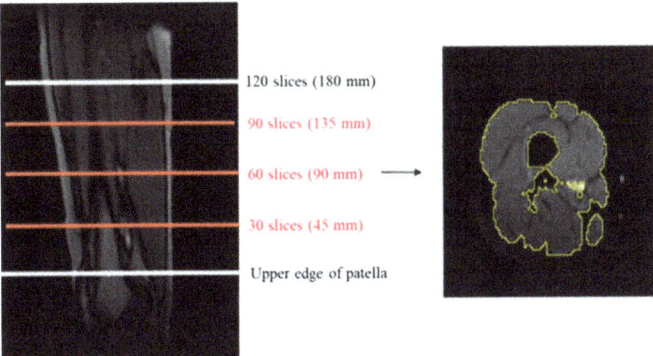

Figure 2. Cross-sectional muscle area of the thigh for segmentation and a sample segmented image.

2.5. Statistical Analysis

The sample size was calculated using G*Power software (version 3.1.9.2) based on a previous study [27], which demonstrated that at least 28 participants were needed for each group to detect a 15% increase in physical functioning. We included 20% more patients in each group because of dropouts observed in our previous studies. The alpha error was defined as 0.05, with a power of 80%. Data have been presented as mean ± standard deviation (SD). All outcome data including physical function and muscle mass were assessed as normally distribution using the Kolmogorov–Smirnov test. Analysis of the intervention effects on outcomes was conducted according to the intention-to-treat principle, with the expectation-maximization algorithm estimation to substitute missing data. Outcome changes were verified by the Student's t-test for paired data in each group. The repeated-measures analysis of variance (ANOVA), with group-by-time interaction, was used to evaluate the intervention effects. Data entry and analysis were performed using IBM SPSS Statistics for Windows (version 25.0). A p-value of <0.05 was considered statistically significant.

3. Results

3.1. Participant Characteristics at Baseline

Figure 1 summarizes the study flow. We screened 72 participants who were eligible and randomized. Participant characteristics and comparisons of baseline assessments between participants in the exercise and the control groups have been presented in Table 1. There were no significant differences in any of the characteristics and outcome measures between the exercise and control groups.

Table 1. Participant characteristics at baseline.

	All (n = 72)	Control Group (n = 36)	Exercise Group (n = 36)	p
Age, y, mean ± SD	75.0 ± 6.9	75.8 ± 7.3	74.1 ± 6.6	0.304
Sex, n (%)				
Female	51 (70.8%)	25 (69.4%)	26 (72.2%)	0.795
BMI, kg/m^2, mean ± SD	20.7 ± 2.4	20.6 ± 2.1	20.9 ± 2.7	0.628
Fall history in the past year, n (%)	9 (12.5%)	4 (11.1%)	5 (13.9%)	0.722
Medial history, n (%)				
Hypertension	25 (35.2%)	10 (27.8%)	15 (42.9%)	0.184
Heart disease	10 (13.9%)	4 (11.1%)	6 (16.7%)	0.496
Diabetes mellitus	6 (8.3%)	4 (11.1%)	2 (5.6%)	0.394
Arthritis	7 (9.7%)	2 (5.6%)	5 (13.9%)	0.233
Medication [a], no. mean ± SD	2.6 ± 2.5	2.1 ± 2.2	3.0 ± 2.8	0.285
Sarcopenia status, n (%)				
Sarcopenia	20 (27.8%)	11 (30.6%)	9 (25.0%)	0.599
Pre-sarcopenia	52 (72.2%)	25 (69.4%)	27 (75.0%)	
Physical function				
Grip strength, kg, mean ± SD	23.0 ± 5.5	23.2 ± 6.3	22.7 ± 4.6	0.702
Usual gait speed, m/sec, mean ± SD	1.34 ± 0.22	1.35 ± 0.24	1.33 ± 0.18	0.593
Maximum gait speed, m/sec, mean ± SD	1.70 ± 0.28	1.73 ± 0.31	1.67 ± 0.25	0.391
Chair stand [a], sec, mean ± SD	10.3 ± 3.2	9.6 ± 2.9	10.9 ± 3.4	0.086
Timed up and go, sec, mean ± SD	8.7 ± 2.0	8.5 ± 2.0	9.0 ± 2.9	0.285
Muscle mass				
ASMI, kg/m^2, mean ± SD	5.7 ± 0.7	5.7 ± 0.7	5.6 ± 0.8	0.811
Cross-sectional right thigh muscle area [b], cm^2, mean ± SD				
Lower [c]	47.5 ± 8.2	47.6 ± 8.5	47.3 ± 8.0	0.871
Middle [c]	64.3 ± 11.0	65.5 ± 11.3	62.8 ± 10.6	0.342
Upper [c]	79.5 ± 13.9	81.3 ± 14.5	77.4 ± 13.1	0.265
Thigh muscle volume [b], cm^3, mean ± SD	566.1 ± 97.9	574.5 ± 101.9	556.2 ± 93.9	0.455

Data presented as mean ± SD or number (%). There were no significant between-group differences in baseline characteristics. BMI = body mass index; SPPB = short physical performance battery; ASMI = appendicular skeletal muscle mass index. [a] Missing, n =1. [b] Missing, n = 7. [c] Lower, a 30-slice section from the upper edge of the patella; middle, a 60-slice section from the upper edge of the patella; upper, a 90-slice section from the upper edge of the patella (1 slice = 1.5 mm thickness).

3.2. Exercise Program Adherence and Adverse Events

Among the 72 randomized participants, 67 (93.1%) completed the trial. The mean participation rate was 81% for the 12 exercise sessions. No adverse events related to the intervention were reported.

3.3. Sarcopenia-Related Physical Function

Table 2 and Figure 3 show the pre- and post-intervention changes in sarcopenia-related physical function in the control and exercise groups. The Student's *t*-test for paired data in each group showed that grip strength declined significantly post intervention in the control group ($p = 0.01$), but no change was found in the exercise group. There were no significant changes in normal and maximum gait speeds in the control group, while maximum gait speed showed significant improvement in the exercise group post-intervention ($p < 0.01$). The chair stand performance improved in both groups. The exercise group showed significantly better performance on the TUG test post intervention ($p < 0.01$); no changes were seen in the control group. In the repeated-measures ANOVA, significant group-by-time interactions were observed on the chair stand ($F = 5.85$, $p = 0.02$) and TUG ($F = 6.33$, $p = 0.01$) tests, with increases in the exercise group. There were no significant group-by-time interactions in the other physical function assessments.

Table 2. Changes in sarcopenia-related physical function during the 12-week intervention period.

	Within-Group Differences						Between-Group Differences			
	Control Group (n = 36)			Exercise Training Group (n = 36)			Control Difference	Intervention Difference	Time by Group Interaction	
	Baseline	At 12 Weeks	p	Baseline	At 12 Weeks	p			F-Value	p
Grip strength, kg	23.2 ± 6.3	22.0 ± 6.3	0.01	22.7 ± 4.6	22.0 ± 4.2	0.09	−1.2 ± 2.2	−0.7 ± 2.4	0.83	0.37
Usual gait speed, m/sec	1.35 ± 0.24	1.39 ± 0.23	0.18	1.33 ± 0.18	1.37 ± 0.14	0.08	0.04 ± 0.15	0.04 ± 0.15	0.10	0.76
Maximum gait speed, m/sec	1.73 ± 0.31	1.75 ± 0.32	0.56	1.67 ± 0.25	1.75 ± 0.24	<0.01	0.02 ± 0.15	0.07 ± 0.12	3.41	0.07
Chair stand [a], sec	9.6 ± 2.9	7.6 ± 2.3	<0.01	10.9 ± 3.4	7.9 ± 2.3	<0.01	−1.9 ± 2.0	−3.0 ± 1.7	5.85	0.02
Timed up and go, sec	8.5 ± 2.0	8.2 ± 2.1	0.13	9.0 ± 2.9	8.0 ± 1.5	<0.01	−0.3 ± 1.2	−1.0 ± 1.0	6.33	0.01

Data presented as mean ± SD. [a] Missing, n = 1 (control group, n = 35).

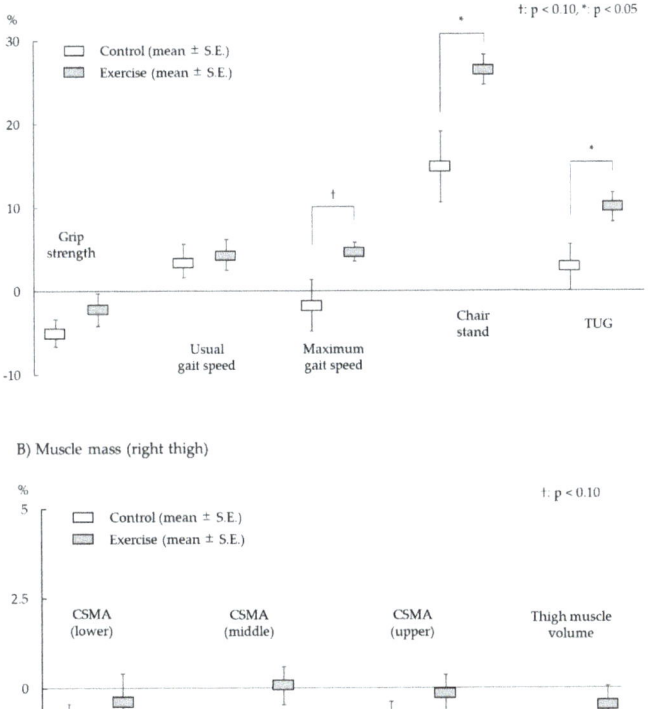

Figure 3. Improvement percentage of sarcopenia-related physical function and muscle mass after intervention.

3.4. Cross-Sectional Muscle Area/Muscle Volume

Table 3 and Figure 3 show the pre- and post-intervention changes in muscle mass outcomes. There were no significant changes in cross-sectional muscle area and muscle volume in the exercise group. However, the cross-sectional muscle area in the middle ($p = 0.01$) and upper levels ($p = 0.06$)

and the muscle volume of the right thigh ($p < 0.01$) declined in the control group post-intervention. Although there was a tendency to prevent loss of muscle mass in the exercise group, no significant interaction effects were detected for cross-sectional muscle area (lower level: F = 0.28, p = 0.60; middle level: F = 2.70, p = 0.11; upper level: F = 1.05, p = 0.31) and muscle volume (F = 1.90, p = 0.17). The ASMI also showed no significant group-by-time interaction (F = 1.71, p = 0.20).

Table 3. Changes in muscle mass outcomes during the 12-week intervention period.

	Within-Group Differences						Between-Group Differences			
	Control Group (n = 36)			Exercise Training Group (n = 36)			Control Difference	Intervention Difference	Time by Group Interaction	
	Baseline	At 12 Weeks	p	Baseline	At 12 Weeks	p			F-Value	p
Cross-sectional right thigh muscle area [a], cm^2										
Lower [b]	47.6 ± 8.5	47.1 ± 8.5	0.10	47.3 ± 8.0	47.0 ± 7.6	0.49	−0.5 ± 1.9	−0.3 ± 2.1	0.28	0.60
Middle [b]	65.5 ± 11.3	64.6 ± 11.1	0.01	62.8 ± 10.6	62.8 ± 10.1	0.82	−0.9 ± 1.9	−0.1 ± 2.0	2.70	0.11
Upper [b]	81.3 ± 14.5	80.5 ± 13.7	0.06	77.4 ± 13.1	77.1 ± 12.6	0.53	−0.8 ± 2.6	−0.3 ± 2.3	1.05	0.31
Thigh muscle volume [a], cm^3	574.5 ± 101.9	565.0 ± 100.5	<0.01	556.2 ± 93.9	552.6 ± 89.3	0.29	−9.5 ± 17.2	−3.5 ± 17.7	1.90	0.17

Data presented as mean ± SD. [a] Missing, n = 7 (control group, n = 35; exercise training group, n = 30). [b] Lower, a 30-slice section from the upper edge of the patella; middle, a 60-slice section from the upper edge of the patella; upper, a 90-slice section from the upper edge of the patella (1 slice = 1.5 mm thickness).

4. Discussion

This RCT indicated that a standardized multicomponent exercise program, including progressive resistance training, improved physical function, especially chair rise and TUG performance, in community-dwelling older adults with sarcopenia or pre-sarcopenia. No adverse events related to the intervention were reported and there was a higher than 80% mean participation rate for the 12 exercise sessions.

Sarcopenia-related physical function and muscle mass decrease with age. Cross-sectional data have indicated an age-associated decline in handgrip strength and muscle mass [28]. In adults aged ≥85 years, as compared with young adults aged 20–29 years, handgrip strength was over 50% lower, and calf muscle cross-sectional area was 15% lower in women and 30% in men [28]. Longitudinal studies also showed that, in individuals aged 75 years, muscle mass decreased at a rate of 0.64%–0.7% in women and 0.8%–0.98% in men per year [29]. Strength was lost more rapidly, at a rate of 3% –4% in men and 2.5%–3% in women per year [29]. Although reduced muscle mass may be an important factor in limited mobility and strength [7], muscle strength as a marker of muscle quality could be more important in estimating mortality risk than is muscle quantity [30]. Therefore, intervention programs are needed to be highly effective at counteracting the decline in physical function, muscle mass and strength associated with ageing. The current RCT indicated useful for improvement of physical function, even for older individuals with sarcopenia.

Handgrip strength is a good predictor of poor health outcomes, including mortality [30], through mechanisms other than those leading from disease to muscle impairment. Gait speed, chair stand, and TUG tests, is also associated with future adverse outcomes including disability [31,32], hospitalization [33], and mortality [34,35]. A previous intervention study involving eight weeks of high-resistance weight training indicated significant gains in muscle strength and functional mobility among frail residents of nursing homes up to 96 years of age (mean age, 90 ± 1 years) [36]. Thus, it is never too late to start resistance exercise to improve muscle function. Multimodal training is an effective intervention to increase physical capacity among frail older individuals [37]. Integrated care including exercise, nutrition, and psychological interventions improved frailty and sarcopenia status among community-dwelling older adults, with high-intensity training yielding greater improvements [38]. Resistance training, based on the percentage of a maximum of one-repetition maximum showed significant effects on physical variables, whereas resistance training based on the rate of perceived effort presented lower effects [37]. Although a training prescription based on a one-repetition maximum practice could be better for gaining muscle, it is not realistic for determining exercise intensity in the community setting. In the current RCT study, a multicomponent exercise program, including progressive resistance training, mainly used resistance bands, which was not a required prescription based on a one-repetition maximum practice improved physical function in older adults with loss of muscle mass, and could be useful to prevent and improve sarcopenia. However, it did not change muscle volume in older adults with sarcopenia. In order to change muscle volume, stricter exercise protocol may be needed.

A systematic review and meta-analysis that aimed to identify dose-response relationships of resistance training variables to improve muscle strength and morphology in healthy older adults indicated that 50–53 weeks of training is most effective [39]. Our multicomponent exercise program of 12 weekly sessions with a progressive protocol using a resistance band was conducted considering its feasibility in the community. Positive effects on physical function could be expected from our program for older adults with sarcopenia, but it may not be enough (e.g., intensity, frequency, and duration) for increasing muscle mass.

Nutrition may be another key element of multimodal interventions for sarcopenia [39,40]. Malnutrition and dietary patterns contribute to progressive, adverse changes in aging muscle [41,42]. Amino acids, β-hydroxyl β-methyl butyrate, energy, and vitamin D are required for muscle synthesis, so it is possible that nutritional intake influences sarcopenia [43,44]. A review suggested that the benefits of exercise could be enhanced with nutritional supplements (energy, protein, and vitamin D) [44]. On the other hand, previous reviews highlighted the importance of exercise interventions with or without nutritional supplements to improve physical function in community-dwelling older adults with sarcopenia [45]. Our program showed little evidence for increase in muscle mass in those with sarcopenia. A combination of a multicomponent exercise program and nutrition may have positive effects on both physical function and muscle mass among older adults with sarcopenia.

Several factors may mediate the associations of exercise with improvements in muscle strength and mass. For instance, genotypes (e.g., α-actinin-3 gene), endocrine, and lifestyle factors could be associated with age-related decline in muscle function [46,47]. Additional analyses are required to determine the mediation factors that support or limit the effects of exercise on muscle function.

Several limitations of this study should be noted. There was more than 80% of mean participation rate for the 12 exercise sessions. Participants were asked to exercise daily using a booklet and exercise calendar, but their adherence to this was not analyzed. Future studies would greatly benefit from the incorporation of activity monitors on the participants. Although our program mainly focused on resistance training with progressive resistance every two weeks, intensity was determined by perceived exertion, and the process was not standardized. Additionally, although other components, such as aerobic and balance exercises, were included to increase difficulty levels, these progress processes were not constant.

In conclusion, the current RCT suggests that a 12-week multicomponent exercise program with progressive resistance training generally improves physical function in community-dwelling older adults with sarcopenia or pre-sarcopenia. Multicomponent exercise could be effective at counteracting the decline in physical function for sarcopenia. However, it is unclear whether this exercise program is effective in increasing muscle mass among those with sarcopenia. Further studies might be needed to clarify the effect of treatment and prevention for the decline of muscle mass and strength related to aging and sarcopenia.

Author Contributions: Conceptualization, H.M.; methodology, H.M., Y.N., K.T. (Kazutoshi Tomioka), and Y.T.; formal analysis, H.M. and K.T. (Kota Tsutsumimoto); investigation, Y.N., K.T. (Kazutoshi Tomioka), Y.T., N.S., A.W., R.K., and Y.K.; resources, M.O., T.K., and T.T.; data curation, Y.N., K.T. (Kazutoshi Tomioka), Y.T., N.S., A.W., R.K., and Y.K.; writing—original draft preparation, H.M.; writing—review and editing, H.M., Y.N., K.T. (Kazutoshi Tomioka), Y.T., N.S., A.W., R.K., and K.T. (Kota Tsutsumimoto); supervision, M.O. and T.T.; project administration, H.M., M.O., T.K., and T.T.; funding acquisition, H.M. All authors have read and agreed to the published version of the manuscript.

Funding: This work was supported by JSPS KAKENHI (Grant-in-Aid for Scientific Research [B]), Grant Number 19H03978 and the Daiwa Securities Health Foundation.

Acknowledgments: We thank Yukitaka Nagata, Sueharu Shimago, and Junji Ichizono, and Tamizu Chuo Hospital for their help with MRI examinations; Daisuke Hirahara, concurrent assistant professor, School Corporation Harada Gakuen, Management Planning Division, Kagoshima Medical Professional College, for his contribution to the determination of assessment methods using MRI, and Tarumizu City Office for their contributions to the study. We also thank all participants who participated in the study.

Conflicts of Interest: The authors declare no conflicts of interest. The funders had no role in the design of the study; in the collection, analyses, or interpretation of data; in the writing of the manuscript, or in the decision to publish the results.

References

1. Cruz-Jentoft, A.J.; Landi, F. Sarcopenia. *Clin. Med.* **2014**, *14*, 183–186. [CrossRef] [PubMed]
2. Reginster, J.Y.; Cooper, C.; Rizzoli, R.; Kanis, J.A.; Appelboom, G.; Bautmans, I.; Bischoff-Ferrari, H.A.; Boers, M.; Brandi, M.L.; Bruyere, O.; et al. Recommendations for the conduct of clinical trials for drugs to treat or prevent sarcopenia. *Aging Clin. Exp. Res.* **2016**, *28*, 47–58. [CrossRef] [PubMed]
3. Cao, L.; Morley, J.E. Sarcopenia is recognized as an independent condition by an International Classification of Disease, tenth revision, Clinical Modification (ICD-10-CM) Code. *J. Am. Med. Dir. Assoc.* **2016**, *17*, 675–677. [CrossRef]
4. Cruz-Jentoft, A.J.; Baeyens, J.P.; Bauer, J.M.; Boirie, Y.; Cederholm, T.; Landi, F.; Martin, F.C.; Michel, J.P.; Rolland, Y.; Schneider, S.M.; et al. Sarcopenia: European consensus on definition and diagnosis: Report of the European Working Group on Sarcopenia in Older People. *Age Ageing* **2010**, *39*, 412–423. [CrossRef]
5. Muscaritoli, M.; Anker, S.D.; Argilés, J.; Aversa, Z.; Bauer, J.M.; Biolo, G.; Boirie, Y.; Bosaeus, I.; Cederholm, T.; Costelli, P.; et al. Consensus definition of sarcopenia, cachexia and pre-cachexia: Joint document elaborated by Special Interest Groups (SIG) "cachexia-anorexia in chronic wasting diseases" and "nutrition in geriatrics". *Clin. Nutr.* **2010**, *29*, 154–159. [CrossRef] [PubMed]
6. Fielding, R.A.; Vellas, B.; Evans, W.J.; Bhasin, S.; Morley, J.E.; Newman, A.B.; van Kan, G.A.; Andrieu, S.; Bauer, J.; Breuille, D.; et al. Sarcopenia: An undiagnosed condition in older adults. Current consensus definition: Prevalence, etiology, and consequences. International working group on sarcopenia. *J. Am. Med. Dir. Assoc.* **2011**, *12*, 249–256. [CrossRef] [PubMed]
7. Morley, J.E.; Abbatecola, A.M.; Argiles, J.M.; Baracos, V.; Bauer, J.; Bhasin, S.; Cederholm, T.; Coats, A.J.; Cummings, S.R.; Evans, W.J.; et al. Sarcopenia with limited mobility: An international consensus. *J. Am. Med. Dir. Assoc.* **2011**, *12*, 403–409. [CrossRef]
8. Chen, L.K.; Liu, L.K.; Woo, J.; Assantachai, P.; Auyeung, T.W.; Bahyah, K.S.; Chou, M.Y.; Chen, L.Y.; Hsu, P.S.; Krairit, O.; et al. Sarcopenia in Asia: Consensus report of the Asian Working Group for Sarcopenia. *J. Am. Med. Dir. Assoc.* **2014**, *15*, 95–101. [CrossRef]
9. McLean, R.R.; Shardell, M.D.; Alley, D.E.; Cawthon, P.E.; Fragala, M.S.; Harris, T.B.; Kenny, A.M.; Peters, K.W.; Ferrucci, L.; Guralnik, J.M.; et al. Criteria for clinically relevant weakness and low lean mass and their longitudinal association with incident mobility impairment and mortality: The foundation for the National Institutes of Health (FNIH) sarcopenia project. *J. Gerontol. A Biol. Sci. Med. Sci.* **2014**, *69*, 576–583. [CrossRef]
10. Shafiee, G.; Keshtkar, A.; Soltani, A.; Ahadi, Z.; Larijani, B.; Heshmat, R. Prevalence of sarcopenia in the world: A systematic review and meta- analysis of general population studies. *J. Diabetes Metab. Disord.* **2017**, *16*, 21. [CrossRef]
11. Shen, Y.; Chen, J.; Chen, X.; Hou, L.; Lin, X.; Yang, M. Prevalence and Associated Factors of Sarcopenia in Nursing Home Residents: A Systematic Review and Meta-analysis. *J. Am. Med. Dir. Assoc.* **2019**, *20*, 5–13. [CrossRef] [PubMed]
12. Cruz-Jentoft, A.J.; Landi, F.; Schneider, S.M.; Zúñiga, C.; Arai, H.; Boirie, Y.; Chen, L.K.; Fielding, R.A.; Martin, F.C.; Michel, J.P.; et al. Prevalence of and interventions for sarcopenia in ageing adults: A systematic review. Report of the International Sarcopenia Initiative (EWGSOP and IWGS). *Age Ageing* **2014**, *43*, 748–759. [CrossRef]

13. Wu, I.C.; Lin, C.C.; Hsiung, C.A.; Wang, C.Y.; Wu, C.H.; Chan, D.C.; Li, T.C.; Lin, W.Y.; Huang, K.C.; Chen, C.Y.; et al. Epidemiology of sarcopenia among community-dwelling older adults in Taiwan: A pooled analysis for a broader adoption of sarcopenia assessments. *Geriatr. Gerontol. Int.* **2014**, *14* (Suppl. 1), 52–60. [CrossRef] [PubMed]
14. Chen, L.K.; Lee, W.J.; Peng, L.N.; Liu, L.K.; Arai, H.; Akishita, M.; Asian Working Group for Sarcopenia. Recent advances in sarcopenia research in Asia: 2016 update from the Asian Working Group for Sarcopenia. *J. Am. Med. Dir. Assoc.* **2016**, *17*, 761–767. [CrossRef] [PubMed]
15. Makizako, H.; Nakai, Y.; Tomioka, K.; Taniguchi, Y. Prevalence of sarcopenia defined using the Asia Working Group for Sarcopenia criteria in Japanese community-dwelling older adults: A systematic review and meta-analysis. *Phys. Ther. Res.* **2019**, *22*, 53–57. [CrossRef] [PubMed]
16. von Haehling, S.; Morley, J.E.; Anker, S.D. An overview of sarcopenia: Facts and numbers on prevalence and clinical impact. *J. Cachexia Sarcopenia Muscle* **2010**, *1*, 129–133. [CrossRef]
17. Patel, H.P.; Syddall, H.E.; Jameson, K.; Robinson, S.; Denison, H.; Roberts, H.C.; Edwards, M.; Dennison, E.; Cooper, C.; Aihie Sayer, A. Prevalence of sarcopenia in community-dwelling older people in the UK using the European Working Group on Sarcopenia in Older People (EWGSOP) definition: Findings from the Hertfordshire Cohort Study (HCS). *Age Ageing* **2013**, *42*, 378–384. [CrossRef]
18. Brown, J.C.; Harhay, M.O.; Harhay, M.N. Sarcopenia and mortality among a population-based sample of community-dwelling older adults. *J. Cachexia Sarcopenia Muscle* **2016**, *7*, 290–298. [CrossRef]
19. Yoshimura, Y.; Wakabayashi, H.; Yamada, M.; Kim, H.; Harada, A.; Arai, H. Interventions for Treating Sarcopenia: A Systematic Review and Meta-Analysis of Randomized Controlled Studies. *J. Am. Med. Dir. Assoc.* **2017**, *18*, 553.e1–553.e16. [CrossRef]
20. Yamada, M.; Kimura, Y.; Ishiyama, D.; Nishio, N.; Abe, Y.; Kakehi, T.; Fujimoto, J.; Tanaka, T.; Ohji, S.; Otobe, Y.; et al. Differential Characteristics of Skeletal Muscle in Community-Dwelling Older Adults. *J. Am. Med. Dir. Assoc.* **2017**, *18*, 807.e9–807.e16. [CrossRef]
21. Borg, G.A. Psychophysical bases of perceived exertion. *Med. Sci. Sports Exerc.* **1982**, *14*, 377–381. [CrossRef] [PubMed]
22. Cruz-Jentoft, A.J.; Bahat, G.; Bauer, J.; Boirie, Y.; Bruyère, O.; Cederholm, T.; Cooper, C.; Landi, F.; Rolland, Y.; Sayer, A.A.; et al. Sarcopenia: Revised European consensus on definition and diagnosis. *Age Ageing* **2019**, *48*, 16–31. [CrossRef] [PubMed]
23. Chen, L.; Woo, J.; Assantachai, P.; Auyeung, T.W.; Chou, M.Y.; Iijimia, K.; Jang, H.C.; Kang, L.; Kim, M.; Kim, S.; et al. Asian Working Group for Sarcopenia: 2019 consensus update on sarcopenia diagnosis and treatment. *J. Am. Med. Dir. Assoc.* **2020**, *21*, 300–307. [CrossRef] [PubMed]
24. Makizako, H.; Shimada, H.; Doi, T.; Tsutsumimoto, K.; Lee, S.; Lee, S.C.; Harada, K.; Hotta, R.; Nakakubo, S.; Bae, S.; et al. Age-dependent changes in physical performance and body composition in community-dwelling Japanese older adults. *J. Cachexia Sarcopenia Muscle* **2017**, *8*, 607–614. [CrossRef]
25. Whitney, S.L.; Wrisley, D.M.; Marchetti, G.F.; Gee, M.A.; Redfern, M.S.; Furman, J.M. Clinical measurement of sit-to-stand performance in people with balance disorders: Validity of data for the Five-Times-Sit-to-Stand Test. *Phys. Ther.* **2005**, *85*, 1034–1045. [CrossRef]
26. Podsiadlo, D.; Richardson, S. The timed "Up & Go": A test of basic functional mobility for frail elderly persons. *J. Am. Geriatr. Soc.* **1991**, *39*, 142–148.
27. Kim, H.K.; Suzuki, T.; Saito, K.; Yoshida, H.; Kobayashi, H.; Kato, H.; Katayama, M. Effects of exercise and amino acid supplementation on body composition and physical function in community-dwelling elderly Japanese sarcopenic women: A randomized controlled trial. *J. Am. Geriatr. Soc.* **2012**, *60*, 16–23. [CrossRef]
28. Lauretani, F.; Russo, C.R.; Bandinelli, S.; Bartali, B.; Cavazzini, C.; Di Iorio, A.; Corsi, A.M.; Rantanen, T.; Guralnik, J.M.; Ferrucci, L. Age-associated changes in skeletal muscles and their effect on mobility: An operational diagnosis of sarcopenia. *J. Appl. Physiol.* **2003**, *95*, 1851–1860. [CrossRef]
29. Mitchell, W.K.; Williams, J.; Atherton, P.; Larvin, M.; Lund, J.; Narici, M. Sarcopenia, dynapenia, and the impact of advancing age on human skeletal muscle size and strength; a quantitative review. *Front. Physiol.* **2012**, *3*, 260. [CrossRef]
30. Newman, A.B.; Kupelian, V.; Visser, M.; Simonsick, E.M.; Goodpaster, B.H.; Kritchevsky, S.B.; Tylavsky, F.A.; Rubin, S.M.; Harris, T.B. Strength, but not muscle mass, is associated with mortality in the health, aging and body composition study cohort. *J. Gerontol. A Biol. Sci. Med. Sci.* **2006**, *61*, 72–77. [CrossRef]

31. Perera, S.; Patel, K.V.; Rosano, C.; Rubin, S.M.; Satterfield, S.; Harris, T.; Ensrud, K.; Orwoll, E.; Lee, C.G.; Chandler, J.M.; et al. Gait speed predicts incident disability: A pooled analysis. *J. Gerontol. A Biol. Sci. Med. Sci.* **2016**, *71*, 63–71. [CrossRef] [PubMed]
32. Makizako, H.; Shimada, H.; Doi, T.; Tsutsumimoto, K.; Nakakubo, S.; Hotta, R.; Suzuki, T. Predictive cutoff values of the five-times sit-to-stand test and the timed "up & go" test for disability incidence in older people dwelling in the community. *Phys. Ther.* **2017**, *97*, 417–424. [PubMed]
33. Duan-Porter, W.; Vo, T.N.; Ullman, K.; Langsetmo, L.; Strotmeyer, E.S.; Taylor, B.C.; Santanasto, A.J.; Cawthon, P.M.; Newman, A.B.; Simonsick, E.M.; et al. Hospitalization-associated change in gait speed and risk of functional limitations for older adults. *J. Gerontol. A Biol. Sci. Med. Sci.* **2019**, *74*, 1657–1663. [CrossRef] [PubMed]
34. Studenski, S.; Perera, S.; Patel, K.; Rosano, C.; Faulkner, K.; Inzitari, M.; Brach, J.; Chandler, J.; Cawthon, P.; Connor, E.B.; et al. Gait speed and survival in older adults. *JAMA* **2011**, *305*, 50–58. [CrossRef]
35. Eekhoff, E.M.W.; van Schoor, N.M.; Biedermann, J.S.; Oosterwerff, M.M.; de Jongh, R.; Bravenboer, N.; van Poppel, M.N.M.; Deeg, D.J.H. Relative importance of four functional measures as predictors of 15-year mortality in the older Dutch population. *BMC Geriatr.* **2019**, *19*, 92. [CrossRef]
36. Fiatarone, M.A.; Marks, E.C.; Ryan, N.D.; Meredith, C.N.; Lipsitz, L.A.; Evans, W.J. High-intensity strength training in nonagenarians. Effects on skeletal muscle. *JAMA* **1990**, *263*, 3029–3034. [CrossRef]
37. Lopez, P.; Izquierdo, M.; Radaelli, R.; Sbruzzi, G.; Grazioloi, R.; Pinto, R.S.; Cadore, E.L. Effectiveness of multimodal training on functional capacity in frail older people: A meta-analysis of randomized controlled trials. *J. Aging Phys. Act.* **2018**, *26*, 407–418. [CrossRef]
38. Chan, D.D.; Tsou, H.H.; Chang, C.B.; Yang, R.S.; Tsauo, J.Y.; Chen, C.Y.; Hsiao, C.F.; Hsu, Y.T.; Chen, C.H.; Chang, S.F.; et al. Integrated care for geriatric frailty and sarcopenia: A randomized control trial. *J. Cachexia Sarcopenia Muscle* **2017**, *8*, 78–88. [CrossRef]
39. Borde, R.; Hortobagyi, T.; Granacher, U. Dose-response relationships of resistance training in healthy old adults: A systematic review and meta-analysis. *Sports Med.* **2015**, *45*, 1693–1720. [CrossRef]
40. Cruz-Jentoft, A.J.; Kiesswetter, E.; Drey, M.; Sieber, C.C. Nutrition, frailty, and sarcopenia. *Aging Clin. Exp. Res.* **2017**, *29*, 43–48. [CrossRef]
41. Mithal, A.; Bonjour, J.P.; Boonen, S.; Burckhardt, P.; Degens, H.; El Hajj Fuleihan, G.; Josse, R.; Lips, P.; Morales Torres, J.; Rizzoli, R.; et al. Impact of nutrition on muscle mass, strength, and performance in older adults. *Osteoporos. Int.* **2013**, *24*, 1555–1566. [CrossRef] [PubMed]
42. Granic, A.; Sayer, A.A.; Robinson, S.M. Dietary patterns, skeletal muscle health, and sarcopenia in older adults. *Nutrients* **2019**, *11*, 745. [CrossRef] [PubMed]
43. Hickson, M. Nutritional interventions in sarcopenia: A critical review. *Proc. Nutr. Soc.* **2015**, *74*, 378–386. [CrossRef] [PubMed]
44. Woo, J. Nutritional interventions in sarcopenia: Where do we stand? *Curr. Opin. Clin. Nutr. Metab. Care* **2018**, *21*, 19–23. [CrossRef]
45. Lozano-Montoya, I.; Correa-Perez, A.; Abraha, I.; Soiza, R.L.; Cherubini, A.; O'Mahony, D.; Cruz-Jentoft, A.J. Nonpharmacological interventions to treat physical frailty and sarcopenia in older patients: A systematic overview - the SENATOR Project ONTOP Series. *Clin. Interv. Aging* **2017**, *12*, 721–740. [CrossRef]
46. Curtis, E.; Litwic, A.; Cooper, C.; Dennison, E. Determinants of muscle and bone aging. *J. Cell. Physiol.* **2015**, *230*, 2618–2625. [CrossRef]
47. Kikuchi, N.; Yoshida, S.; Min, S.K.; Lee, K.; Sakamaki-Sunaga, M.; Okamoto, T.; Nakazato, K. The ACTN3 R577X genotype is associated with muscle function in a Japanese population. *Appl. Physiol. Nutr. Metab.* **2015**, *40*, 316–322. [CrossRef]

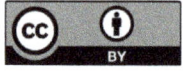

© 2020 by the authors. Licensee MDPI, Basel, Switzerland. This article is an open access article distributed under the terms and conditions of the Creative Commons Attribution (CC BY) license (http://creativecommons.org/licenses/by/4.0/).

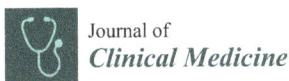 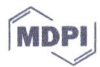

Article

Impact of Decorin on the Physical Function and Prognosis of Patients with Hepatocellular Carcinoma

Takumi Kawaguchi [1,*], Sachiyo Yoshio [2], Yuzuru Sakamoto [2,3], Ryuki Hashida [4,5], Shunji Koya [5], Keisuke Hirota [5], Dan Nakano [1], Sakura Yamamura [1], Takashi Niizeki [1], Hiroo Matsuse [4,5] and Takuji Torimura [1]

1. Division of Gastroenterology, Department of Medicine, Kurume University School of Medicine, Kurume 830-0011, Japan; nakano_dan@med.kurume-u.ac.jp (D.N.); yamamura_sakura@med.kurume-u.ac.jp (S.Y.); niizeki_takashi@kurume-u.ac.jp (T.N.); tori@med.kurume-u.ac.jp (T.T.)
2. Department of Liver Disease, Research Center for Hepatitis and Immunology, National Center for Global Health and Medicine, Kohnodai, Ichikawa 272-8516, Japan; sachiyo@hospk.ncgm.go.jp (S.Y.); yuzurusakamoto18@gmail.com (Y.S.)
3. Department of Gastroenterological Surgery I, Hokkaido University Graduate School of Medicine, Sapporo 060-8638, Japan
4. Department of Orthopedics, School of Medicine, Kurume University, Kurume 830-0011, Japan; hashida_ryuuki@med.kurume-u.ac.jp (R.H.); matsuse_hiroh@kurume-u.ac.jp (H.M.)
5. Division of Rehabilitation, Kurume University Hospital, Kurume 830-0011, Japan; kouya_shunji@kurume-u.ac.jp (S.K.); hirota_keisuke@kurume-u.ac.jp (K.H.)
* Correspondence: takumi@med.kurume-u.ac.jp; Tel.: +81-942-31-7627

Received: 15 February 2020; Accepted: 25 March 2020; Published: 28 March 2020

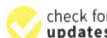

Abstract: The outcome of patients with hepatocellular carcinoma (HCC) is still poor. Decorin is a small leucine-rich proteoglycan, which exerts antiproliferative and antiangiogenic properties in vitro. We aimed to investigate the associations of decorin with physical function and prognosis in patients with HCC. We enrolled 65 patients with HCC treated with transcatheter arterial chemoembolization (median age, 75 years; female/male, 25/40). Serum decorin levels were measured using enzyme-linked immunosorbent assays; patients were classified into the High or Low decorin groups by median levels. Associations of decorin with physical function and prognosis were evaluated by multivariate correlation and Cox regression analyses, respectively. Age and skeletal muscle indices were not significantly different between the High and Low decorin groups. In the High decorin group, the 6-min walking distance was significantly longer than the Low decorin group and was significantly correlated with serum decorin levels ($r = 0.2927$, $p = 0.0353$). In multivariate analysis, the High decorin group was independently associated with overall survival (hazard ratio 2.808, 95% confidence interval 1.016–8.018, $p = 0.0498$). In the High decorin group, overall survival rate was significantly higher than in the Low decorin group (median 732 days vs. 463 days, $p = 0.010$). In conclusion, decorin may be associated with physical function and prognosis in patients with HCC.

Keywords: hepatoma; myokine; decorin; walking distance; survival

1. Introduction

Hepatocellular carcinoma (HCC) is a common cancer and the fourth leading cause of death due to cancer worldwide [1]. The incidence of HCC is predicted to continuously increase in both sexes and all age groups, since risk factors for HCC such as obesity, non-alcoholic steatohepatitis, and type 2 diabetes mellitus have become more prevalent worldwide [2]. In addition, the mortality rate of HCC has increased since 2000 [3], although there has been remarkable progresses in treatment for HCC, including the use of tyrosine kinase inhibitors [4]. The age-adjusted incidence and mortality rates of HCC are reported to be the highest in Eastern Asia [2]. The average 5-year survival rate is less than 15% in patients with HCC [5]. Thus, the prognosis of patients with HCC remains poor.

Skeletal muscle mass is known to be associated with the prognosis of patients with HCC [6]. Muscle atrophy is an independent factor associated with poor prognosis in patients with HCC treated with surgical resection and radiofrequency ablation [7]. Muscle atrophy is also a prognostic factor in patients with HCC treated with transarterial chemoembolization (TACE) and sorafenib [8,9]. In addition, muscle atrophy is associated with treatment tolerability and additional or subsequent therapies in patients with HCC treated with sorafenib [10]. In contrast, physical activity is associated with a reduced risk of HCC [11]. Moreover, exercise is reported to improve the prognosis of patients with HCC, regardless of changes in skeletal muscle mass [12].

Skeletal muscle is known as an endocrine organ [13]. By muscle contraction, myocytes release small peptides and cytokines, called myokines, and regulate muscle mass [13]. Myostatin is a myokine, which suppresses skeletal muscle growth and causes muscle atrophy [14]. Meanwhile, decorin is an exercise-induced myokine that suppresses muscle atrophy via inhibition of myostatin [15]. We previously reported that serum decorin levels are positively correlated with skeletal muscle mass in patients with HCC [16]. Decorin is also reported to interact with transforming growth factor-β and receptors of tyrosine kinase such as epidermal and insulin-like growth factors [17], leading to suppression of proliferation of various tumor cell lines, including HCC cell lines [18–20]. In addition, decorin is known to be expressed in various tissues including intestinal tissue, cardiac tissue, and adipose tissue and is known to regulate autophagy, inflammation, and glucose homeostasis [21–24]. Thus, accumulated evidence from basic studies suggests that decorin has an impact on the prognosis of patients with HCC. However, there has been no clinical study investigating the prognostic impact of decorin in patients with HCC.

The aim of this study was to investigate the association of serum decorin levels with physical function and prognosis in patients with HCC.

2. Materials and Methods

2.1. Study Design

This was a retrospective study to investigate the impact of serum decorin levels on the physical function and prognosis of patients with HCC.

2.2. Ethics

The study protocol conformed to the ethical guidelines of the Declaration of Helsinki and was approved by the institutional review board of Kurume University. We employed an opt-out approach to obtain informed consent from patients.

2.3. Subjects

We registered 339 consecutive patients with HCC between November 2014 and March 2018. Of these patients, 165 patients were excluded because of radiofrequency ablation ($n = 43$), hepatic arterial infusion chemotherapy ($n = 91$), tyrosine-kinase inhibitor ($n = 23$), or radiation ($n = 8$), and the remaining 174 patients with HCC who underwent TACE were selected. Of the 174 patients with HCC who underwent TACE, 105 patients were excluded because of hepatic encephalopathy ($n = 27$), HCC rupture ($n = 17$), renal failure ($n = 7$), or lack of data for physical function tests ($n = 54$). Finally, a total of 69 patients with HCC were analyzed in this study (Figure 1). We classified all patients into the High or Low decorin group per the median decorin level.

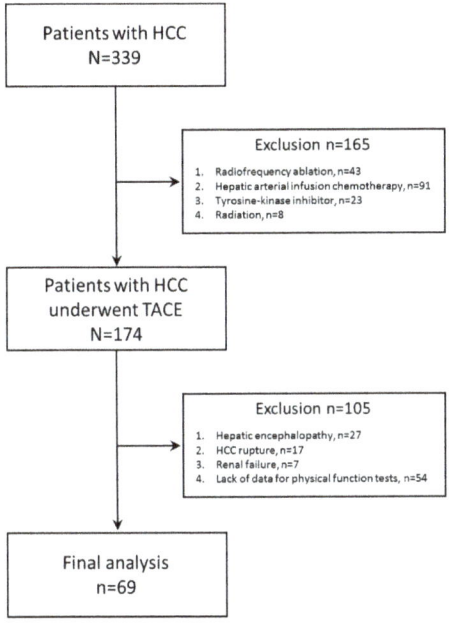

Figure 1. A flow diagram of analyzed subjects.

2.4. Diagnosis, Barcelona Clinic Liver Cancer (BCLC) Staging, and Treatment of HCC

HCC was diagnosed and treated according to the guidelines for HCC of the Japan Society of Hepatology [25]. The clinical stage of HCC was evaluated using the BCLC staging system [26].

2.5. Measurement of Skeletal Muscle Index (SMI) and Visceral Fat Area

The SMI was evaluated using computed tomography (CT) images obtained at the diagnosis of HCC as previously described [27,28]. The skeletal muscle mass was measured by manual tracings on CT images, and their sum was calculated using ImageJ Version 1.50 software (National Institutes of Health, Bethesda, MD, USA) [29]. The skeletal muscle mass was evaluated by the SMI.

2.6. Measurement of Physical Function

Grip strength and the 6-min walking distance were evaluated by qualified physical therapists. Handgrip was measured on the non-dominant hand using a dynamometer (TKK5401; Takei Scientific Instruments Co., Ltd., Niigata, Japan) [6]. The 6-minute walking distance was measured by evaluating the total ambulated distance [30].

2.7. Diagnosis of Sarcopenia

The diagnosis of sarcopenia was based on the Japan Society of Hepatology diagnostic criteria for sarcopenia in patients with liver disease [6]. Patients who showed both a decrease in grip strength (the cut-off value is 26 kg for men and 18 kg for women) and a decrease in skeletal muscle mass (the cut-off value of SMI is 42 cm^2/m^2 for men and 38 cm^2/m^2 for women) were diagnosed with sarcopenia. The other patients were classified as non-sarcopenia [6].

2.8. Biochemical Tests

Blood samples were obtained at the baseline in the early morning after an overnight fast. The blood biochemical tests performed were for serum levels of alpha-fetoprotein, des-γ-carboxy prothrombin, liver function tests, renal function tests, total cholesterol, creatine kinase, and hemoglobin A1c. We also measured the complete blood cell count.

2.9. Measurement of Serum Levels of Myostatin, FGF-21 and Decorin

Serum levels of myostatin, FGF-21, and decorin were measured using a Myostatin Quantikine enzyme-linked immunosorbent assay (ELISA) Kit (R&D Systems, Inc., Minneapolis, MN, USA), Human FGF-21 ELISA Kit (BioVendor—Laboratorni medicina a.s., Brno, Czech Republic), and Human Decorin ELISA Kit (Abcam plc., Cambridge, UK) according to the manufacturers' instructions, respectively.

2.10. Follow-Up and Definition of Survival Term

After treatment with TACE, patients were followed up until death or the study censor date through routine physical examinations, biochemical tests, and abdominal imaging including ultrasonography, CT, or magnetic resonance imaging according to the HCC guidelines of the Japan Society of Hepatology [25]. The median observational period was 617 days (range, 52–2068 days). The survival term was defined as the period from the diagnosis of HCC to death or the study censor date.

2.11. Statistical Analysis

Data are expressed as the median (interquartile range), range, or number. The differences between the High and Low decorin groups were analyzed using Wilcoxon rank sum tests. Factors correlated with serum decorin levels were evaluated by pairwise correlations [31]. In addition, independent factors associated with survival were analyzed using Cox regression analysis, as previously described [27]. The overall survival in the High and Low decorin groups was estimated using the Kaplan–Meier method, and differences in survival between the groups were analyzed using the log-rank test. All the statistical analyses were performed using JMP Pro® 14 (SAS Institute Inc., Cary, NC, USA). Values of $p < 0.05$ were considered to indicate statistically significant differences.

3. Results

3.1. Patient Characteristics

The patient characteristics are summarized in Table 1. There was no significant difference in age and body mass index. The prevalence of men was significantly higher in the High decorin group than that in the Low decorin group. There was no significant difference in the hospitalization period between the two groups.

In the High decorin group, the prevalence of sarcopenia was significantly lower than that in the Low decorin group. Although no significant differences were noted in the SMI and serum creatine kinase level between the two groups, the 6-min walking distance in the High decorin group was significantly longer than that in the Low decorin group (Table 1).

Although there was no significant difference in the serum fibroblast growth factor (FGF)-21 level between the two groups, the serum level of myostatin was significantly higher in the High decorin group than that in the Low decorin group (Table 1).

There was no significant difference in the BCLC classification between the High and Low decorin groups. No significant difference in the serum alpha-fetoprotein level was also observed between the two groups; however, in the High decorin group, the serum des-γ-carboxy prothrombin level was significantly lower than that in the Low decorin group (Table 1).

There was no significant difference in the prevalence of Child–Pugh class B and use of branched-chain amino acid supplementation between the two groups. Serum levels of aspartate aminotransferase, alanine aminotransferase, and estimated glomerular filtration rate were significantly higher in the High decorin group than those in the Low decorin group. In the High decorin group, serum levels of blood urea nitrogen, creatinine, and triglycerides and the hemoglobin A1c value were significantly lower than those in the Low decorin group (Table 1).

Table 1. Patients' characteristics.

	All Subjects			High Decorin			Low Decorin			
	Median (IQR)	Range (min-max)		Median (IQR)	Range (min-max)		Median (IQR)	Range (min-max)		p
Number (n)	65			33			32			N/A
Age (years)	75 (71–80)	60–90		76 (72–80)	60–89		75 (71–80)	63–90		0.9528
Sex (women/men)	38.5%/61.5% (25/40)	N/A		54.5%/45.5% (18/15)	N/A		21.9%/78.1% (7/25)	N/A		0.0068
Body mass index (kg/m^2)	23.9 (21.2–26.0)	16.7–37.8		23.0 (21.5–26.3)	19.6–30.3		24.1 (20.5–25.8)	16.7–37.8		0.6227
Hospitalization period (days)	14 (11–21)	7–55		13 (11.5–17.5)	7–55		17 (11–21)	7–34		0.3076
Grip strength (kg)	24.2 (20.3–31.3)	13.3–42.8		24.1 (19.25–30.63)	13.3–42.8		25.0 (21.5–32.1)	14.9–39		0.8045
Skeletal muscle index (cm^2/m^2)	29.69 (23.94–35.20)	11.85–51.18		28.50 (23.21–34.22)	11.85–41.79		31.53 (24.33–36.82)	12.45–51.18		0.3758
Sarcopenia (Presence/Absence)	18.5%/81.5% (12/53)	N/A		6.1%/93.9% (2/31)	N/A		31.3%/68.7% (10/22)	N/A		0.0089
Visceral fat area (cm^2)	61.7 (39.8–84.6)	4.4–240.8		59.2 (39.8–78.1)	24.2–240.8		61.9 (36.5–95.9)	4.4–197.8		0.7578
Serum creatine kinase (U/L)	95 (70.5–132.5)	17–374		99 (77–133)	44–246		90.5 (63.75–129.5)	17–374		0.3558
6-minute walking distance (m)	379 (302–420)	26–621		391 (365–433)	228–621		334 (255–407)	26–501		0.0093
Decorin (pg/mL)	17,322 (13,499–21,866)	7400–32,102		21,799 (18,990–27,033)	17,322–32,102		13,499 (11,939–14,726)	7400–16,838		<0.0001
Myostatin (pg/mL)	1699 (1180–3658)	245–7788		3056 (1313–4610)	501–6350		1500 (1154–3214)	246–7788		0.0426
FGF-21 (pg/mL)	160 (116–344)	13–2150		174 (140–340)	39–2150		156 (96–357)	13–1328		0.4197
BCLC stage (A/B)	10.8%/89.2% (7/58)	N/A		15.2%/84.8%(5/28)	N/A		6.2%/93.8%(2/30)	N/A		0.2471
AFP (ng/mL)	32.75 (6.83–275.18)	1.4–67,036		20 (8.25–72.27)	3.9–1594		93 (5.5–1613)	1.4–67,036		0.2218
DCP (mAU/mL)	76 (28–888.5)	9–30,844		36 (24–211.5)	12–17,353		144 (43–6753)	9–30,844		0.0253
Child–Pugh class (A/B)	69.2%/30.8% (45/20)	N/A		75.8%/24.2% (25/8)	N/A		62.5%/37.5% (20/12)	N/A		0.2469
BCAA supplementation (With/Without)	52.3%/47.7% (34/31)	N/A		51.5%/48.5% (17/16)	N/A		53.1%/46.9% (17/15)	N/A		0.8966
AST (IU/L)	43 (32–55.5)	19–158		45 (40–65.5)	23–158		34 (26–48)	19–99		0.0009
ALT (IU/L)	28 (21–37.5)	7–186		32 (24.5–41)	24–186		23 (17.5–32.5)	7–87		0.0031
ALP (IU/L)	351 (291–479)	180–854		356 (309.5–541.5)	200–854		325 (275.75–455)	180–659		0.2299
GGT (IU/L)	44 (26–73.5)	9–551		45 (26.5–79.5)	15–551		42 (26–66.5)	9–252		0.6088
Total protein (g/dL)	7.28 (6.72–7.78)	5.94–8.89		7.36 (6.62–7.81)	5.94–8.15		7.28 (6.82–7.62)	6.04–8.89		0.9477
Albumin (g/dL)	3.5 (3.1–3.7)	2.5–4.3		3.4 (3.1–3.7)	2.5–4.3		3.5 (3.0–3.8)	2.8–4.2		1.0000
Total bilirubin (mg/dL)	0.9 (0.6–1.3)	0.3–2.8		0.9 (0.6–1.3)	0.4–2.8		0.9 (0.6–1.2)	0.3–1.6		0.5996
Prothrombin activity (%)	80 (68–88)	38–117		81 (65.5–90)	42–117		79 (69–85.5)	38–108		0.6365
Blood urea nitrogen (mg/dL)	17 (14–19.6)	5.9–47.6		14.9 (13–18.9)	5.9–28.1		17.45 (15–20.18)	11.5–47.6		0.0253
Creatinine (mg/dL)	0.74 (0.61–0.92)	0.43–1.91		0.66 (0.55–0.77)	0.43–1.52		0.81 (0.66–1.03)	0.56–1.91		0.0013
eGFR (mL/min/1.73 m^2)	73.2 (54.3–84.85)	27.3–121.3		78.6 (62.15–89.95)	34.3–121.3		65.7 (52.63–75.8)	27.3–102.4		0.0107
Total cholesterol (mg/dL)	144 (126–162)	79–233		138 (121–156)	84–197		147 (128–163)	79–233		0.3154
Triglyceride (mg/dL)	82 (70–108)	28–249		75 (64–94)	28–249		91 (78–130)	54–179		0.0237
HbA1c (%)	5.8 (5.5–6.4)	4.3–13.4		5.7 (5.25–6.1)	4.3–8.3		6.1 (5.7–6.8)	4.7–13.4		0.0268
Red blood cell count (×10^4/μL)	389 (355–420)	249–615		385 (356–416)	310–455		393 (347–442)	249–615		0.7528
Hemoglobin (g/dL)	11.9 (10.4–12.75)	7.3–15.4		11.9 (10.6–12.8)	7.3–15.4		11.9 (9.8–12.7)	7.3–14.9		0.7083
White blood cell count (/μL)	3800 (3100–5050)	1800–7900		3700 (3050–5560)	1900–6600		4150 (3125–5525)	1800–7900		0.2270
Platelet count (×10^3/mm^3)	10.9 (8.35–15.1)	3.2–31.8		9.4 (7.8–13.0)	3.2–22.6		11.8 (8.6–16.1)	4.0–31.8		0.0881

Note: Data are expressed as median (interquartile range (IQR)), range, or number. Abbreviations: AFP, alpha-fetoprotein; ALP, alkaline phosphatase; ALT, alanine aminotransferase; AST, aspartate aminotransferase; BCAA, branched-chain amino acid; BCLC, Barcelona Clinic Liver Cancer; DCP, des-γ-carboxy prothrombin; eGFR, estimated glomerular filtration rate; FGF-21, fibroblast growth factor-21; GGT, gamma-glutamyl transpeptidase; HbA1c, hemoglobin A1c; N/A, not applicable

3.2. Multivariate Correlation Analysis Between Serum Decorin Levels and Each Variable

No significant correlation was seen between serum decorin levels and age, body mass index, grip strength, SMI, levels of alpha-fetoprotein, albumin, total bilirubin, creatine kinase, hemoglobin A1c, and estimated glomerular filtration rate. Serum decorin levels showed a significant negative correlation with serum des-γ-carboxy prothrombin levels. Serum decorin levels demonstrated a significant positive correlation between the 6-min walking distance and serum myostatin levels (Table 2).

Table 2. Multivariate correlation analysis between serum decorin levels and each variable.

Variable	Correlation Coefficient	p
Age	−0.0250	0.8750
Body mass index	0.0415	0.7942
Grip strength	−0.0532	0.7380
Skeletal muscle index	−0.1362	0.3898
Visceral fat area	0.0278	0.861
6-min walking distance	0.2927	0.0353
Creatine kinase	−0.0062	0.9690
Myostatin	0.3200	0.0389
FGF-21	−0.0352	0.8249
AFP	−0.2270	0.1482
DCP	−0.3476	0.0241
AST	0.2453	0.0992
ALT	0.2734	0.0798
ALP	0.1260	0.4266
GGT	0.0042	0.979
Total protein	−0.0197	0.9015
Albumin	−0.1754	0.2664
Total bilirubin	0.1054	0.5063
Prothrombin activity	0.1078	0.4968
Blood urea nitrogen	−0.1606	0.3095
Creatinine	−0.1650	0.2965
eGFR	0.0695	0.6617
Total cholesterol	−0.0914	0.5650
Triglyceride	−0.0594	0.7089
HbA1c	−0.2748	0.0782
Red blood cell count	−0.1337	0.3984
Hemoglobin	−0.0384	0.8091
White blood cell count	−0.233	0.1376
Platelet count	−0.2261	0.15

Abbreviations: FGF-21, fibroblast growth factor-21; AFP, alpha-fetoprotein; DCP, des-γ-carboxy prothrombin; AST, aspartate aminotransferase; ALT, alanine aminotransferase; ALP, alkaline phosphatase; GGT, gamma-glutamyl transpeptidase; eGFR, estimated glomerular filtration rate; HbA1c, hemoglobin A1c.

3.3. Independent Factors Associated with Survival

We examined independent factors associated with survival and found that high decorin levels were identified as an independent factor of better overall survival. Meanwhile, the BCLC stage and Child–Pugh class were not identified as independent factors associated with overall survival (Table 3).

Table 3. Multivariate Cox regression analysis for overall survival.

Factors	Hazard Ratio	95% Confidence Interval	p-Value
Decorin (High/Low)	2.808	1.016–8.018	0.0498
BCLC stage (A/B–C)	6.720	0.707–73.877	0.0553
Child–Pugh class (A/B)	1.436	0.461–4.473	0.5308

Abbreviations: BCLC, Barcelona Clinic Liver Cancer.

3.4. Kaplan–Meier Analysis for Survival

In the High decorin group, the overall survival rate was significantly higher compared to that in the Low decorin group (median 732 days vs. 463 days; log-rank test $p = 0.0498$) (Figure 2A). In the subgroup analysis of BCLC stage B, the difference in overall survival rates between the High and Low decorin groups became more significant than that in the analysis in all subjects (BCLC stages A and B) (Figure 2B).

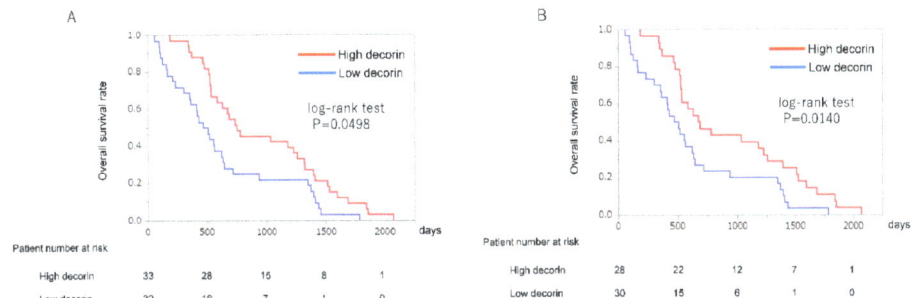

Figure 2. Kaplan–Meier analysis between the High decorin and Low decorin groups. (**A**) All patients; (**B**) Patients with BCLC stage B HCC. BCLC, Barcelona Clinic Liver Cancer; HCC, hepatocellular carcinoma.

4. Discussion

In this study, we demonstrated that serum decorin levels were positively correlated with the 6-min walking distance, an index of cardiopulmonary function in patients with HCC. In addition, we found that serum decorin levels were an independent prognostic factor in patients with HCC. Although more research is needed and our data are preliminary in essence, these data suggest that decorin may be associated with physical function and prognosis in patients with HCC.

TACE is a standard treatment for intermediate-stage HCC [26,32]. In this study, we enrolled patients with HCC treated with TACE, and the median survival period was 617 days, which is comparable to that reported previously [26,33]. The prognosis of patients with HCC is dependent on the BCLC stage [26]. However, the BCLC stage was not identified as an independent prognostic factor in this study, and the reason for this remains unclear. However, all enrolled patients with HCC were treated with TACE, and patients with the BCLC stage B accounted for about 90% of the enrolled patients. Therefore, the narrow distribution of the BCLC stage may be a possible explanation.

Although myostatin and FGF-21 are myokines, the levels of these myokines were not identified as independent prognostic factors in patients with HCC. Nishikawa et al. reported that elevated serum myostatin levels are associated with worse survival in patients with liver cirrhosis [34]. Hyperammonemia has been reported to transcriptionally upregulate myostatin through nuclear transport of p65 nuclear factor-κB, resulting in sarcopenia and poor prognosis [35]. Meanwhile, patients with hepatic encephalopathy (West Haven criteria grade II–IV) were excluded, and the prevalence of hyperammonemia was thought to be low in this study. Therefore, myostatin may not be identified as a prognostic factor. Deficiency of FGF-21 is reported to promote HCC in mice receiving a long-term obesogenic diet [36]. Long-term administration of FGF-21 prevents chemically induced hepatocarcinogenesis in mice [37]. However, FGF-21 is known to be expressed in several tissues, including those of the liver, fat, and pancreas [38]. Serum FGF-21 levels are affected by various tissues expressing FGF-21, and, therefore, FGF-21 was not identified as an independent prognostic factor in patients with HCC.

Serum decorin levels were positively correlated with the 6-min walking distance, an index of cardiopulmonary function in patients with HCC. Overexpression of decorin is reported to ameliorate diabetic cardiomyopathy and cardiac function in rats [39]. N-terminal cleavage of decorin confers an inhibitory effect against myostatin, suppressing the atrophy of cardiomyocytes [40]. In fact, serum decorin level was positively correlated with serum myostatin level in this study. One would think that decorin may be up regulated to suppress muscle atrophy in response to an increase in serum myostatin level. In addition, C-terminal truncation of decorin interacts with the connective tissue growth factor, leading to suppression of myocardial fibrosis through down-regulation of cardiac extracellular matrix production [40]. Furthermore, Kwon et al. reported that decorin causes macrophage polarization via cluster of differentiation-44, resulting in an amelioration of pulmonary function in a rat model of hypertoxic lung damage [41]. These previous basic studies, along with our results, may suggest that decorin may be associated with cardiopulmonary function in patients with HCC (Figure 3). However, the correlation between serum decorin level and the 6-min walking distance could not lead to the conclusion that the high decorin level is a cause of high cardiovascular fitness, in such a small number of subjects.

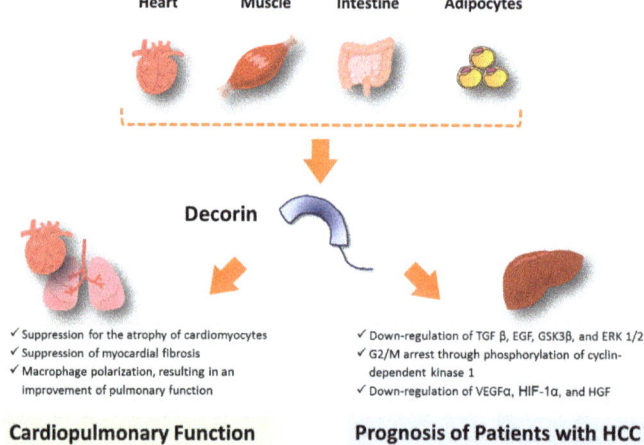

Figure 3. A scheme for the proposed hypothesis of this study. Decorin is expressed in various tissues including skeletal muscle, heart, intestine, and adipocytes. In this study, it remains unclear where decorin comes from. Decorin may be associated with cardiopulmonary function, because decorin suppresses the atrophy of cardiomyocytes, myocardial fibrosis, and causes macrophage polarization. In addition, decorin may be associated with prognosis of patients with HCC, because decorin downregulates transforming growth factor-β1, epidermal growth factor receptor, glycogen synthase kinase 3β, and extracellular signal-regulated kinase 1/2, G2/M arrest through phosphorylation of cyclin-dependent kinase 1, downregulation of vascular endothelial growth factor A, hypoxia-inducible factor 1-α, and hepatocyte growth factor. Abbreviations: TGF β, transforming growth factor-β1; EGF, epidermal growth factor receptor; GSK3β, glycogen synthase kinase 3β; and ERK, extracellular signal-regulated kinase; VEGF, vascular endothelial growth factor; HIF-1α, hypoxia-inducible factor 1-α; HGF, hepatocyte growth factor.

In this study, we first examined the impact of the serum decorin level in patients with HCC and found that serum decorin levels were identified as an independent prognostic factor in patients with HCC. Moreover, in the stratification analysis according to the BCLC stage, the prognostic impact of decorin was more evident in patients with HCC with the BCLC stage B. Horváth et al. reported that genetic ablation of decorin leads to enhanced hepatocarcinogenesis compared to that in wild-type animals [42]. Meanwhile, recombinant human decorin inhibits the proliferation of HepG2 cells [43,44]. Several mechanisms for decorin-induced inhibition of cell proliferation have been reported. Decorin is reported to reduce the secretion of transforming growth factor-β1 in HCC cell lines [20]. Decorin is also reported to downregulate the phosphorylation of epidermal growth factor receptor, glycogen synthase kinase 3β, and extracellular signal-regulated kinase 1/2 [20]. In addition, decorin suppresses the ATR/Chk1/Wee1 axis, leading to inhibition of the cell cycle in the G2/M phase via phosphorylation of cyclin-dependent kinase 1 [20]. Moreover, decorin is known to decrease the expression of pro-angiogenic factors, vascular endothelial growth factor A, and hypoxia-inducible factor 1-α, resulting in downregulation of the hepatocyte growth factor and epidermal growth factor receptor signaling axes [45]. In fact, the serum decorin level was negatively correlated with the serum des-γ-carboxy prothrombin level, which is a tumor maker for HCC in this study. Thus, decorin may suppress the proliferation of HCC through direct and indirect tumor inhibitory effects and may be associated with prognosis in patients with HCC (Figure 3). However, decorin is known to be expressed not only in skeletal muscle [15], but also in various tissues including intestinal tissue, cardiac tissue, and adipose tissue [21–24]. Accordingly, it remains unclear where decorin comes from in the present study (Figure 3). In addition, we have to be cautious of the interpretation of our data. Expression of decorin is recently reported to be seen in the tumor cell such as glioblastoma and is negatively associated with the overall survival rate of patients with glioblastoma multiforme [46]. Thus, further research is required to investigate the expression of decorin in HCC tissue and a causal relationship between decorin and prognosis of the patients with HCC.

Limitations of this study are the following: First, this was a retrospective study conducted in a single center. Second, the number of enrolled subjects is very limited to examine independent prognostic factors. Third, we enrolled patients with HCC treated with TACE. It remains unclear if serum decorin levels have a prognostic impact in patients with HCC treated with hepatic resection or tyrosine kinase inhibitors. Fourth, no patient underwent liver transplantation during the observation period, suggesting the selection bias. Thus, a multicenter prospective cohort study should be conducted with various HCC stages and treatments for HCC including liver transplantation.

5. Conclusions

In conclusion, we demonstrated that serum decorin levels were positively correlated with cardiopulmonary function in patients with HCC. In addition, serum decorin levels were an independent prognostic factor in patients with HCC. Although more research is needed and our data are preliminary in essence, the results of this study may suggest that decorin may be associated with physical function and prognosis in patients with HCC.

Author Contributions: Author Contributions: T.K., S.Y. (Sachiyo Yoshio), and R.H. participated in the study conception and design, data acquisition and interpretation, and manuscript drafting. Y.S. participated in data analysis and manuscript drafting. S.K., K.H., D.N., S.Y. (Sakura Yamamura), and T.N. participated in data acquisition and interpretation and manuscript drafting. H.M. and T.T. participated in the study conception and design, interpretation, and critical revision. All authors have read and agreed to the published version of the manuscript.

Funding: This research was supported by the Program for Basic and Clinical Research on Hepatitis (AMED) under JP19fk0210045.

Acknowledgments: We would like to thank Editage for English language editing.

Conflicts of Interest: T.K. received lecture fees from MSD K.K., Mitsubishi Tanabe Pharma Corporation and Otsuka Pharmaceutical Co., Ltd. The other authors have no conflicts of interest.

References

1. Weinmann, A.; Koch, S.; Niederle, I.M.; Schulze-Bergkamen, H.; Konig, J.; Hoppe-Lotichius, M.; Hansen, T.; Pitton, M.B.; Duber, C.; Otto, G.; et al. Trends in epidemiology, treatment, and survival of hepatocellular carcinoma patients between 1998 and 2009: An analysis of 1066 cases of a German HCC Registry. *J. Clin. Gastroenterol.* **2014**, *48*, 279–289. [CrossRef]
2. Younossi, Z.M.; Golabi, P.; de Avila, L.; Paik, J.M.; Srishord, M.; Fukui, N.; Qiu, Y.; Burns, L.; Afendy, A.; Nader, F. The global epidemiology of NAFLD and NASH in patients with type 2 diabetes: A systematic review and meta-analysis. *J. Hepatol.* **2019**, *71*, 793–801. [CrossRef]

3. Xu, J. Trends in Liver Cancer Mortality among Adults Aged 25 and Over in the United States, 2000–2016. *NCHS Data Brief.* **2018**, *314*, 1–8.
4. Ikeda, K. Recent advances in medical management of hepatocellular carcinoma. *Hepatol. Res.* **2019**, *49*, 14–32. [CrossRef] [PubMed]
5. El-Serag, H.B. Hepatocellular carcinoma. *N. Engl. J. Med.* **2011**, *365*, 1118–1127. [CrossRef] [PubMed]
6. Nishikawa, H.; Shiraki, M.; Hiramatsu, A.; Moriya, K.; Hino, K.; Nishiguchi, S. Japan Society of Hepatology guidelines for sarcopenia in liver disease (1st edition): Recommendation from the working group for creation of sarcopenia assessment criteria. *Hepatol. Res.* **2016**, *46*, 951–963. [CrossRef] [PubMed]
7. Hiraoka, A.; Otsuka, Y.; Kawasaki, H.; Izumoto, H.; Ueki, H.; Kitahata, S.; Aibiki, T.; Okudaira, T.; Yamago, H.; Miyamoto, Y.; et al. Impact of muscle volume and muscle function decline in patients undergoing surgical resection for hepatocellular carcinoma. *J. Gastroenterol. Hepatol.* **2018**, *33*, 1271–1276. [CrossRef]
8. Fujita, M.; Takahashi, A.; Hayashi, M.; Okai, K.; Abe, K.; Ohira, H. Skeletal muscle volume loss during transarterial chemoembolization predicts poor prognosis in patients with hepatocellular carcinoma. *Hepatol. Res.* **2019**, *49*, 778–786. [CrossRef]
9. Takada, H.; Kurosaki, M.; Nakanishi, H.; Takahashi, Y.; Itakura, J.; Tsuchiya, K.; Yasui, Y.; Tamaki, N.; Takaura, K.; Komiyama, Y.; et al. Impact of pre-sarcopenia in sorafenib treatment for advanced hepatocellular carcinoma. *PLoS ONE* **2018**, *13*, e0198812. [CrossRef]
10. Sawada, K.; Saitho, Y.; Hayashi, H.; Hasebe, T.; Nakajima, S.; Ikuta, K.; Fujiya, M.; Okumura, T. Skeletal muscle mass is associated with toxicity, treatment tolerability, and additional or subsequent therapies in patients with hepatocellular carcinoma receiving sorafenib treatment. *JGH Open.* **2019**, *3*, 329–337. [CrossRef]
11. Baumeister, S.E.; Schlesinger, S.; Aleksandrova, K.; Jochem, C.; Jenab, M.; Gunter, M.J.; Overvad, K.; Tjonneland, A.; Boutron-Ruault, M.C.; Carbonnel, F.; et al. Association between physical activity and risk of hepatobiliary cancers: A multinational cohort study. *J. Hepatol.* **2019**, *70*, 885–892. [CrossRef] [PubMed]
12. Hashida, R.; Kawaguchi, T.; Koya, S.; Hirota, K.; Goshima, N.; Yoshiyama, T.; Otsuka, T.; Bekki, M.; Iwanaga, S.; Nakano, D.; et al. Impact of Cancer Rehabilitation on the Prognosis of Patients with Hepatocellular Carcinoma. *Oncol. Lett.* **2020**, in press. [CrossRef] [PubMed]
13. Pedersen, B.K.; Febbraio, M.A. Muscles, exercise and obesity: Skeletal muscle as a secretory organ. *Nat. Rev. Endocrinol.* **2012**, *8*, 457–465. [CrossRef] [PubMed]
14. Dasarathy, S.; Dodig, M.; Muc, S.M.; Kalhan, S.C.; McCullough, A.J. Skeletal muscle atrophy is associated with an increased expression of myostatin and impaired satellite cell function in the portacaval anastamosis rat. *Am. J. Physiol. Gastrointest Liver Physiol.* **2004**, *287*, G1124–G1130. [CrossRef]
15. Kanzleiter, T.; Rath, M.; Gorgens, S.W.; Jensen, J.; Tangen, D.S.; Kolnes, A.J.; Kolnes, K.J.; Lee, S.; Eckel, J.; Schurmann, A.; et al. The myokine decorin is regulated by contraction and involved in muscle hypertrophy. *Biochem. Biophys. Res. Commun.* **2014**, *450*, 1089–1094. [CrossRef] [PubMed]
16. Bekki, M.; Hashida, R.; Kawaguchi, T.; Goshima, N.; Yoshiyama, T.; Otsuka, T.; Koya, S.; Hirota, K.; Matsuse, H.; Niizeki, T.; et al. The association between sarcopenia and decorin, an exercise-induced myokine, in patients with liver cirrhosis: A pilot study. *J. Cachexia Sarcopenia Muscle Rapid Commun.* **2018**, *1*, e00068. [CrossRef]
17. Tanaka, Y.; Tateishi, R.; Koike, K. Proteoglycans Are Attractive Biomarkers and Therapeutic Targets in Hepatocellular Carcinoma. *Int. J. Mol. Sci.* **2018**, *19*, E3070. [CrossRef]
18. Shi, X.; Liang, W.; Yang, W.; Xia, R.; Song, Y. Decorin is responsible for progression of non-small-cell lung cancer by promoting cell proliferation and metastasis. *Tumour Biol.* **2015**, *36*, 3345–3354. [CrossRef]
19. Dawoody Nejad, L.; Biglari, A.; Annese, T.; Ribatti, D. Recombinant fibromodulin and decorin effects on NF-kappaB and TGFbeta1 in the 4T1 breast cancer cell line. *Oncol. Lett.* **2017**, *13*, 4475–4480. [CrossRef]
20. Horvath, Z.; Reszegi, A.; Szilak, L.; Danko, T.; Kovalszky, I.; Baghy, K. Tumor-specific inhibitory action of decorin on different hepatoma cell lines. *Cell Signal.* **2019**, *62*, 109354. [CrossRef]
21. Svard, J.; Rost, T.H.; Sommervoll, C.E.N.; Haugen, C.; Gudbrandsen, O.A.; Mellgren, A.E.; Rodahl, E.; Ferno, J.; Dankel, S.N.; Sagen, J.V.; et al. Absence of the proteoglycan decorin reduces glucose tolerance in overfed male mice. *Sci. Rep.* **2019**, *9*, 4614. [CrossRef] [PubMed]
22. Zhao, H.; Xi, H.; Wei, B.; Cai, A.; Wang, T.; Wang, Y.; Zhao, X.; Song, Y.; Chen, L. Expression of decorin in intestinal tissues of mice with inflammatory bowel disease and its correlation with autophagy. *Exp. Ther. Med.* **2016**, *12*, 3885–3892. [CrossRef] [PubMed]

23. Gubbiotti, M.A.; Neill, T.; Frey, H.; Schaefer, L.; Iozzo, R.V. Decorin is an autophagy-inducible proteoglycan and is required for proper in vivo autophagy. *Matrix Biol.* **2015**, *48*, 14–25. [CrossRef] [PubMed]
24. Pohle, T.; Altenburger, M.; Shahin, M.; Konturek, J.W.; Kresse, H.; Domschke, W. Expression of decorin and biglycan in rat gastric tissue: Effects of ulceration and basic fibroblast growth factor. *Scand. J. Gastroenterol.* **2001**, *36*, 683–689. [CrossRef] [PubMed]
25. Arii, S.; Sata, M.; Sakamoto, M.; Shimada, M.; Kumada, T.; Shiina, S.; Yamashita, T.; Kokudo, N.; Tanaka, M.; Takayama, T.; et al. Management of hepatocellular carcinoma: Report of Consensus Meeting in the 45th Annual Meeting of the Japan Society of Hepatology (2009). *Hepatol. Res.* **2010**, *40*, 667–685. [CrossRef] [PubMed]
26. European Association for the Study of the Liver. Electronic address, e.e.e., European Association for the Study of the, L. EASL Clinical Practice Guidelines: Management of hepatocellular carcinoma. *J. Hepatol.* **2018**, *69*, 182–236. [CrossRef]
27. Koya, S.; Kawaguchi, T.; Hashida, R.; Goto, E.; Matsuse, H.; Saito, H.; Hirota, K.; Taira, R.; Matsushita, Y.; Imanaga, M.; et al. Effects of in-hospital exercise on liver function, physical ability, and muscle mass during treatment of hepatoma in patients with chronic liver disease. *Hepatol. Res.* **2017**, *47*, E22–E34. [CrossRef]
28. Hirota, K.; Kawaguchi, T.; Koya, S.; Nagamatsu, A.; Tomita, M.; Hashida, R.; Nakano, D.; Niizeki, T.; Matsuse, H.; Shiba, N.; et al. Clinical utility of the Liver Frailty Index for predicting muscle atrophy in chronic liver disease patients with hepatocellular carcinoma. *Hepatol. Res.* **2019**, *50*, 330–341. [CrossRef]
29. Schneider, C.A.; Rasband, W.S.; Eliceiri, K.W. NIH Image to ImageJ: 25 years of image analysis. *Nat. Methods* **2012**, *9*, 671–675. [CrossRef]
30. Brooks, D.; Solway, S.; Gibbons, W.J. ATS statement on six-minute walk test. *Am. J. Respir Crit. Care Med.* **2003**, *167*, 1287. [CrossRef]
31. Chong, C.D.; Dumkrieger, G.M.; Schwedt, T.J. Structural Co-Variance Patterns in Migraine: A Cross-Sectional Study Exploring the Role of the Hippocampus. *Headache* **2017**, *57*, 1522–1531. [CrossRef] [PubMed]
32. Forner, A.; Gilabert, M.; Bruix, J.; Raoul, J.L. Treatment of intermediate-stage hepatocellular carcinoma. *Nat. Rev. Clin. Oncol.* **2014**, *11*, 525–535. [CrossRef] [PubMed]
33. Shimose, S.; Tanaka, M.; Iwamoto, H.; Niizeki, T.; Shirono, T.; Aino, H.; Noda, Y.; Kamachi, N.; Okamura, S.; Nakano, M.; et al. Prognostic impact of transcatheter arterial chemoembolization (TACE) combined with radiofrequency ablation in patients with unresectable hepatocellular carcinoma: Comparison with TACE alone using decision-tree analysis after propensity score matching. *Hepatol. Res.* **2019**, *49*, 919–928. [CrossRef] [PubMed]
34. Nishikawa, H.; Enomoto, H.; Ishii, A.; Iwata, Y.; Miyamoto, Y.; Ishii, N.; Yuri, Y.; Hasegawa, K.; Nakano, C.; Nishimura, T.; et al. Elevated serum myostatin level is associated with worse survival in patients with liver cirrhosis. *J. Cachexia Sarcopenia Muscle.* **2017**, *8*, 915–925. [CrossRef]
35. Dasarathy, S.; Merli, M. Sarcopenia from mechanism to diagnosis and treatment in liver disease. *J. Hepatol.* **2016**, *65*, 1232–1244. [CrossRef]
36. Singhal, G.; Kumar, G.; Chan, S.; Fisher, F.M.; Ma, Y.; Vardeh, H.G.; Nasser, I.A.; Flier, J.S.; Maratos-Flier, E. Deficiency of fibroblast growth factor 21 (FGF21) promotes hepatocellular carcinoma (HCC) in mice on a long term obesogenic diet. *Mol. Metab.* **2018**, *13*, 56–66. [CrossRef]
37. Xu, P.; Zhang, Y.; Wang, W.; Yuan, Q.; Liu, Z.; Rasoul, L.M.; Wu, Q.; Liu, M.; Ye, X.; Li, D.; et al. Long-Term Administration of Fibroblast Growth Factor 21 Prevents Chemically-Induced Hepatocarcinogenesis in Mice. *Dig. Dis. Sci.* **2015**, *60*, 3032–3043. [CrossRef]
38. Watanabe, M.; Singhal, G.; Fisher, F.M.; Beck, T.C.; Morgan, D.A.; Socciarelli, F.; Mather, M.L.; Risi, R.; Bourke, J.; Rahmouni, K.; et al. Liver-derived FGF21 is essential for full adaptation to ketogenic diet but does not regulate glucose homeostasis. *Endocrine* **2020**, *67*, 95–108. [CrossRef]
39. Lai, J.; Chen, F.; Chen, J.; Ruan, G.; He, M.; Chen, C.; Tang, J.; Wang, D.W. Overexpression of decorin promoted angiogenesis in diabetic cardiomyopathy via IGF1R-AKT-VEGF signaling. *Sci. Rep.* **2017**, *7*, 44473. [CrossRef]
40. Barallobre-Barreiro, J.; Gupta, S.K.; Zoccarato, A.; Kitazume-Taneike, R.; Fava, M.; Yin, X.; Werner, T.; Hirt, M.N.; Zampetaki, A.; Viviano, A.; et al. Glycoproteomics Reveals Decorin Peptides With Anti-Myostatin Activity in Human Atrial Fibrillation. *Circulation* **2016**, *134*, 817–832. [CrossRef]
41. Kwon, J.H.; Kim, M.; Bae, Y.K.; Kim, G.H.; Choi, S.J.; Oh, W.; Um, S.; Jin, H.J. Decorin Secreted by Human Umbilical Cord Blood-Derived Mesenchymal Stem Cells Induces Macrophage Polarization via CD44 to Repair Hyperoxic Lung Injury. *Int. J. Mol. Sci.* **2019**, *20*, E4815. [CrossRef] [PubMed]

42. Horvath, Z.; Kovalszky, I.; Fullar, A.; Kiss, K.; Schaff, Z.; Iozzo, R.V.; Baghy, K. Decorin deficiency promotes hepatic carcinogenesis. *Matrix Biol.* **2014**, *35*, 194–205. [CrossRef] [PubMed]
43. Zhang, Y.; Wang, Y.; Du, Z.; Wang, Q.; Wu, M.; Wang, X.; Wang, L.; Cao, L.; Hamid, A.S.; Zhang, G. Recombinant human decorin suppresses liver HepG2 carcinoma cells by p21 upregulation. *Onco Targets Ther.* **2012**, *5*, 143–152. [CrossRef] [PubMed]
44. Hamid, A.S.; Li, J.; Wang, Y.; Wu, X.; Ali, H.A.; Du, Z.; Bo, L.; Zhang, Y.; Zhang, G. Recombinant human decorin upregulates p57KIP (2) expression in HepG2 hepatoma cell lines. *Mol. Med. Rep.* **2013**, *8*, 511–516. [CrossRef]
45. Appunni, S.; Anand, V.; Khandelwal, M.; Gupta, N.; Rubens, M.; Sharma, A. Small Leucine Rich Proteoglycans (decorin, biglycan and lumican) in cancer. *Clin. Chim. Acta.* **2019**, *491*, 1–7. [CrossRef]
46. Tsidulko, A.Y.; Kazanskaya, G.M.; Volkov, A.M.; Suhovskih, A.V.; Kiselev, R.S.; Kobozev, V.V.; Gaytan, A.S.; Krivoshapkin, A.L.; Aidagulova, S.V.; Grigorieva, E.V. Chondroitin sulfate content and decorin expression in glioblastoma are associated with proliferative activity of glioma cells and disease prognosis. *Cell Tissue Res.* **2020**, *379*, 147–155. [CrossRef]

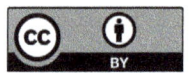

© 2020 by the authors. Licensee MDPI, Basel, Switzerland. This article is an open access article distributed under the terms and conditions of the Creative Commons Attribution (CC BY) license (http://creativecommons.org/licenses/by/4.0/).

MDPI
St. Alban-Anlage 66
4052 Basel
Switzerland
Tel. +41 61 683 77 34
Fax +41 61 302 89 18
www.mdpi.com

Journal of Clinical Medicine Editorial Office
E-mail: jcm@mdpi.com
www.mdpi.com/journal/jcm

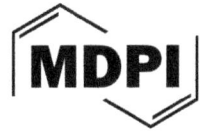

www.ingramcontent.com/pod-product-compliance
Lightning Source LLC
LaVergne TN
LVHW070144100526
838202LV00015B/1891